DEPRESSION IN THE MEDICALLY ILL

An Integrated Approach

Gary Rodin, M.D.
John Craven, M.D.
Christine Littlefield, PH.D

BRUNNER/MAZEL, Publishers • New York

Library of Congress Cataloging-in-Publication Data

Rodin, Gary.
    Depression in the medically ill ; an integrated approach / Gary
Rodin, John Craven, Christine Littlefield.
        p.   cm.
    Includes bibliographical references and index.
    ISBN 0-87630-596-6
    1. Depression, Mental.   2. Sick—Mental health.   I. Craven, John.
II. Littlefield, Christine.   III. Title.
RC537.R82   1991
616.85′27—dc20   90-26064
                                                                        CIP

Published by
BRUNNER/MAZEL, Inc.
19 Union Square West
New York, New York 10003

Designed by Tere LoPrete

Manufactured in the United States of America

10   9   8   7   6   5   4   3   2   1

For
Ilana, Danielle, and Rebecca
Karen and Emily
Jim

Contents

Acknowledgments

The authors extend their heartfelt appreciation to the many people who contributed so much to the preparation of this book. Anne Rydall's tireless and meticulous efforts in coordinating all aspects of the book were invaluable. The final manuscript has benefitted enormously from her initiative and from her cheerful attention to the smallest details. Debby Proctor's loyalty to the project and careful preparation of the manuscript contributed greatly to its final form. The patience and ingenuity of Lori Turner and Pierrette Buklis in tracking down references, and the fine help of Lynn Kukay in manuscript preparation are also reflected in the finished product. We are extremely grateful to all of these individuals for their enthusiastic involvement in this project.

The authors would also like to express their gratitude to the Ontario Mental Health Foundation and the Canadian Psychiatric Research Foundation for their generous support of our work.

Introduction

*"Everyone who is born holds dual citizenship, in the kingdom
of the well and in the kingdom of the sick. Although we all
prefer to use only the good passport, sooner or later each of
us is obliged, at least for a spell, to identify ourselves as
citizens of that other place"* (SONTAG, 1977, p. 3).

Medical illness and depression are common experiences during the
lifetime of many individuals. When these states coexist, it may be that
depression is a complication of the medical illness, a cause of it, or a
coincidental occurrence. Attempts to understand the relationships between depression and medical illness bring into bold relief all of the
conundrums and controversies that persist regarding the nature of
depressive affect, the etiologic mechanisms of depression, the validity
of psychiatric diagnoses, and the implications of tragic life events for
the diagnosis and management of psychiatric disorders.

That depression is associated with medical illness is consistent with
the general literature on life events and depression. Paykel et al. (1969)
reported that undesirable life events, including changes in physical
health, are common occurrences during the six months before the onset
of clinical depression. This association between life events and depression has been confirmed by a number of subsequent investigators
(Brown & Harris, 1978; Benjaminsen, 1981; Fava et al., 1981; Roy et
al., 1985; Hammen et al., 1986). Akiskal (1982) also reported that the
co-occurrence of a medical illness is associated with incomplete recovery
from primary depression. However, these studies do not fully elucidate
the mechanisms by which medical illness is associated with depression.
This issue is of considerable theoretical and practical importance since
it has been shown that depression is common among those with chronic
medical illness (Taube et al., 1988; Wells, Golding, & Burnam, 1988).
Further, treatment of depression and other psychiatric conditions in
such patients benefits from an understanding of etiologic mechanisms

and may contribute significantly to a reduction in nonpsychiatric health care utilization (Mumford et al., 1984).

A major factor that has complicated the study of the prevalence and mechanisms of depression in the physically ill is the difficulty in establishing valid diagnostic criteria for depression in these patients. The precise boundary between normality and pathology is always difficult to demarcate. However, this distinction becomes even more problematic in the face of the unusually stressful life circumstances that are often associated with a medical illness. A variety of perplexing questions arise in this regard. For example, when are the depressive symptoms that occur in this context manifestations of a serious psychiatric disorder, and when are they simply part of a nonpathological psychological response? Are there valid criteria to differentiate normal and adaptive psychological reactions from dysfunctional states and overt psychiatric disorders? When does a desire to discontinue life-sustaining medical treatment represent a rational decision and when does it signal clinical depression? When are symptoms such as apathy, anhedonia, fatigue or insomnia manifestations of a physical disease, and when do they reflect a depressive disorder? These questions and the diagnostic criteria for depressive disorders in the medically ill are a major emphasis of the first two chapters of this text.

We have ventured into the area of depression in the medically ill for a variety of reasons. We were certainly impelled by a wish to understand and better treat patients in the medical setting who presented with vague, puzzling, depresssion-like symptoms. We recall the apathetic, lethargic patient with diabetes, blindness, and renal failure who regarded his pessimism about the future as a realistic response to his life situation rather than as a manifestation of depression. We struggled with the appropriate psychiatric response to the elderly woman with a minor physical illness who attempted suicide to avoid the possibility of disability and helplessness in her declining years. We were perplexed by the young woman with persistent and unexplained fatigue who denied subjective feelings of depression. Such patients forced us to examine our biases and assumptions regarding depression and medical illness. We became aware that there were few definitive criteria and no "gold standard" to diagnose depression in this context. Furthermore, the response to antidepressant treatment in many such conditions has been insufficiently tested. We hoped that a systematic evaluation of studies of depression in different medical conditions would help to provide some clarity and precision regarding the diagnosis, etiology and treatment of depression in the medically ill.

Ultimately, our intrigue with the problem of depression in this population likely stems from a basic interest common to most mental health professionals, namely the desire to understand varieties of human experience and forms of adaptation. Depression is central in this regard, not only because it commonly accompanies physical illness, but because it emanates from the core of human psychological experience during both normal and pathological adjustment.

We also hoped to generate interest in this subject among health professionals because we became aware that many do not identify, treat, or refer depressed medical patients for psychiatric assessment and intervention. Further, mental health professionals accustomed to treating the physically well are often unnecessarily reluctant to accept into their clinical practices, patients with serious medical illness. This reluctance is sometimes related to justifiable worry about the expertise and ability required to deal with the special demands and needs of these patients. However, hesitancy to undertake psychological treatments in the medically ill may also be related to a number of common myths, particularly about depression in these patients. Common misconceptions include the belief that most patients with a serious medical illness are depressed, that depression which is understandable as a reaction to severe circumstances does not require treatment, and/or that conventional treatments for depression are either ineffective or hazardous with such patients. Such false assumptions lead to unwarranted therapeutic nihilism regarding depression and other psychological disturbances in patients with physical illnesses. These misconceptions may lead clinicians not only to ignore potentially effective treatments for their medical patients who are depressed, but also to pay insufficient attention to the investigation and treatment of specific causes of depression in this context.

Although depression in nonmedical populations has been investigated extensively, from every conceivable point of view, the systematic study of mood disturbances among patients with a medical illness did not begin until the past decade. In fact, most earlier studies of mood disorders specifically excluded patients with serious physical illness, in order to preserve sample homogeneity. In recent years, depression has been studied systematically in numerous medical conditions and settings, but much of this research is fraught with conceptual and methodological problems and is complicated by numerous confounding variables. Indeed, the multiple manifestations of medical disease and the complex interactions among biological, psychological, and social variables pose formidable obstacles for systematic research. There is also still considerable confusion about a number of basic issues, such as the validity of standardized measures and diagnostic criteria for depression in the medically ill, the actual prevalence of depressive disorders, the psychological mechanisms by which depression may occur in context, the protective value of social supports and personality traits, and the response to antidepressant treatment. Because of these unresolved questions, it has been a formidable task either to conduct or to interpret research on depression in the medically ill. In addition, knowledge has been fragmented in this field because most studies have focused on selected aspects of depression without integrating findings from related areas of study including neurobiology, psychoanalysis, and social psychology.

The present text is directed toward an integration and critical evaluation of the literature in this field from several perspectives. At the core of the book are five main issues:

1. The prevalence and effects of mood disorders in general medical samples and in patients with specific medical disorders.
2. Methodological issues related to the assessment and diagnosis of depression in the medically ill. This includes a discussion of the validity of psychiatric rating scales, structured diagnostic interviews, and diagnostic categories.
3. The psychological, social, and biological factors that may be associated with or contribute to depression in this population.
4. Psychotherapeutic approaches to the prevention and treatment of depressive disorders in the medically ill.
5. The efficacy and use of pharmacological approaches and electroconvulsive therapy in the treatment of depression in the medically ill.

There are a number of important aspects of depression in this population that we have not specifically addressed. These include depression in medically ill children, adolescents, and the elderly. In addition, we have not discussed depression in pregnancy and the post-partum period, or depression in association with other conditions or states that are not clearly related to medical illness. Finally, we have not specifically discussed depression secondary to other psychiatric disorders (e.g., dementia, eating disorders and addictions), although we recognize that these may commonly be associated with physical conditions and may often be seen in the general hospital setting. The primary focus of this text is the relationship of depression to chronic medical illness.

The organization of this text is based primarily on conceptual issues, rather than on medical diagnoses. Although we have drawn from research undertaken on patients with a wide variety of medical conditions, we have not attempted to present an exhaustive review of the psychiatric and psychosocial literature regarding any one medical disorder. For clarity, we have divided some of the discussion according to biological, psychological, and social perspectives. However, although such divisions may help in presentation, we concur with those who consider each of these perspectives to be alternative and complementary, rather than competing approaches to the understanding of psychiatric disorders (e.g., Nemiah, 1989).

Throughout the book, and particularly in the first two chapters on diagnosis and classification, we attend to the distinction between psychiatric depressive disorders and nonpathological depressive symptoms. However, we have assumed that there is some similarity, if not a continuum, between clinical and subclinical depression. In addition, to have focused exclusively on strictly defined psychiatric disorders would have excluded subclinical states of dysphoria and distress experienced by medical patients that could well benefit from therapeutic intervention.

In assessing published research, we have given greater weight to studies that are methodologically rigorous. For example, in the section on the prevalence and epidemiology of depressive disorders, we have based our conclusions only upon studies that described diagnostic criteria in detail. Studies with less rigorous methodology are discussed separately in a section reviewing the occurrence of depressive symptoms, not necessarily associated with depressive disorders. Overall, stricter criteria were applied to those sections in which there is a considerable body of empirical research (e.g., the assessment and diagnosis of depression) compared with those areas in which there is relatively little empirical research (e.g., the psychodynamics and psychotherapy of depression in the medically ill).

We are keenly aware that a comprehensive approach to the understanding of depression must include not only reliable methods of measurement and diagnosis but also an understanding of the underlying phenomena that are being measured. As Faust and Miner (1986) observed, although measurement and precision are important in science, "in the long run, there is little to be gained by attempting to measure poorly understood things precisely and then multiplying our observations of them" (p. 966). Unfortunately, although psychiatric methodology has become more sophisticated in recent years, clinical concepts of affect and its disturbances have still tended to be somewhat reductionistic (Berrios, 1985). Although recent studies of depression in the medically ill tend to be more rigorous, research in this area has been particularly hampered by studies that have applied measurement techniques without establishing either their conceptual basis or validity in the sample studied. Unfortunately, such limitations persist in much of the literature on depression in the physically ill. While a primary goal of this text is to summarize the best available research literature on the relevant topics, we are also interested in conveying to the reader, an appreciation of the human experience of depression in the context of physical illness.

Clinical and research investigations into depression and other psychiatric disturbances in the medically ill have too often been limited by approaches that are narrow and compartmentalized. One kind of compartmentalization, disease-specific research, tends not to take into account findings based on other medical conditions. Such research is important and necessary to understand the variability between illnesses, but its utility is enhanced when it is well grounded in concepts that are generalizable to other types of physical illness. Unfortunately, approaches to a broad range of medical illness in the literature have tended to be anecdotal, impressionistic, or else based upon observations of general medical samples in which documentation or quantification of the medical variables is minimal or absent.

Another kind of compartmentalization that affects investigations of depression in the medically ill involves what has been characterized as "hard" versus "soft" science. This distinction is typically dependent on whether or not observations are quantitative and/or theories are exact. We applaud the "hard" empirical research that has contributed to the refinement of diagnostic and assessment methods and to the evaluation of treatment modalities for depression. Without the strict application of this methodology, clinical observations could not be tested and refinement of knowledge would cease. However, an exclusive emphasis on empirical methods has led too often in psychiatry and psychology to neglect of the human drama and of the individual, interpersonal, and social contexts in which symptoms are found. In this regard, Kleinman (1988) has recently suggested that the narrow technological bias of modern biomedicine has led practitioners away from what he argues ought to be important aspects of medical care. He emphasizes that one of the most important functions of health care providers ought to be the "empathic witnessing" of the patient's existential experience and his or her practical efforts to cope with the major psychosocial crises of illness. We are in sympathy with this point of view. However, humanistic practitioners and theorists who have focused on the experiential aspects of medical illness have too often neglected scientific methods and ignored biological contributions to psychopathology. This bias has led to erroneous generalizations based upon limited observations, and, unwittingly, to the discreditation of humanistic approaches within some quarters of the scientific community.

We hope that we have not fallen victim to the temptations of compartmentalized thinking regarding our subject. We have attempted to synthesize some of the vast literature on depression in the medically ill, to organize the discussion along conceptual lines, and to present a balanced and accurate perspective regarding the contribution of psychosocial and somatic contributions to depression in these patients. Our goal has been to present a scientific perspective on depression in the medically ill without neglecting the human dilemma involved. The reader must judge our success in this task.

REFERENCES

Akiskal, H.S. (1982). Factors associated with incomplete recovery in primary depressive illness. *Journal of Clinical Psychiatry, 43,* 266-271.

Benjaminsen, S. (1981). Stressful life events preceding the onset of neurotic depression. *Psychological Medicine, 11,* 369-378.

Berrios, G.E. (1985). The Psychopathology of affectivity: Conceptual and historical aspects. *Psychological Medicine, 15,* 745-758.

Brown, G.W. & Harris, T.O. (1978). *Social Origins of Depression: A Study of Psychiatric Disorder in Women.* London: Tavistock Publications.

Faust, D. & Miner, R.A. (1986). The empiricist and his new clothes: DSM-III in perspective. *American Journal of Psychiatry, 143,* 962-967.

Fava, G.A., Munari, F., Pavan, L., & Kellner, R. (1981). Life events and depression: A replication. *Journal of Affective Disorders, 3,* 159-165.

Hammen, C., Mayol, A., deMayo, R., & Marks, T. (1986). Initial symptom levels and the life-event-depression relationship. *Journal of Abnormal Psychology, 95,* 114-122.

Kleinman, A. (1988). *The Illness Narrative: Suffering, Healing and the Human Condition.* New York: Basic Books, Inc.

Mumford, E., Schlesinger, H.J., Glass, G.V., Patrick, C., & Cuerdon, T. (1984). A new look at evidence about reduced cost of medical utilization following mental health treatment. *American Journal of Psychiatry, 141,* 1145-1158.

Nemiah, J. (1989). The varieties of human experience. *British Journal of Psychiatry, 154,* 459-465.

Paykel, E.S., Myers, J.K., Dienelt, M.N., Klerman, G.L., Lindenthal, J.J., & Pepper, M.P. (1969). Life events and depression: A controlled study. *Archives of General Psychiatry, 21,* 753-760.

Roy, A., Breier, A., Doran, A.R., & Pickar, D. (1985). Life events in depression: Relationship to subtypes. *Journal of Affective Disorders, 9,* 143-148.

Sontag, S. (1977). *Illness as Metaphor.* New York: Random House.

Taube, C.A., Goldman, H.H., Burns, B.J., & Kessler, L.G. (1988). High users of outpatient mental health services: I. Definition and characteristics. *American Journal of Psychiatry, 145,* 19-24.

Wells, K.B., Golding, J.M., & Burnam, M.A. (1988). Psychiatric disorder in a sample of the general population with and without chronic medical conditions. *American Journal of Psychiatry, 145,* 976-981.

PART I

CLINICAL PRESENTATION

1

Assessment and Diagnosis: I

The assessment of depression is fraught with difficulty because of the uncertain, and at times, arbitrary, boundaries among its clinical, sub-clinical, and nonpathological forms. Controversies about the conditions under which mood changes should be regarded as pathological (see Klerman, 1981) are heightened in the medically ill. In that context, clinicians are called upon to differentiate symptoms of major depression not only from those of less severe adjustment disorders and nonpath-ological reactions to illness, but also from those symptoms that are more direct manifestations of physical disease. These distinctions are problematic both because there is a realistic basis for feelings of sadness associated with a serious medical illness, and because vegetative symptoms such as anorexia or loss of energy may be the result of the physical illness.

It has been repeatedly demonstrated that the somatic symptoms that are used to diagnose depression are reported frequently by patients in general medical settings (Moffic & Paykel, 1975; Clark, Cavanaugh, & Gibbons, 1983) and with specific medical conditions including cancer (Bukberg, Penman, & Holland, 1984), endstage renal disease (Smith, Hong, & Robson, 1985; Craven et al., 1987), diabetes mellitus with metabolic dyscontrol (Lustman et al., 1986a), rheumatoid arthritis (Frank et al., 1988), Parkinson's disease (Starkstein & Robinson, 1989) and multiple sclerosis (Krupp et al., 1988). Each of these illnesses is as-sociated with a different constellation of symptoms that may confound the diagnosis of depression. For this reason, a substantial body of recent research has been directed toward identifying features that discriminate major depression from somatic symptoms that are produced directly by different physical illnesses. Some of this research is reviewed in this chapter and in the two which follow. The latter are devoted to the assessment and diagnosis of depression in the physically ill. This topic has been given extensive attention, not only because it is multifaceted, but also because diagnosing depression in this population remains a difficult task, even for experienced clinicians and researchers in the field.

DEPRESSIVE SYMPTOMS IN THE MEDICALLY ILL

Description of Measures

Due to their ease of administration and scoring, self-report measures of depressive symptoms are commonly used to study depression in the medically ill. In general, these instruments are composed of a standardized series of statements or questions based upon characteristic or typical symptoms of depression. The responses are scored either by the patient (self-report) or, less commonly, by the interviewer (observer-rated). These instruments have been termed "dimensional" measures because their scoring system usually allows a simple addition of items and the score reflects the overall severity of depressive symptoms on a continuous scale ranging from absent to severe. An assumption upon which these scales are founded is that depression is a continuous variable extending through their range (House, 1988). However, for many of the instruments, one or more cutoffs or threshold scores have also been defined to identify subgroups of patients (e.g., not depressed, mildly depressed).

Compared with unstructured clinical interviews, self-report inventories may be more reliable indicators of the presence and severity of depressive symptoms. The reliability of these instruments derives from the standardization of the questions or statements, their order of presentation, the wording and choices of answers, and the method of scoring. Unfortunately, these measures are of limited usefulness in the diagnosis of clinical depression (Boyle, 1985). Before discussing in more detail the general shortcomings and limitations of self-report instruments, we will describe the three instruments most frequently used to study depression in the medically ill—the Beck Depression Inventory (BDI), the Zung Self-Rating Depression Scale (SDS) and the Center for Epidemiologic Studies Depression Scale (CES-D).

Beck Depression Inventory (BDI)

The Beck Depression Inventory (Beck et al., 1961; Beck, Steer, & Garbin, 1988) is one of the most commonly used measures of depressive symptoms in medically ill samples. It is a 21-item, self-report questionnaire that includes 14 cognitive-affective symptoms and seven somatic ones. Each item (e.g., I feel like I am being punished) describes a symptom of depression with four accompanying descriptive statements ranging in intensity from absent, mild, moderate to severe. The respondent indicates which statement for each item best applies to him or her over the past seven days. Scoring the instrument involves the simple addition of the answers for the 21 items to give a total score ranging between 0 and 63. In addition to this summation score reflecting overall severity, Beck, Steer, and Garbin (1988) have provided cutoff scores for use in medically well samples. These cutoffs have been validated to define the following four groups: no depression (0-9); mild-moderate (10-18); moderate-severe (19-29); and severe (30-63) depressive symptoms.

The BDI has adequate reliability and validity (Beck, Steer, & Garbin, 1988) in medically well samples and has been used in several hundred studies since its inception (Steer, Beck, & Garrison, 1986). However, the evidence that the BDI can be used to quantify the construct of depressed mood with reasonable consistency should not be considered equivalent to its utility in identifying major depression. From an examination of the factor structure of the BDI, Louks, Hayne, and Smith (1989) found that whereas the instrument appears to measure the cognitive aspects of depression, its total score was not strongly related to the vegetative symptoms of depression that are an important clinical aspect of a major depressive episode.

The BDI has been widely used in medical settings, but only a small number of studies have examined the validity of this measure in these patients. One study by Clark, Cavanaugh, and Gibbons (1983) demonstrated adequate internal consistency for the BDI in a sample of general medical inpatients. In order to determine its diagnostic validity in 153 general medical inpatients, Schwab et al. (1967a) compared the BDI scores with results from clinical interviews and from an observer-rated measure of depressive symptoms, the Hamilton Rating Scale for Depression (HAM-D). They concluded that the BDI cutoff (i.e., >9) used in the general population to indicate at least mild depressive symptoms was also useful in their sample. Subsequent investigators have most commonly suggested that the threshold for case definition of depression should be increased in the physically ill. The need for a higher threshold is suggested by the increased frequency of both somatic symptoms (e.g., loss of energy), and of nonpathological depressive symptoms associated with adjustment to illness in physically ill patients. Unfortunately, there has been little agreement about what is the most appropriate cutoff score to screen for severe or clinical depression. Thresholds of >9 (e.g., Smith, Hong, & Robson, 1985), >13 (e.g., Moffic & Paykel, 1975), and >17 (e.g., Rodin & Voshart, 1987) have been used to identify significant depression. The use of a similar cutoff by different investigators would certainly improve the comparability of studies, but little evidence exists to support strongly the use of any particular cutoff. Some investigators have wisely reported the case rates found using several different BDI cutoffs (e.g., Nielsen & Williams, 1980).

Zung Self-Rating Depression Scale (SDS)

The Zung Self-Rating Depression Scale (Zung, 1965, 1986) was con-structed from verbatim reports of depressed patients. Statements most representative of the depressive symptoms were included in the 20-item scale (e.g., I feel downhearted, blue, and sad). When administered, the patient is asked to rate each item according to how often this symptom was experienced during the week prior to completing the questionnaire. The possible answers include: none or little of the time; some of the time; a good part of the time; and most of the time. The maximum possible raw score is 80.

The SDS has been found to have adequate concurrent validity com-pared with several other dimensional scales of depression. Construct validity has been demonstrated in studies that have shown a reduction in scores as patients recover from major depression (Zung, 1986). The average score on the scale in nondepressed samples drawn from the general population is 39 (Zung, 1986). A series of studies, which together include more than 1500 patients with depressive disorders, showed that the mean score of these patients is most commonly between 55 and 70 (Zung, 1986). These and other data led to the establishment of a cutoff score of either >50 or >55 to indicate significant depression, although Okimoto et al. (1982) provided evidence to support a cutoff of >60 to detect depression in elderly medical patients. The psycho-metric properties of the SDS have not been clearly established in patients with physical illness.

Center for Epidemiologic Studies Depression Scale (CES-D)

The Center for Epidemiologic Studies Depression Scale (Comstock & Helsing, 1976; Craig & Van Natta, 1976) is a self-administered 20-item questionnaire that contains statements, as do the BDI and SDS, corresponding to characteristic symptoms of depression experienced over the week prior to completing the scale. Each item in the questionnaire has a range of four response options based on how often during the past week the respondent experienced a symptom (e.g., rarely or none of the time, some or little of the time, occasionally or a moderate amount of the time, and most or all of the time). The score, which may range from 0 to 60, indicates the severity of depressive symptoms.

The CES-D has been most commonly used to screen for depressive symptoms in the general population. From these studies, it has been determined that a cutoff of >15 is suggestive of at least mild depression. For example, Radloff (1977) has shown that the mean score in a normal population is approximately 8, and that about 20 percent of a normal population and 70 percent of a psychiatric population score above 15. In both normal and psychiatric samples, the instrument has been demonstrated to have very high internal consistency and adequate test-retest reliability. The diagnostic validity of this scale has not been stringently tested in medical samples.

Nonspecific Measures of Psychologic Morbidity

Several other measures have also been used to measure emotional distress in medical patients. The General Health Questionnaire (GHQ) (Goldberg, 1972) has been widely applied in medical settings. However, the GHQ is a measure of overall emotional distress and does not selectively focus on depressive symptoms. Similarly, the Symptom Distress Checklist (SCL-90-R) (Derogatis, 1983) has been used in medical inpatients. Although this inventory includes a depression subscale, the total score is most frequently reported, and the findings of the depression subscale are seldom described in full. Some have argued that measures of generalized distress are the most appropriate for use in the medical setting (Mayou & Hawton, 1986). This may be true, depending upon the purpose for which they are used. Studies using these less specific measures of psychologic morbidity are occasionally referred to in this text, but for the most part, we discuss in detail only those studies and measures that selectively focus on depression and depressive symptoms in the physically ill.

Limitations of Self-Report Measures

The absence of adequate validation of self-report measures in medically ill patients is a major limitation to their use in medical settings. Most problematic, when these measures are used with physically ill patients, is that they include somatic symptoms of depression that are confounded by the physical illness. For example, the Minnesota Multiphasic Personality Inventory (MMPI), which includes a depression subscale, has been used frequently in studies of patients with rheumatoid arthritis. Pincus et al. (1986) found that 70 randomly selected rheumatoid arthritis patients attending an arthritis treatment center had elevated scores on depression, hypochondriasis, and hysteria, three subscales of the MMPI. However, these authors also reported that the elevations on these subscales were almost entirely accounted for by a small number of items (e.g., loss of energy) which two-thirds of 117 rheumatologists rated as highly consistent with active rheumatoid arthritis itself. The investigators concluded that depressive and other symptoms measured by the MMPI were likely to be falsely elevated in patients with rheumatoid arthritis and suggested that similar false positives might be found with other chronic diseases.

Several studies have shown that somatic symptoms that represent specific diagnostic criteria for major depression (e.g., fatigue, anorexia, weight loss, insomnia, sleep disturbance, and loss of sexual interest) are common in both depressed and nondepressed medical patients (Clark, Cavanaugh, & Gibbons, 1983; Plumb & Holland, 1977). Schwab et al. (1967b) found that loss of sexual interest, sleep disturbance, and fatigue were present in from 34 percent to 66 percent of nondepressed mixed medical inpatients with BDI scores of less than 10. Thus, somatic symptoms such as these may be less useful in distinguishing depressed from euthymic medical patients (Schwab et al., 1967a; Moffic & Paykel, 1975; Plumb & Holland, 1977; Gibbons et al., 1985; Emmons, Fetting, & Zonderman, 1987). However, the above studies of mixed medical samples do not identify which somatic symptoms, in which specific medical illnesses are useful in discriminating major depression. Symptoms such as weight loss may have little diagnostic value in conditions such as cancer, but may be more specific for depression in other medical diseases such as rheumatoid arthritis and endstage renal disease.

In their review of depression and physical illness, Mayou and Hawton (1986) concluded that most rating scales lead to the overdiagnosis of depression in medical patients. These and other authors have expressed concern that the somatic items (e.g., anorexia) included on measures of depressive symptoms likely contribute directly to this overdiagnosis because they also directly measure symptoms of physical illness. This concern led to the suggestion that depression inventories contain fewer somatic items (Mayou & Hawton, 1986) or, alternatively, that scales be developed that eliminate somatic items altogether (Aylard et al., 1987).

Mayou and Hawton (1986) suggested that some available measures such as the Beck Depression Inventory and the General Health Questionnaire-30 are well suited to assess depression in the medically ill, as they are already heavily weighted for cognitive-affective disturbances. Zigmond and Snaith (1983) designed the Hospital Anxiety and Depression Scale (HAD) specifically for medically ill patients, and they included in this measure a high proportion of psychological rather than somatic items. Others have suggested that "inappropriate" somatic items should be deleted from existing scales (Aylard et al., 1987). However, this latter approach would require extensive investigation prior to its adoption because the psychometric properties of the scales would be altered. Modification of a scale requires revalidation and preferably renaming, as House (1988) suggested. Furthermore, though the deletion of somatic items from questionnaires may avoid overdiagnosing depression in the medical setting, this practice risks underdiagnosing medical depressives who present largely with somatic symptoms. Studies that contribute further to the refinement of diagnostic methodology in the medical setting are discussed in the last section of this chapter.

To avoid overdiagnosing major depression in the physically ill, others have recommended raising the cutoff scores for case identification (Moffic & Paykel, 1975; Cavanaugh, 1983; Bridges & Goldberg, 1984). This approach has merit in that it minimizes the number of false positive cases due to the confounding of illness-related and depressive symptoms without eliminating somatic symptoms from consideration. The latter, we would argue, are common manifestations of depression in the physically ill. However, there is little agreement at present regarding what is an appropriate increase in the threshold for case identification. Only a limited number of studies of depression in the physically ill have used standardized diagnoses of mood disorders to help define appropriate cutoff scores (e.g., Nielson & Williams, 1980; Craven, Rodin, & Littlefield, 1988; Parikh et al., 1988). In addition, most of the studies that have examined the validity of various cutoff scores have self-report measures as screening, rather than diagnostic devices. The utility of self-report measures as screening instruments for depression in the physically ill is discussed in Chapter 2.

Several other factors may also contribute to a high rate of false positive and false negative findings when self-report measures are used to identify clinical depression in the medically ill (Myers & Weissman, 1980; Boyle, 1985). First, psychological symptoms are not specific for depression and may occur both in normal states and in other psychological conditions (Gotlib, 1984). Thus, elevated scores on depression measures can occur with normal adjustment processes or with other psychiatric conditions (e.g., anxiety disorders) whose symptoms overlap with depressive disorders. Second, elevated depression scores may occur due to normal fluctuations in mood state and/or to relatively transient psychological reactions to physical symptoms such as pain or nausea. Third, the diagnostic specificity of most self-report measures is diminished by the lack of weighting of particular items. In most cases, each item is weighted equally, with the total score being a simple addition of all recorded symptoms. However, it is not necessarily accurate to assume that all items should be granted equal status in the diagnosis of depression. For example, anhedonia is considered by some to be pathognomic of depression (Snaith, 1987) and might warrant greater weighting than a less specific symptom such as insomnia. In fact, a high score on a self-report measure can be obtained even if the specific complaints of depressed mood or loss of interest are absent.

These and other limitations raise serious concern about the utility of self-report measures to define cases of depression in the medically ill (Blumenthal, 1975; Plumb & Holland, 1977; Glass et al., 1978; Boyd et al., 1982; Bukberg, Penman, & Holland, 1984; Craven, Rodin, & Littlefield, 1988). Overall, studies that have examined the validity of self-report measures of depressive symptoms have found that, when used alone, they are not adequate to diagnose depressive disorders. In fact, these measures were not originally designed for this purpose, although some investigators have used them in this way. In this text we distinguish studies of depressive symptoms (e.g., based on self-report symptom inventories) from studies of depressive disorders. With these limitations in mind, studies based upon self-report measures may still add to our understanding of depression in the physically ill.

Prevalence of Depressive Symptoms

Tables 1.1, 1.2, and 1.3 represent a comprehensive selection of English language reports of studies whose primary purpose was to estimate the prevalence of depressive symptoms in medically ill patients. Table 1.1 lists those studies that report the prevalence of depressive symptoms in outpatients in either primary care or general medical settings. Table 1.2 lists studies of depressive symptoms in general medical inpatients. Table 1.3 summarizes those studies in which there is a specific medical disorder common to the sample, although the sample may include either inpatients or outpatients. For the most part, studies were included only if the samples consisted of subjects with medical disorders with a clearly defined organic basis. Not included were studies undertaken in patients with conditions in which the pathophysiology was ill-defined (e.g., tinnitus or chronic fatigue syndrome), and studies designed primarily to assess the prevalence of depressive symptoms following a medical or surgical intervention (e.g., depression following hysterectomy). Conditions in which there is unresolved ambiguity regarding both medical diagnosis and mood symptoms are described in Chapter 3.

Certain minimal methodological criteria were used in selecting the studies included here. Only those studies in which the depression measure was administered to the entire sample, and in which the sample size was large enough to allow reasonable confidence in interpreting the results were included. Studies had to specify either the cutoff or threshold used to define cases of depression, or provide the raw data from which a prevalence estimate could be derived. Preference was given to studies that used a measure specifically designed to assess depressive symptoms. However, this rule was relaxed when the majority of studies in an area of interest used less specific measures of emotional distress (e.g., the General Health Questionnaire has been commonly administered in studies in primary care settings).

Our decision to exclude most surveys of general psychological distress may have led to an underestimation of the prevalence of emotional distress in medical samples. Indeed, Mayou and Hawton (1986) have argued that the most common emotional disorder in the medically ill is an "undifferentiated neurotic pattern" consisting of symptoms of both depression and anxiety, and corresponding most closely to the DSM-III diagnosis of adjustment disorder with mixed emotional features. For this reason, they have argued that a general symptom questionnaire such as the General Health Questionnaire is most appropriate for use in the medical setting. This is a valid argument, particularly in the primary care setting where physicians should be aware of nonspecific emotional distress and are in an ideal position to investigate further and to implement some form of intervention. Our focus in this text is on the more specific construct of depression, although we hope that such an approach will contribute to an improved understanding of the broader range of emotional problems that occur in medical patients.

It should be noted that many of the studies listed in Table 1.1 are based on primary care patients in which the presence of physical illness

TABLE 1.1. *Prevalence of Depressive Symptoms in Primary Care or General Medical Outpatient Settings*

Author(s) and Year	n	Subject Characteristics	Instrument	Cut-off Point	Prevalence
Salkind (1969)	80	general practice	Beck Depression Inventory	≥11 ≥23	48.0% 8.0%
Moore, Silimperi, & Bobula (1978)	212	general practice	Zung Self-Rating Depression Scale	≥50 ≥60	45.3% 19.3%
Linn & Yager (1980)	100	internal medicine	Zung Self-Rating Depression Scale	≥50 ≥60 ≥70	42.0% 21.0% 7.0%
MacDonald & Bouchier (1980)	100	gastroenterology and general medicine	General Health Questionnaire–60, & Standard Psychiatric Interview	≥10 and depression	26.0%
Nielsen & Williams (1980)	526	general practice	Beck Depression Inventory	≥10 ≥13 ≥15 ≥17 ≥20 ≥30	19.8% 12.2% 8.4% 5.5% 3.0% 0.4%
Wright et al. (1980)	199	general practice	Zung Self-Rating Depression Scale	≥50 ≥60	41.0% 17.0%
Seller, Blascovich, & Lenkei (1981)	222	general practice	Beck Depression Inventory	≥11 ≥21	34.7% 14.4%
Okimoto et al. (1982)	55	elderly general medical patients	Zung Self-Rating Depression Scale	≥60	23.6%

Author (year)	N	Setting	Instrument	Criterion	Percentage
Dhadphale, Ellison, & Griffin (1983)	388	general practice	Self Reporting Questionnaire, & Standard Psychiatric Interview	ICD-8 depression	9.3%
Hankin & Locke (1983)	1,921	internal medicine & obstetrics-gynecology	Center for Epidemiologic Studies Depression Scale	≥ 16	21.6%
Zung et al. (1983)	1,086	general practice	Zung Self-Rating Depression Scale	≥ 55	13.2%
Barnes & Prosen (1984)	1,250	general practice	Center for Epidemiologic Studies Depression Scale	≥ 16 ≥ 21 ≥ 31	33.2% 21.4% 8.1%
Borson et al. (1986)	406	elderly medical	Zung Self-Rating Depression Scale	> 60	24.4%
Katon et al. (1986)	147	general practice	Beck Depression Inventory - Short Form, & Zung Self-Rating Depression Scale	≥ 8 ≥ 60	17.0% 11.6%
Rose et al. (1986)	100	gastroenterology outpatients	Beck Depression Inventory - Short Form	≥ 8 > 15	29.0% 9.0%
Rucker, Frye, & Cygan (1986)	375	general practice	Beck Depression Inventory - Short Form	at least moderate symptoms	32.5%
Williamson (1987)	354	general practice	Beck Depression Inventory	≥ 13	15.5%

TABLE 1.2. *Prevalence of Depressive Symptoms in General Medical Inpatients*

Author(s) and Year	n	Subject Characteristics	Instrument	Cut-off Point	Prevalence
Schwab et al. (1967a)	153	general medical	Beck Depression Inventory, & Hamilton Rating Scale for Depression	≥14 >42	21.6% 22.9%
Maguire et al. (1974)	230	general medical	General Health Questionnaire–60, & Standardized Psychiatric Interview	>11 and depression	10.8%
Moffic & Paykel (1975)	150	general medical	Beck Depression Inventory	≥14 ≥26	24.0% 2.0%
Knights & Folstein (1977)	57	general medical	General Health Questionnaire–30	>4	46.0%
Fava et al. (1982a)	325	general medical	Center for Epidemiologic Studies Depression Scale	≥16 ≥23 ≥28	58.0% 35.5% 25.2%
Fava et al. (1982b)	325	oncology	Center for Epidemiologic Studies Depression Scale	≥16 ≥23	57.8% 33.5%
Cavanaugh (1983)	335	general medical	Beck Depression Inventory	≥10 ≥14 ≥18 ≥21	51.0% 32.0% 18.0% 14.0%

Study	N	Setting	Instrument	Cutoff	Percentage
Magni, De Leo, & Schifano (1985)	379	general medical geriatric (n=178) adult (n=201)	Zung Self-Rating Depression Scale	≥50 (geriatric) (adult)	42.1% 20.4%
Levenson et al. (1986)	80	general medical	Hopkins Symptom Checklist (SCL-90-R)	>28	21.3%
Feldman et al. (1987)	382	general medical	General Health Questionnaire–30, & Present State Examination	CATEGO depression >4	6.8%
Hengeveld, Ancion, & Rooijmans (1987)	220	general medical	Beck Depression Inventory	≥13	32.0%
Johnston et al. (1987)	113	general medical (geriatric)	General Health Questionnaire–28, & Clinical Interview	>4 and depression ?	43.0% 17.0%
Yang et al. (1987)	251	general medical	Beck Depression Inventory	≥13 ≥25	47.8% 13.5%
Koenig et al. (1988)	128	neurology & medicine (geriatric)	Geriatric Depression Scale, & Brief Carroll Depression Rating Scale (n=64)	≥11 ≥14 ≥6	19.5% 15.6% 17.2%
Rosenberg et al. (1988)	71	general medical	Beck Depression Inventory	≥14	38.0%

TABLE 1.3. *Prevalence of Depressive Symptoms in Patients with Specific Medical Illness*

Author(s) and Year	n	Subject Characteristics	Instrument	Cut-off Point	Prevalence
Endstage Renal Disease					
Rodin et al. (1984)	85	ESRD	Beck Depression Inventory	≥18	26.0%
Kutner, Fair, & Kutner (1985)	128	ESRD	Zung Self-Rating Depression Scale	≥56	26.6%
Rodin & Voshart (1987)	115	ESRD	Beck Depression Inventory	≥17 >30	25.7% 6.2%
Neurological Diseases					
Kirk & Saunders (1979)	342	neurology outpatients	General Health Questionnaire–60	>11 >26	48.0% 21.0%
Bridges & Goldberg (1984)	100	neurology inpatients	General Health Questionnaire–28, & Clinical Interview Schedule	≥12 and "minor depression"	24.0%
Robinson & Price (1982)	103	poststroke	General Health Questionnaire–28	≥5	29.1%
Sinyor et al. (1986)	64	poststroke	Zung Self-Rating Depression Scale	≥50 ≥60	47.0% 22.0%
Wade, Legh-Smith, & Hewer (1987)	976	poststroke (six months)	Wakefield Self-Assessment Depression Inventory	≥15 ≥19	32.0% 20.0%

Study	N	Diagnosis	Instrument	Cutoff	%
Ebrahim, Barer, & Nouri (1987)	149	poststroke	General Health Questionnaire–28	≥12	22.8%
Warburton (1967)	140	Parkinson's disease	Warburton Criteria	Grades I, II, III	63.0%
Celesia & Wanamaker (1972)	153	Parkinson's disease	Warburton Criteria	Grade I Grade II Grade III	12.4% 15.0% 9.8%
Mayeux et al. (1981)	55	Parkinson's disease	Beck Depression Inventory	≥10 ≥18 ≥25	47.2% 16.3% 3.6%
Gotham, Brown, & Marsden (1986)	189	Parkinson's disease	Beck Depression Inventory	≥10 ≥18 ≥25	69.0% 29.0% 12.0%
Frochtengarten et al. (1987)	56	Parkinson's disease	Hamilton Rating Scale for Depression (modified-max.40)	≥9 ≥13	62.5% 27.0%
Folstein, Folstein, & McHugh (1979)	11	Huntington's Chorea	General Health Questionnaire–30	>4	72.7%
Whitlock & Siskind (1980)	30	multiple sclerosis	Beck Depression Inventory	≥15 ≥25	26.7% 10.0%
Comings & Comings (1987)	246	Tourette syndrome	Beck Depression Inventory	≥9	20.7%
Jahanshahi & Marsden (1988)	85	torticollis	Beck Depression Inventory	≥10 ≥18 >24	53.6% 28.6% 11.9%
"	49	cervical spondylosis	Beck Depression Inventory	≥10 ≥18 >24	38.5% 15.4% 2.6%

TABLE 1.3. (continued)

Author(s) and Year	n	Subject Characteristics	Instrument	Cut-off Point	Prevalence
Oncology					
Koenig, Levin, & Brennan (1967)	36	oncology	Minnesota Multiphasic Personality Inventory-Depression Subscale	≥70 (D30 raw score of ≥14)	25.0%
Craig & Abeloff (1974)	30	oncology inpatients	Hopkins Symptom Checklist (SCL-90)	Depression Dimension >2.0	13.3%
Plumb & Holland (1977)	97	oncology	Beck Depression Inventory	≥14 ≥25	23.0% 4.0%
Silberfarb, Maurer, & Crouthamel (1980)	146	oncology: breast cancer	Psychiatric Status Schedule	depressed affect	15.0%
Cain et al. (1983)	60	gynecological oncology	Hamilton Rating Scale for Depression	≥18 ≥25	36.7% 3.3%
Bukberg, Penman, & Holland (1984)	62	oncology inpatients	Hamilton Rating Scale for Depression, & Beck Depression Inventory	>21 ≥14	15.0% 33.0%

Study	n	Population	Instrument	Cutoff	%
Lansky et al. (1985)	505	oncology	Zung Self-Rating Depression Scale, & Hamilton Rating Scale for Depression	≥50	5.3%
Davies, Davies, & Delpo (1986)	38	head & neck oncology	Leeds Scale for Assessment of Depression	≥20 >6	28.9%
Bisno & Richardson (1987)	53	oncology receiving radiotherapy	Beck Depression Inventory	≥14 ≥25	22.6% 1.9%
Lasry et al. (1987)	123	breast cancer i) lumpectomy (n=44) ii) mastectomy (n=43) iii) lumpectomy & radiotherapy (n=36)	Center for Epidemiologic Studies Depression Scale	>15	i) 41.0% ii) 50.0% iii) 50.0%
Other					
Zaphiropoulos & Burry (1974)	50	rheumatoid arthritis	Beck Depression Inventory	≥15 ≥25	46.0% 16.0%
Bishop et al. (1987)	39	rheumatoid arthritis	Beck Depression Inventory	≥17	11.0%
Mayou (1975)	94	venereal disease	Clinical Interview Schedule	>20 (depression) (depression & anxiety)	5.3% 16.0%
Stern, Pascale, & Ackerman (1977)	68	myocardial infarction	Zung Self-Rating Depression Scale	≥40	22.0%

TABLE 1.3. *(continued)*

Author(s) and Year	n	Subject Characteristics	Instrument	Cut-off Point	Prevalence
Teiramaa (1979)	100	asthma	Beck Depression Inventory	≥15	21.0%
McSweeney et al. (1982)	203	COPD outpatients	Minnesota Multiphasic Personality Inventory— Depression Subscale	T score >60	42.0%
Light et al. (1985)	45	COPD outpatients	Beck Depression Inventory	≥15	42.0%
Hughes et al. (1983)	196	dermatology outpatients	General Health Questionnaire–30, & Wakefield Self-Assessment Depression Scale	≥5 ≥14	30.1% 15.0%
Byrne (1984)	211	gynecology outpatients	General Health Questionnaire–60	≥12	45.5%
Lalinec-Michaud, Engelsmann, & Marino (1988)	152	gynecology	Zung Self-Rating Depression Scale, & Hamilton Rating Scale for Depression	≥64 ≥13	7.2% 13.2%

Study	N	Population	Scale	Cutoff	%
Chamberlain & Chamberlain (1985)	120	denture prosthodontics	Beck Depression Inventory	≥10 ≥13	10.7% 6.6%
Ward et al. (1987)	139	post-burn patients	Beck Depression Inventory	≥10 ≥15	22.3% 12.9%
Wulsin et al. (1988)	49	ER patients with atypical chest pain	Center for Epidemiologic Studies Depression Scale	≥16	38.8%
Lyons et al. (1989)	69	elderly patients with Hip fracture	Hamilton Rating Scale for Depression, & Geriatric Depression Scale	≥17 ≥25 ≥15	34.7% 6.1% 47.4%
Millman et al. (1989)	55	obstructive sleep apnea	Zung Self-Rating Depression Scale	≥50	45.0%
Mossey et al. (1989)	219	post-hip fracture	Center for Epidemiologic Studies Depression Scale	≥16 (post surgery) ≥8 (12 month follow-up)	51.2% 20.0%

is sometimes not clearly documented. In addition, the relationship between depression and physical illness is least clear in this setting because the primary care patients with more depressive symptoms tend to be those who do not have a medical diagnosis (Kirk & Saunders, 1979; MacDonald & Bouchier, 1980; Vazquez-Barquero et al., 1985). It may be that such patients present to their general practitioners primarily for psychological rather than physical assistance. On the other hand, Henley and Coussens (1988) found that depressive symptoms were more frequent in 297 general practice patients with a medical diagnosis than in the remainder of the sample without a defined illness. Further work is required, in a wider range of samples, to clarify the relationship between depression and physical illness in the primary care setting.

Depressive symptoms based on self-report measures occur in from less than 10 percent of some samples (Lansky et al., 1985; Rose et al., 1986; Johnston et al., 1987; Feldman et al., 1987) to over 50 percent of other samples (Fava et al., 1982a, 1982b; Lasry et al., 1987). The majority of studies have found at least mild symptoms of depression in one-fifth to one-third of medical patients studied. These figures support the contention that depressive symptoms are common in the physically ill. However, a striking feature of the findings summarized in these tables is the wide variation in the prevalence rates reported. The confounding of depressive and illness-related symptoms may contribute to this variability, as may variations in the cutoff scores used for case definition. Other factors that influence the results include demographic or clinical differences among the samples, and the time of measurement in relation to the longitudinal course of the medical illness. For example, in patients with endstage renal disease, more severe depressive symptoms may be expected during the first one to two years following the initiation of dialysis than at other times during the course of this condition (Kutner, Fair, & Kutner, 1985).

Other trends are evident from the summary tables of these studies. Most cases defined as depressed using symptom thresholds show mild to moderate, rather than severe depression. This is most obvious in studies reporting prevalence rates based on multiple cutoff scores (Zaphiropoulos & Burry, 1974; Moffic & Paykel, 1975; Nielsen & Williams, 1980; Cavanaugh, 1983; Barnes & Prosen, 1984). As higher cutoffs are used for case definition, the prevalence of "depression" drops dramatically. Moffic and Paykel (1975) found that 24 percent of their medical inpatients demonstrated at least mild symptoms of depression (BDI ≥ 14) whereas only 2 percent were found to be severely depressed (BDI ≥ 26). An additional trend is that although depressive symptoms are relatively common in medical patients, more than one-half of the patients in most of the samples reported no significant depressive symptoms. Even studies undertaken in patients with severe and potentially disabling physical illness have consistently found that one-half or more of the sample reported no symptoms of depression (e.g., Holland, 1977; Robinson & Price, 1982; Comings & Comings, 1987). Apparently, even mild depression is not universal in the medically ill. Thus, the occurrence of depressive symptoms cannot be explained entirely by the presence or absence of medical illness, but must also depend upon other factors. The assumption that a patient is "understandably" depressed solely due to the presence of a physical illness is not necessarily justified. Additional and more specific factors must be identified to account for depression in these patients.

Factors Associated with Depressive Symptoms

Illness Severity

A frequent finding in this literature is that increased disease severity or disability is associated with greater severity of depressive symptoms (Moffic & Paykel, 1975; Massie et al., 1979; Bukberg & Holland, 1980; Wright et al., 1980; Zung et al., 1983; Bukberg, Penman, & Holland, 1984; Cassileth et al., 1984; Lansky et al., 1985; Rodin & Voshart, 1987; Yang et al., 1987; Littlefield et al., 1990). Several factors may contribute to this association, including the multiple stressors that are likely to occur with a more severe medical condition. Unfortunately, the severity of the illness is difficult to assess accurately in many medical disorders. Further, as Stein et al. (1987) have noted, many published studies have not adequately standardized or described their methods of measuring severity of illness. Where available, the use of a standardized severity classification can facilitate a more exact test of the relationship between severity of illness and depression. For example, a grading system with operationalized criteria has been developed to document severity of illness in patients with Tourette syndrome (TS). Using the BDI in a sample of 247 patients, Comings and Comings (1987) found a significant association between severity of TS and the proportion of patients with at least mild symptoms of depression. The frequency of patients with BDI >8 at different degrees of illness severity was: grade I TS, 9.3 percent; grade II TS, 17.7 percent; and grade III TS, 34.3 percent. The frequency of BDI scores >8 in 47 normal control patients was 6.4 percent. In another example, Harris et al. (1988) found that not only was depression correlated with level of disability in a study of elderly medical rehabilitation patients, but that depression was most likely to persist in those who failed to regain their premorbid level of physical functioning. The strength of the findings in these studies arises largely from the standardized descriptions of the illness severity measures which were applied.

What is not clear from these and many similar studies is which factor(s) accounts for the relationship between depression and illness severity. Because the assessment of depressive symptoms is often confounded by symptoms of the physical illness (e.g., anorexia and insomnia), elevated depression scores might be expected on this basis with more severe medical disease. Hawley and Wolfe (1988) reported a comprehensive and careful study of the association of depression with rheumatoid arthritis. After following 400 patients for a mean of 3.1 years, they found that depression was closely associated with active rheumatic disease. In a study of depressive symptoms in patients with endstage renal disease, Rodin and Voshart (1987) demonstrated that a relationship between severity of depressive symptoms and severity of disability occurred at mild but not high levels of depressive symptomatology. These authors concluded that overlap of illness severity and depressive symptom measures accounted for the association between the two factors at mild levels of depression. However, individual vulnerabilities and other factors were likely necessary for more severe depression to occur.

We assume that psychological and social mechanisms also mediate the association between depressive symptoms and disease severity. Greater disability is more likely to be associated with loss of vocational, family, and other social roles. In addition, both financial resources and the patient's social support network are more likely to be strained with greater illness severity. These secondary consequences of more severe medical disease may increase the likelihood of depression. We have shown that social support is an important moderating or "buffering" factor for depressive symptoms as illness severity increases (Littlefield et al., 1990). Therefore, with increased disease severity, depressive symptoms may be greater in patients with inadequate social support than in those who feel adequately supported. An individual's cognitive appraisal of illness severity may also determine the degree of depression, although this individual appraisal has been found to relate only moderately to objective measurements of disease severity (Rosenberg et al., 1988). Finally, physical discomfort is likely to be greatest and most prolonged when illness is severe, and this discomfort may also contribute to more severe depression.

The elimination of somatic criteria from depressive symptom measures would entirely circumvent the problem of confounding variables. However, this strategy would lead to an underestimation, not only of the prevalence of depression, but also of psychological distress. It seems likely that somatic complaints are, in some cases, psychological manifestations of depression that are preferentially reported in medical settings (Cadoret, Widmer, & Troughton, 1980). To eliminate these symptoms from depression inventories would remove physical complaints that are, in fact, manifestations of the psychological disturbance of depression. For example, Lustman, Clouse, and Carney (1988) have shown that the physical symptoms associated with the same level of diabetic dyscontrol are greater in depressed than nondepressed diabetic patients. Thus, the somatic symptoms usually considered to be characteristic of the medical illness may actually be manifestations of depression. One way to confirm this possibility would be to administer several measures of depression, some with no somatic symptoms and others which include an extended list of physical symptoms. The contribution of somatic symptoms to depression could then be determined in a single sample. As noted later in this chapter, this design has been used to study physical symptoms which confound the diagnosis of depressive disorders in medical patients.

Valid and standardized measures of disease severity are necessary to accurately determine the correlation between illness severity and depressive symptoms, and to establish the factors that contribute to their association. This is easier said than done. Standardized indicators of disease severity are available for some medical conditions (e.g., cardiovascular disease, Tourette syndrome), but not for most others. Also, comparing illness severity among patients with different symptoms or different illnesses is inherently difficult. For example, how should the severity of a nonlethal but persistent and distressing symptom such as chronic pain or nausea be compared with one that is less symptomatic but which may affect longevity and survival (e.g., hypertension). Also, in measuring disease severity, it is important to distinguish among indices of functional impairment, symptomatic distress, objective prognosis, laboratory indices, and so forth. A study that operationalizes disease severity in terms of functional disability may not be comparable to one that uses biochemical indices to determine severity of disease. The method chosen to assess illness severity is crucial in studies testing the correlation between illness severity and depressive symptoms. Although each type of comparison has academic merit, very different results may be found, depending on whether a depressive symptom measure is correlated with a measure of functional disability or a biochemical indicator of illness severity.

Stein et al. (1987), in a discussion of the difficulties in measuring the severity of illness, offered four recommendations. They suggested that investigators:

1. Specify the nature of the construct that is being assessed (i.e., physiological, morphological, functional, aspects of illness), the reference interval, and the purpose of the measure.
2. Use more than one measure whenever possible.
3. Consider which factors may alter the physiological indices.
4. Compare the severity of different conditions in terms of functional status or burden of illness.

Several investigators have examined the influence of depression and other psychological states on the medical course of patients with end-stage renal disease (Foster, Cohn, & McKegney, 1973; Farmer et al., 1979; Wai et al., 1981; Burton et al., 1986; Shulman, Price, & Spinelli, 1989). However, the measurement of illness severity has not been adequately standardized in these reports. Following the guidelines provided by Stein et al. (1987), we have recently devised the Endstage Renal Disease Severity Index (ESRD-SI) as a measure of physical and morphologic illness severity for use as an experimental and control variable in medical-psychiatric research (Craven et al., 1990). Preliminary analyses demonstrate adequate inter-rater reliability, test-retest reliability, construct and predictive validity for this measure.

Not all studies have found that depressive symptoms increase with increased severity of physical illness. Starkstein and Robinson (1989) found that the degree of depression in patients with stage I Parkinson's disease (mild) was similar to those with more severe disease (stages IV or V). In stroke patients, Robinson, Lipsey, and Pearlson (1984) found that severity of illness accounted for only a small proportion of depressive symptom severity. These and other similar findings suggest that factors other than the severity of illness also contribute to the development of depression, at least in some patients. Factors that may have an effect independent of illness severity include biological predisposition to depression, and illness characteristics unrelated to severity of illness (e.g., location of stroke lesion). The biological mechanisms by which physical illness may lead to depression are further discussed in Chapter 8.

Other recent research may provide an additional perspective on the relationship of illness severity to depression. In a study of 99 renal dialysis patients, our group found that severity of depressive symptoms, as measured by the Beck Depression Inventory, was positively correlated

with several indices of illness severity including: total number of concurrent physical illnesses (r=.35, p<.01), total number of medications
prescribed (r=.36, p<.01); and level of disability as measured by the
Agerholm Disability Scale (r=.33, p<.01) (Craven, Rodin, & Littlefield,
unpublished data). These findings suggest that disease severity is related
to depressive symptoms, although not necessarily to clinically significant
depressive disorders. In another analysis conducted in this same sample,
patients with major depression and dysthymic disorder were compared
to the remainder of the sample. No differences were found between
these two groups in any of the indices of illness severity (Craven et
al., 1987). Factors that did distinguish patients with mood disorders
included female gender, single marital status, and living alone. Together,
these findings suggest that illness severity influences the number of
depression-like symptoms reported by dialysis patients, but that the
occurrence of mood disorders is also determined by individual factors
not associated with illness severity.

Other Factors

A number of studies have found that increased depressive symptoms
are associated with lower socioeconomic status in medical samples
(Schwab et al., 1967b; Nielsen & Williams, 1980; Wright et al., 1980;
Barnes & Prosen, 1984; Magni, De Leo, & Schifano, 1985; Yang et
al., 1987), although some have not found this association (Moffic &
Paykel, 1975). Gender may also play a role in determining depressive
symptoms. Blacker and Clare (1988) administered the General Health
Questionnaire to a sample of 2,308 general practice patients, and a
subsequent screening interview to those patients who scored above a
particular threshold. They found that four times as many women as
men showed evidence of depressive disorders. Other studies also report
more depressive symptoms in female medical patients (Culpan, Davies,
& Oppenheim, 1960; Porter, 1970; Nielsen & Williams, 1980; Fava et
al., 1982a; Barnes & Prosen, 1984; Magni, De Leo, & Schifano, 1985).
However, a sizable number of studies have found no such association
(Schwab et al., 1967b; Moffic & Paykel, 1975; Wright et al., 1980;
Cavanaugh, 1983; Hengeveld, Ancion, & Rooijmans, 1987; Rodin &
Voshart, 1987; Yang et al., 1987; Rosenberg et al., 1988). These findings
leave in question the issue of whether or not depressive symptoms are
more common in female medical patients.

Finally, some studies have found an association between increased
age and depression in the physically ill (Fava et al., 1982a; Magni, De
Leo, & Schifano, 1985; Rosen et al., 1987). However, the majority of

studies have found no relationship between age and severity of depressive symptoms (Schwab et al., 1967b; Moffic & Paykel, 1975; Nielsen & Williams, 1980; Wright et al., 1980; Cavanaugh, 1983; Zung et al., 1983; Barnes & Prosen, 1984; Hengeveld, Ancion, & Rooijmans, 1987; Rodin & Voshart, 1987; Yang et al., 1987; Rosenberg et al., 1988).

Distinguishing Symptoms of Depression in the Medically Ill

A number of investigators have suggested that particular symptoms may best distinguish depressed from euthymic medical patients (Cassidy et al., 1957; Beck et al., 1961; Stewart, Drake, & Winokur, 1965; Moffic & Paykel, 1975; Plumb & Holland, 1981; Katon, 1982; Katon, Kleinman, & Rosen, 1982). A design commonly employed to test this hypothesis has been to compare the frequency and types of symptoms reported by medical patients who score high on self-report depression measures with those who have low scores. For example, Schwab et al. (1967a) compared the relative frequency of depressive symptoms in patients who scored >13 on the BDI with those in the same sample who scored 13 or less. Symptoms that were found more often in the high scorers included guilt, pessimism, sense of failure, and dissatisfaction with body image. Moffic and Paykel (1975), using similar methodology and a BDI cutoff of >13, found that the group scoring above this threshold more often reported guilt, pessimism, sadness, somatic preoccupation, irritability, suicidal ideation, anorexia, and insomnia. Plumb and Holland (1977) studied oncology patients who scored >13 on the BDI. They found that low self-esteem was the core indicator of depression in this sample. Other characteristic symptoms were marked guilt, loss of self-regard, and feelings of worthlessness. These authors concluded that cancer patients who were not depressed reported that they loathed their situation, but not themselves. Also, depressed patients were much more likely to report a negative self-image.

Clark, Cavanaugh, and Gibbons (1983) reported one of the more extensive investigations of this type. They administered the BDI to 335 general hospital inpatients, 101 psychiatric patients with major depression, and 101 normal controls. Latent trait analysis was used to examine the discriminative ability, fit to the model, and commonality of each symptom, based on the most severely depressed patients in the sample. The following symptoms were found to best discriminate medical patients with the most severe depression: feeling like a failure, feeling punished, suicidal ideation, and frequent crying. Unlike previous reports, guilt, self-hate, and self-blame were not good discriminators of depressive severity in this study. From this same sample, Cavanaugh (1983) also reported a list of symptoms that were significantly more common in the medically ill group as a whole than in the normal controls—irritability, crying, sadness, dissatisfaction, discouragement about the future, and difficulty with decisions. These symptoms were considered to be manifestations of a normal psychological reaction to acute illness or hospitalization and, unless persistent or severe, not indicative of depression. Similarly, Schwab et al. (1966) previously reported that irritability, crying, and sadness were very common among nondepressed, hospitalized medical patients.

Overall, studies using self-report measures in general medical samples have found that psychological symptoms are more useful than somatic ones to distinguish depressed from euthymic patients. The characteristic psychological symptoms of depression in medical patients include low self-esteem, dissatisfaction with one's self, and self-recrimination. However, the methodological limitations of these studies limit their generalizability. The most serious limitation is the method of case definition which, in each of the studies cited, was a self-report inventory of depressive symptoms. As previously discussed, these measures are nonspecific, so that "cases" identified by higher scores do not necessarily represent patients with depressive disorders. Furthermore, investigators that used the BDI did not necessarily report the presence or absence of specific symptoms (e.g., anhedonia) which may be more pathognomonic of depression, at least in psychiatric samples. It is unclear whether these or other symptoms have any particular specificity for depression in the physically ill.

DEPRESSIVE DISORDERS IN THE MEDICALLY ILL

Most systems of classifying mental disorders are based on the assumption that psychiatric conditions such as depression are discrete categorical states. This contrasts with the assumption on which many self-report measures are based, namely that symptoms such as depression are continuous variables and that clinical disorders represent one end of the continuum. The respective validity of these alternate conceptualizations has been the subject of a longstanding, still unresolved, debate regarding the nature of depression and other psychiatric disorders. In fact, much of the recent research on mood disorders has tried to define valid clinical categories of depression. Although some (Kleinman, 1988) have criticized the cultural biases and biological determinism that may affect the assignment of such categories, improved reliability, communicability, and generalizability of research findings have resulted from this development.

The most longstanding debate regarding the classification of depression has been whether depression can be categorized as either "endogenous" or "reactive." Endogenous depression refers to a state that develops without an apparent external factor, and is considered to arise largely as a result of vulnerabilities within the person (e.g., genetic predisposition). Reactive depression refers to a reaction or complication of some other illness or event. For example, a first episode of major depression soon after the onset of a severe physical illness might be considered to be reactive to the illness. Early on, Gillespie (1929) and Lewis (1934), respectively, argued most cogently for and against the validity of the endogenous-reactive dichotomy. However, a major impediment to testing this question empirically was the lack of agreement about criteria by which an external stressor could be judged to be related etiologically to the depressed state.

More recently, the Feighner Criteria (Feighner et al., 1972) specified operational diagnostic criteria for depression and other psychiatric disorders. This system, and the Research Diagnostic Criteria (Spitzer, Endicott, & Robins, 1978) that followed, included several improvements in diagnostic methodology that have increased the reliability and validity of psychiatric diagnoses. Within these systems, depression is classified into primary and secondary types. Primary depression refers to a depressive syndrome occurring prior to the onset of any other psychiatric disorder, whereas secondary depression implies a depressive syndrome beginning after the onset of another illness. According to this classification, secondary depression may be diagnosed following a nonaffective psychiatric disorder (e.g., anorexia nervosa) or a severe or life-threatening physical illness. This distinction avoids the necessity for judgments about whether or not an external event "caused" the depression. Primary versus secondary subtypes are distinguished simply by whether or not a psychiatric or medical illness preceded the depression. Several investigations have found differences between primary and secondary depression. These differences include the familial incidence of psychiatric disease (Andreasen & Winokur, 1979), age and sex distribution (Guze, Woodruff, & Clayton, 1971; Wood et al., 1977), rapid eye movement activity (Kupfer, Foster, & Coble, 1977), and dexamethasone response (Schlesser, Winokur, & Sherman, 1980). However, few systematic differences have been found to justify the primary-secondary distinction on clinical grounds (Wood et al., 1977; Andreasen & Winokur, 1979; Akiskal et al., 1979). Andreasen and Winokur (1979) have argued that including depression following medical illness in the category of secondary depression would so dilute the category as to render it meaningless. Winokur, Black, and Nasrallah (1988) have also pointed out that depression secondary to medical illness remains much less well characterized than other secondary depressions. Major depression that occurs following a severe physical illness is included in some studies of secondary depression (e.g., Stancer et al., 1984), but not in others (Guze, Woodruff, & Clayton, 1971; Wood et al., 1977). Because of these inconsistencies, findings from studies of secondary depression cannot necessarily be generalized to patients with depression following physical illness.

One study that systematically compared depression secondary to physical illness with that following other psychiatric disorders, found that the latter group more closely resembled patients with "neurotic" or characterological depression (Winokur, Black, & Nasrallah, 1988). Those with depression secondary to psychiatric illness were more likely to have made suicide attempts, to relapse, to have more family history of alcoholism, and were less likely to improve with treatment than were patients with depression secondary to medical illness. Similarly, Stewart, Drake, and Winokur (1965) found that compared with a depressed psychiatric control group, depressed medical patients reported fewer depressive symptoms, fewer thoughts of suicide and suicide attempts, and a less frequent history of depression. Similarly, Lipsey et al. (1986) found that 43 poststroke patients with major depression were less likely to report either a personal or a family history of depression than were 43 nonmedical patients with major depression. These findings suggest that depression secondary to physical illness is not identical either to primary depression or to depression secondary to other psychiatric disorders. However, the similarities between depression in these different contexts far outweigh the differences. Although the distinctions may be significant in terms of some research, a distinct diagnosis of depression secondary to physical illness is likely not warranted.

The term "situational depression" has been used to refer to a depressive episode which, in the clinician's judgment, is temporally and etiologically related to a stressful event. Hirschfeld et al. (1985), in a review of the concept of situational major depression, concluded that though stress and distress were important in the pathogenesis of depression, situational MDE did not represent a discrete diagnostic category. In a subsequent commentary on these findings, Glass (1985) also concluded that although the nature and meaning of a precipitant may be clinically relevant, its presence or absence does not appear to lead to a valid subclassification of patients with major depression.

Rosen et al. (1987) have suggested that the DSM-III be adjusted to include a "V" code for "depressive reactions secondary to physical illness." This approach was proposed to avoid the arbitrary assignment of a psychiatric diagnosis to distressed medical patients, while permitting the descriptive labelling of depressive symptoms that occur during the process of adjustment to physical illness. We consider this to be a useful category for depressive symptoms that do not meet the criteria for major depressive episode, as well as for other psychological reactions that are not necessarily maladaptive or pathological. Indeed, there is considerable individual variation in the experience of depression in the course of normal adjustment to major life stress. Others have noted that nonpathological mood states in the medically ill correspond closely to fluctuations in medical symptoms over time (Popkin, Callies, & Colon, 1987). However, when mood symptoms are severe, multiple, or persist in spite of fluctuations in medical symptoms, the clinician should consider the possibility that a mood disorder has now developed. We do not agree with Rosen et al. (1987) that a "V" code diagnosis should be applied to patients who meet criteria for major depressive episode. As will be discussed further in this chapter, there is little consistent data to support the view that a medical patient with a major depressive episode should be given a clinical diagnosis which is distinct from any other patient with this disorder.

DSM-III and DSM-III-R

At present, the most widely used classification system in North America is the revised Third Edition of the Diagnostic and Statistical Manual of Mental Disorders (DSM-III-R) (American Psychiatric Association, 1987). The DSM-III-R, which categorizes depression into several disorders (listed in Table 1.4), has found wide application in both research and clinical settings. In the DSM-III, mood disorders are largely differentiated by clinical criteria that have been clearly operationalized according to the severity and duration of symptoms. In the absence of convincing evidence to support the clinical distinction between primary versus secondary depressive disorders, these categories have not been included in either the DSM-III or the DSM-III-R.

Standard Diagnostic Interviews

The DSM-III-R and other classification systems permit clinical diagnoses to be made with relative ease by trained clinicians using a comprehensive clinical interview. However, of importance to research

TABLE 1.4. *DSM-III-R Disorders with Depression as a Predominant Feature*

Mood Disorders

Major depression
single episode
recurrent

Bipolar disorder
depressed
mixed

Other Specific Affective Disorders

Dysthymia
Cyclothymia

Organic Brain Syndromes

Organic mood disorder

Adjustment Disorder

With depressed mood

in this area, structured and semi-structured diagnostic interviews have been devised specifically for the various diagnostic classifications to increase further the reliability and generalizability of research findings. Such interviews standardize the criteria used both for clinical data collection and for diagnosis. Furthermore, data from these interviews allow other mood disorders in the differential diagnoses to be ruled out. Examples of structured diagnostic interviews include the Schedule for Affective Disorders and Schizophrenia (SADS) (Spitzer, Endicott, & Robins, 1978), designed for use with Research Diagnostic Criteria (RDC), and the Diagnostic Interview Schedule (DIS) (Robins et al., 1981), designed for use with DSM-III criteria. However, structured diagnostic interviews to determine the prevalence of depressive disorders in medical samples are still the exception rather than the rule in the literature. The recent development of these measures, and the sizable investment of time and specialized training to administer them are significant limitations to their use in many settings. However, studies that use diagnostic interviews are the most useful to determine the prevalence, clinical significance, and treatment requirements of depression in the physically ill.

In a unique effort to validate the Diagnostic Interview Schedule in medical patients, Koenig et al. (1989) administered the section of the DIS employed to diagnose affective disorders to a large sample of hospitalized adults. When compared with independent clinical assessment by a psychiatrist, the sensitivity of the DIS for major depressive episode was over 70 percent, and the specificity, 65 percent. As the authors suggested, improved results would likely have been obtained if the structured interview had been used in its entirety.

Some diagnostic interviews discriminate diagnostic criteria based on whether particular symptoms are due to physical illness or to depression. For example, it is specified in the Present State Examination (PSE) that symptoms apparently caused by physical illness should not be recorded as symptoms of depression. Unfortunately, criteria upon which to base this decision are not provided. By contrast, the DIS includes a decision tree to assist in determining which symptoms are the result of a physical illness. For example, particular symptoms do not contribute to a diagnosis of depression if the patient was told by the physician that these symptoms are the result of a physical illness or a medication. Such operationalized criteria add reliability to the decision-making process. However, this method assumes that the patient has been given information about each specific symptom by the physician, and that the patient's interpretation and recall of this information is accurate.

Major Depressive Episode

Major depressive episode (MDE) refers to a clinical syndrome of signs and symptoms that may be best conceptualized as a "final common pathway" for biological, psychological, or social stressors (Akiskal & McKinney, 1975). MDE is diagnosed when a clinically depressed patient meets specified criteria, without reference to whether the depression began "spontaneously" or can be understood as a reaction to a major life event or illness. The DSM-III-R defines MDE as depressed mood or loss of interest associated with at least four additional symptoms that have lasted for two or more weeks (see Table 1.5). The melancholic type is a subgroup with more severe vegetative symptoms for which biological treatments are most indicated. The reliability and validity of DSM-III criteria for MDE have been adequately demonstrated in medically well patients (Mazure, Nelson, & Price, 1986). However, the presence of the diagnostic criteria alone is insufficient for the diagnosis (Carroll, 1984; Fava, Sonino, & Wise, 1988). This caution is particularly applicable in the physically ill, in whom conditions other than a mood disorder may commonly produce symptoms that meet criteria for MDE.

Case Example

■ Mr. S., a 45-year-old married man, suffered from endstage liver disease with secondary pulmonary insufficiency. He was offered a liver transplant but was informed that his postoperative course would be prolonged and complicated because of his pulmonary disease. Mr. S. readily accepted the offer of a transplant, believing that he could become physically active immediately afterward. He tended to deny both his prognosis and the personal relevance of the medical information with which he was provided. He demonstrated magical hopes for recovery and his tolerance for discomfort or disappointment was low.

Mr. S.'s new liver functioned well after the transplant, but his pulmonary function declined so that, three weeks after the surgery, he was

TABLE 1.5. *Diagnostic Criteria for Major Depression (MDE)*

At least five of the following symptoms have been present during the same two-week period:

- Depressed mood
- Loss of interest or pleasure
- Loss of appetite
- Loss of weight (or weight gain)
- Insomnia (or hypersomnia)
- Psychomotor agitation or retardation
- Fatigue or loss of energy
- Feelings of worthlessness, sinfulness, or guilt
- Diminished ability to think or concentrate, indecisiveness
- Recurrent thoughts of death or suicide

Subtypes:

- Mild
- Moderate
- Severe without psychotic features
- Severe with psychotic features

Adapted with permission from the Diagnostic and Statistical Manual of Mental Disorders, Third Edition, Revised. Copyright 1987 American Psychiatric Association.

unable to get out of bed. He was referred for psychiatric assessment because of his persistent requests to discontinue treatment. He stated that he had been depressed since the time of the transplant and said he had no interest in any rehabilitation program or any other post-operative activities. He insisted that he wanted to die and, in fact, threatened to jump out of a hospital window if the opportunity presented itself. Mr. S. also reported poor concentration, nausea, little appetite, and poor sleep. He felt anxious most of the time, hopeless that his circumstances would change, and he believed that his family would be better off without him. On examination, Mr. S. was emotionally labile and slow to respond, but he demonstrated no psychomotor changes and was interactive and engaging during the interview.

A major depressive episode was considered to be the cause of this patient's symptoms, but additional information suggested that other contributing factors were also important. The nurses noted that he reported waking dreams and demonstrated transient confusion during the early morning hours, as is common with liver transplant recipients. It appeared likely that Mr. S.'s concentration difficulties and emotional lability were components of a mild delirium. Gastroparesis was also diagnosed and his symptoms of nausea and anorexia responded well to treatment with metachlopramide. Symptomatic relief of anxiety and insomnia was achieved with low dose perphenazine at bedtime. Following these changes, a rapid improvement in mood occurred; Mr. S. was more amenable to reassurance and to supportive interactions with friends and family and his suicidal ideation disappeared.

At the time of initial assessment, Mr. S. met criteria for major depressive episode. However, on further examination, several of his symptoms were caused, not by a depressive syndrome, but by a com-bination of other organic mental and medical conditions. His inability to cope with the extreme stress of his situation resulted in feelings of hopelessness and a wish to escape by death. A decision was made to defer specific antidepressant treatment and to intervene based on the biological and psychological contributing factors that were identified. ■

The DSM-III-R includes a directive to "not include symptoms which are clearly due to a physical disorder" (p. 222). This proscription is intended to avoid attributing symptoms of physical illness to a de-pressive syndrome. This is relevant to the earlier discussion in this chapter on the specificity of somatic symptoms to diagnose depression in medical patients. Excluding only those somatic symptoms related to the physical illness may be preferable to other suggestions that have been put forward. In particular, proposals to eliminate or to replace somatic symptoms of depression with psychological ones in medically ill patients (Endicott, 1984) have several distinct disadvantages. First, findings from validity studies of the DSM-III-R criteria do not necessarily apply to such modified criteria. Second, it is not clear how severe a medical illness must be to warrant modification of the criteria. This poses a substantial problem since, even in psychiatric facilities, a large proportion of depressed patients also have a medical diagnosis (Eastwood, 1975; Ananth, 1984). For example, Koranyi (1980) found that about one-half of more than 4,000 psychiatric patients had undiagnosed physical illnesses. Others have found that of depressed patients attending a psychiatric facility, over one-third of cases have an associated physical illness (Maguire & Granville-Grossman, 1968; Hall et al., 1980). Third, elimination or replacement of somatic criteria likely would result in underdiagnosis of depression in the physically ill. Depression may present with predominantly somatic symptoms, particularly in patients with a physical illness or attending a medical facility (Cadoret, Widmer, & Troughton, 1980; Williamson & Yates, 1989).

Finally, elimination of somatic criteria from the diagnosis of mood disorders in the medically ill would result in valid manifestations of depression being disregarded in many medical patients. Although it may be difficult in clinical practice to determine whether somatic symptoms are due to a depressive disorder or to a physical condition, somatic complaints may nevertheless be components of depression in the physically ill. Rapp and Vrana (1989) examined the sensitivity, specificity, and diagnostic accuracy of a diagnostic system that replaces somatic with psychological criteria to diagnose major depression. These substitutive criteria were first proposed by Endicott (1984) for use in cancer patients. Rapp and Vrana (1989) found that 96 percent of their sample of elderly medical inpatients were classified similarly by the two systems. However, as we have argued elsewhere, the similarity of results using the two diagnostic methods indicates that there may be no advantage to the substitutive criteria (Craven & Rodin, 1990). Careful clinical judgment may allow certain somatic symptoms to be excluded in some cases without radical changes to existing diagnostic methodology.

Emmons, Fetting, and Zonderman (1987) compared 52 consultation-liaison patients with MDE with 58 psychiatric inpatients having the same diagnosis. They found that cognitive-affective symptoms occurred with greater frequency in the psychiatric patients, but that somatic symptoms were more common in the medical depressives. Depression in the psychiatric patients was characterized by suicidal ideation, loss of interest, a sense of punishment, and feelings of being a burden to others. In the medical patients, depression was characterized by worry and helplessness, loss of energy, insomnia, and loss of appetite accompanied by weight loss. Based on the prominence of somatic symptoms in the depressed medical patients, these investigators concluded that it would be inappropriate to abandon somatic items when diagnosing depression in the medically ill. They suggested that such an approach would inevitably lead to a substantial underdiagnosis of depression in medical patients. This conclusion was supported by a study by Brown et al. (1988) who reported that depression in Parkinson's disease is characterized by dysphoria, pessimism, and somatic complaints.

Rather than systematically eliminating somatic criteria from the diagnosis of major depression, some investigators have compiled systematic information to help determine whether somatic symptoms are due to a particular physical illness or to major depression (see Table 1.6). This information is largely based on studies that compare the prevalence of individual DSM-III criteria in depressed versus nondepressed medical patients. Bukberg, Penman, and Holland (1984) found that anorexia, weight loss, and loss of energy are common symptoms in all acutely ill oncology patients. They proposed a modified DSM-III scale in which anorexia and fatigue are eliminated as criteria for MDE in such patients. Craven et al. (1987) administered the DIS to a sample of 99 renal dialysis patients and found that three diagnostic criteria for depression (e.g., insomnia, loss of energy, and loss of sexual interest) were reported by so many of the nondepressed patients that they were of little value in the diagnosis of depression. Interestingly, this study of dialysis patients and a previous one by Smith, Hong, and Robson (1985), both found that anorexia and weight loss were, in fact, valid discriminators of major depression in well-dialyzed patients with endstage renal disease. Frank et al. (1988) found that 80 percent of a sample of 137 rheumatoid arthritis patients reported loss of energy and insomnia sufficient to meet DSM-III criteria for MDE. This suggests that these symptoms are not specific for depression in this condition. In a sample of 105 consecutive patients with Parkinson's disease, Starkstein and Robinson (1989) found that psychomotor retardation occurred in three-quarters of the sample, and was therefore not useful in diagnosing major depression. However, all other DSM-III criteria did discriminate patients with MDE from the remainder of their sample. Also, it was observed in patients with multiple sclerosis that loss of energy commonly occurs following physical activity (Krupp et al., 1988) and should not be considered a manifestation of depression in these patients (Rabins, 1989). These findings support the argument that certain disease-specific

symptoms should be ignored in the diagnosis of depression, but that
other somatic symptoms retain diagnostic value.

Lustman et al. (1986a) found that loss of energy and difficulty
concentrating are common in all diabetic patients with poor metabolic
control. In an interesting subsequent report, this group demonstrated
how inclusion of somatic criteria influenced the diagnosis of MDE in
diabetic patients (Lustman et al., 1986b). They found that when all
somatic symptoms likely to be secondary to diabetes were excluded,
almost one-third of 114 patients with diabetes could be diagnosed with
major depression, based on the DIS with DSM-III criteria. When these
symptoms were included, an additional five patients were diagnosed
with depression. This study confirms that depression in the medically
ill may be overdiagnosed when all somatic criteria are used for diagnostic purposes. However, when standardized methodology and strict
criteria are used, the rate of misdiagnosis in patients with diabetes
mellitus is not large. Alternatively, in a sample of oncology patients,

TABLE 1.6. *Symptoms Found to be Nonspecific for Major
Depressive Disorder (DSM-III Criteria) in the Presence of
Specific Physical Illnesses*

Study	Illness	Confounding Symptoms
Bukberg, Penman, & Holland (1984)	cancer	Loss of energy Anorexia Weight loss
Lustman et al. (1986a)	diabetes (with metabolic dyscontrol)	Loss of energy Difficulty concentrating
Craven et al. (1987)	endstage renal disease	Loss of energy Insomnia Loss of sexual interest
Frank et al. (1988)	rheumatoid arthritis	Loss of energy Insomnia
Krupp et al. (1988)	multiple sclerosis	Fatigue
Starkstein & Robinson (1989)	Parkinson's disease	Psychomotor retardation

Bukberg, Penman, and Holland (1984) found that the point prevalence of major depressive episode dropped from 42 percent to 24 percent when all somatic symptoms were eliminated as diagnostic criteria for depression. Therefore, the influence of somatic symptoms on the diagnosis of major depression appears to vary widely among illnesses. However, one important difference between these two reports is that the Diagnostic Interview Schedule, which includes a standardized decision tree for excluding somatic symptoms likely to be secondary to physical illness, was used in the former (Lustman et al., 1986a), whereas, in the latter (Bukberg, Penman, & Holland, 1984) the diagnoses were based on clinical interviews and thus likely included more confounding somatic criteria. Also, Lustman et al. (1986a) eliminated disease-specific symptoms and Bukberg, Penman, and Holland (1984) eliminated all somatic symptoms. Similar studies in different samples are required to clarify further these important findings.

Even though particular somatic symptoms may be so common in certain physical illnesses that they are of little utility to diagnose depression, the severity of these symptoms may still fluctuate according to the severity of depression. For example, Bishop et al. (1987) found that low energy, insomnia, and anorexia were common in patients with rheumatoid arthritis, but that the intensity of these symptoms over time corresponded over time to the severity of depressive symptoms. In a similar vein, although anorexia and weight loss may have little diagnostic specificity for depression in cancer patients, Schmale (1979) has postulated a psychological mechanism involving depression and hopelessness to account for changes in these symptoms in at least some situations.

The studies cited above may assist in determining which symptoms contribute to the diagnosis of major depression in patients with an active medical illness. As discussed earlier, studies using self-report instruments are less valuable in this regard because they do not incorporate the same criteria of severity or duration of depression used in the DSM-III-R. Research with specific medical illness groups, rather than with general medical samples, is necessary to delineate which symptoms are useful to diagnose depression in different medical conditions. There is no reason to exclude specific somatic symptoms from the diagnosis of depression, if they are not commonly produced by the associated medical condition. For some illnesses, particular somatic criteria may be acceptable or even excellent discriminators of depression (e.g., Craven et al., 1987).

These considerations suggest that the method proposed by the DSM-III-R is likely the best solution to the problem of somatic symptoms in the physically ill. With this approach, somatic criteria are used for the diagnosis unless clearly produced by a physical disorder. In any one patient, this method most often excludes only one or two symptoms from consideration. This approach balances the risk of underdiagnosis which would probably result from eliminating all somatic criteria, against the risk of overdiagnosis which would result from including all somatic criteria in all cases. The diagnostician can thereby tailor the criteria to individual clinical cases. Systematic studies, such as those described above, will further assist with this decision.

The differential diagnosis for MDE in the medical setting includes adjustment disorder with depressed mood or with mixed emotional features. These diagnoses are applied when symptoms of depression do not meet criteria for MDE. However, differentiating MDE from an adjustment disorder may be a challenging problem in the physically ill patient (Leigh et al., 1982; Grossman, 1982). This distinction is made more difficult when physical symptoms secondary to illness are excluded, leaving a smaller group of criteria to diagnose MDE.

Adjustment Disorder

Adjustment disorder in the DSM-III-R refers to a maladaptive reaction to a recent and identifiable psychosocial stressor. This disorder may present with depressed or anxious mood, mixed emotional features, physical complaints, or social withdrawal. Adjustment disorder with depressed mood (ADDM) may be an appropriate diagnosis to apply to a patient who demonstrates depressive symptoms following a stressful illness-related event, when these symptoms do not meet criteria for MDE. However, adjustment disorder is a problematic diagnosis in patients with severe physical illness since this diagnosis entails a judgment that the response is "maladaptive" (Lipowski & Wolston, 1981). Whether depressive symptoms that do not meet DSM-III criteria for MDE are part of an adaptive reaction, or alternatively, are abnormal or maladaptive, may be difficult to determine (Mackenzie, Popkin, & Callies, 1983). Lindemann (1944) and others have described the emotional turmoil that may follow the discovery of a serious medical diagnosis or prognosis, or the loss of a valued physical function. There is a risk of inappropriate psychiatric labelling of normal processes when patients who are grieving, as the result of a recently diagnosed medical illness, are assigned the diagnosis of adjustment disorder with depressed mood (Rosen et al., 1987). However, while normal grief is often accompanied by anger, withdrawal, tearfulness, and insomnia, it is less often associated with vegetative symptoms or suicidal ideation. Although complicated by the presence of physical illness, these latter symptoms may assist somewhat with the differentiation of normal adjustment from an adjustment disorder or MDE.

Other Mood Disorders

Other DSM-III-R diagnoses may be applied to depressed patients in the medical setting. The diagnosis of a dysthymic disorder may be made when there is depressed mood and other symptoms of depression that persist for the most part of two years or more but do not meet the criteria for MDE. Persons who are characterologically depressed, have a history of untreated or partially treated major depression, or who have an unresolved depressed state secondary to major life stress may be included in this group.

Organic mood disorder is a diagnosis that is applied when there is clinical or laboratory evidence of an organic factor that is etiologically responsible for a depressive disorder. For example, depressive syndromes associated with corticosteroids, reserpine, and other medications would be classified as organic mood disorder-depressed. In some individual cases, it may be difficult to determine whether or not the depressive syndrome is caused by an organic factor. For example, although neurohumoral factors are presumed to contribute to depression in some cancer patients (Brown & Paraskevas, 1982), there may be many other etiologic factors to consider. In poststroke depression, left anterior neurological lesions may play an etiological role in depression (Robinson, Lipsey, & Pearlson, 1984). However, psychological mechanisms in these patients may produce similar results or may act in conjunction with biological factors to produce depression.

Kathol and Petty (1981) found that the diagnosis of organic mood disorder was often interpreted as synonymous with depression secondary to medical illness. However, as these authors have pointed out, it is ncorrect to diagnose depression routinely in a patient with cancer as an organic mood disorder, even though cancer may in some patients produce depression by biological mechanisms. This usage would blur the distinction drawn in the DSM-III-R between depression of organic etiology and that due to other causes, since there may be multiple factors that lead to clinical depression in a cancer patient. Furthermore, to label as organic those depressive syndromes that occur in cancer patients may lead to neglect of psychological and social issues in patient care. Even when it is obvious that a biological agent is directly and solely responsible for the depression, all of the biological, psychological, and social factors involved should be considered as potentially relevant to the management of individual patients.

Fogel (1990) has argued that the distinction between organic factors which are contributory and those which are causally related is often arbitrary. Further, he underscores the difficulty of clearly demarcating organic from other etiologies for depression in the individual patient. For these reasons, he has persuasively argued that organic mood disorder be eliminated as a diagnosis. He has suggested that regardless of etiology, a mood disorder be diagnosed according to phenomenologic criteria on Axis I, and that organic factors which cause or contribute to the disorder listed on Axis III. This practice would avoid the arbitrary classification of depression as either organic or nonorganic and would encourage clinicians to consider other contributing factors, even when an organic etiology is recorded.

The mechanisms by which physical factors may cause or contribute to a depressive disorder are further discussed in Chapter 8.

Limitations of the DSM-III and DSM-III-R

The DSM-III/DSM-III-R diagnostic criteria, when used with the corresponding diagnostic interviews, offer several advantages compared to other methods of assessing depression in the physically ill. This approach identifies patients with depressive disorders in a standardized, reliable fashion allowing comparisons with samples in other studies. However, the question of which somatic symptoms to attribute either to depression or to physical illness is not resolved by these diagnostic methods, and the selective use of specific symptoms may limit somewhat their diagnostic validity. The use of operationalized criteria and the incorporation of specific criteria for MDE in patients with particular physical illnesses may help to resolve these problems, although some authors have suggested that the DSM-III diagnostic categories are less than ideal for diagnosing depression in medical patients (Leigh et al., 1982; Mackenzie, Popkin, & Callies, 1983).

Prevalence of Depressive Disorders

Studies that have reported the prevalence of depressive disorders in samples of primary practice and general medical patients are summarized in Table 1.7. Reports of patients with specific medical illnesses are listed in Table 1.8. These tables are limited to studies that used standardized diagnostic criteria and, preferentially, but not necessarily, semi-structured or structured interview techniques. Studies that did not either specify the method by which diagnoses were determined or use a standardized classification system with operationalized criteria were not included.

TABLE 1.7. *Prevalence of Depressive Disorders in General Medical Patients*

Author(s) and Year	n	Subject Characteristics	Instrument	Criteria	Prevalence
Stewart, Drake, & Winokur (1965)	60	inpatients	semi-structured interview	Specifically defined for study: clinical depression	20.0%
Bergmann & Eastham (1974)	100	inpatients (geriatric)	clinical interview	Glossary of Mental Disorders endogenous depression neurotic depression	5.0% 14.0%
Cheah, Baldridge, & Beard (1979)	136	inpatients (geriatric)	clinical interview	Specifically defined for study: dysphoria-depression mild depression moderate depression severe depression	36.8% 27.2% 7.4% 2.2%
Hoeper et al. (1979)	1,072*	primary practice	Schedule for Affective Disorders and Schizophrenia-Lifetime version (n=247)	RDC and DSM-III major depression minor depression intermittent depression cyclothymic depression	5.8% 3.4% 5.0% 2.0%
Harding et al. (1980)	1,624	primary practice	Present State Examination (following screening with a self-report questionnaire)	ICD-8 depressive neurosis affective psychosis	8.6% 0.3%
Wright et al. (1980)	199	primary practice	clinical interview	Feighner Criteria all depressive disorders	17.0%

Study	N	Setting	Instrument	Criteria	Prevalence
Schulberg et al. (1985)	294	primary practice	Diagnostic Interview Schedule, & Center for Epidemiologic Studies Depression Scale	DSM-III all depressive disorders ≥16	9.2% 47.0%
Von Korff et al. (1987)	1,242*	primary practice	Diagnostic Interview Schedule (n=809)	DSM-III MDE DD	5.0% 3.7%
Coulehan et al. (1988)	294	primary practice	Diagnostic Interview Schedule	DSM-III MDE	7.1%
Koenig et al. (1988)	128	neurology & general medicine	Structured psychiatric interview (from DIS, SADS)	DSM-III MDE	12.0%

*screened with General Health Questionnaire (cutoff ≥5); weighting scheme used for corrected prevalence of DSM-III disorders

TABLE 1.8. *Prevalence of Depressive Disorders in Patients with Specific Medical Illness*

Author(s) and Year	n	Subject Characteristics	Instrument	Criteria	Prevalence
Endstage Renal Disease					
Farmer, Snowden & Parsons (1979)	32	ESRD	Standardized Psychiatric Interview	ICD-9 endogenous depression depressive neurosis	9.4% 3.1%
Lowry & Atcherson (1979)	58	ESRD	Home Dialysis Interview Schedule	DSM-III MDE	22.4%
Smith, Hong, & Robson (1985)	60	ESRD	Schedule for Affective Disorders and Schizophrenia	DSM-III MDE	5.0%
Craven et al. (1987)	99	ESRD	Diagnostic Interview Schedule	DSM-III MDE DD	8.1% 6.1%
Hinrichsen et al. (1989)	124	ESRD	Schedule for Affective Disorders and Schizophrenia	RDC major depression minor depression	6.5% 17.7%
Neurological Disorders					
Finklestein et al. (1982)	25	poststroke	clinical interview, & Hamilton Rating Scale for Depression	RDC definite secondary depression probable secondary depression	24.0% 12.0%
Robinson et al. (1983)	103	poststroke	Present State Examination, Zung Self-Rating Depression Scale, & Hamilton Rating Scale for Depression	DSM-III MDE DD	27.0% 20.0%

Study	N	Condition	Assessment	Criteria/Diagnosis	%
Mayeux et al. (1984)	29	Parkinson's disease	clinical interview	DSM-III MDE	27.6%
				DD	13.8%
Frank et al. (1985)	32	spinal cord injuries	semi-structured clinical interview	DSM-III MDE	37.5%
				DD	6.3%
Pfeiffer et al. (1986)	46	Parkinson's disease	semi-structured clinical interview, & Hamilton Rating Scale for Depression	DSM-III MDE	30.4%
Santamaria, Tolosa, & Valles (1986)	34	Parkinson's disease	clinical interview, & Beck Depression Inventory	DSM-III MDE	2.9%
				DD	29.4%
				≥18	23.5%
Joffe et al. (1987)	100	multiple sclerosis	Schedule for Affective Disorders and Schizophrenia-Lifetime version	DSM-III MDE (current)	14.0%
				MDE (past)	47.0%
				minor depression (current)	1.0%
				minor depression (past)	9.0%
				BAD (past)	13.0%
Minden, Orav, & Reich (1987)	50	multiple sclerosis	Schedule for Affective Disorders and Schizophrenia	RDC major depression (lifetime)	54.0%
				minor depression (lifetime)	52.0%
				intermittent depression (lifetime)	28.0%
				hypomania (lifetime)	16.0%
				mania (lifetime)	2.0%
				major depression (one year prior to assessment)	34.0%
Judd et al. (1989)	71	acute spinal cord injury	structured clinical interview for DSM-III	DSM-III MDE	19.7%

TABLE 1.8. (continued)

Author(s) and Year	n	Subject Characteristics	Instrument	Criteria	Prevalence
Brown & MacCarthy (1990)	40	Parkinson's disease	standardized, semi-structured clinical interview	ICD-9 simple depression	25.0%
Starkstein et al. (1990)	105	Parkinson's disease	structured clinical interview	DSM-III MDE minor depression	21.0% 20.0%
Oncology					
Bukberg & Holland (1980)	62	oncology inpatients	clinical interview, & Beck Depression Inventory	DSM-III MDE ≥14	42.0% 36.0%
Plumb & Holland (1981)	80	oncology	CAPPS (semi-structured interview)	at least moderate depression	45.0%
Derogatis et al. (1983)	215	oncology inpatients	clinical interview	DSM-III MAD-unipolar MAD-bipolar MAD-atypical MAD-dysthymic ADDM	3.7% 0.5% 1.4% 0.5% 12.1%
Bukberg, Penman, & Holland (1984)	62	oncology inpatients	clinical interview	DSM-III MDE somatic criteria eliminated	42.0% 24.0%
Morton et al. (1984)	48	buccopharyngeal carcinoma (geriatric)	Geriatric Mental State Schedule	DSM-III depressive disorder	39.6%

Author (year)	N	Sample	Interview	Criteria	Prevalence
Dean (1987)	113	oncology: breast cancer	Present State Examination	RDC major depression minor depression	9.7% 17.7%
Evans et al. (1986)	83	gynecological oncology inpatients	clinical interview	DSM-III MDE DD ADDM	22.9% 4.8% 16.9%
Weddington, Segraves, & Simon (1986)	33	survivors of sarcoma (with amputation)	Schedule for Affective Disorders and Schizophrenia	RDC major depression (lifetime) minor depression (lifetime)	24.2% 15.2%
Diabetes Mellitus					
Lustman et al. (1986b)	114	diabetes mellitus	Diagnostic Interview Schedule	DSM-III MDE (lifetime) DD	32.5% 17.5%
Popkin et al. (1988)	75	diabetes mellitus applying for pancreatic transplantation	Diagnostic Interview Schedule	DSM-III MDE (lifetime) MDE (6 month) DD (lifetime) DD (6 month)	24.0% 10.7% 4.0% 0.0%
Robinson, Fuller, & Edmeades (1988)	130	diabetes mellitus	Present State Examination	Bedford College Survey Criteria depression current within 5 years	8.5% 17.7%
Other					
Lloyd & Cawley (1978)	100	acute myocardial infarction	Standardized Psychiatric Interview	ICD-8 depressive neurosis	18.0%
Kashani et al. (1983)	65	amputees	semi-structured clinical interview	DSM-III MDE	35.4%
Helzer et al. (1984)	50	Crohn's disease	Renard Research Interview	Feighner Criteria depressive disorder (lifetime)	36.0%

/ 49

TABLE 1.8. *(continued)*

Author(s) and Year	n	Subject Characteristics	Instrument	Criteria	Prevalence
Fava et al. (1985)	37	gastroenterology inpatients i) organic (n=23) ii) functional (n=14)	Paykel's clinical interview	DSM-III MDE	i) 43.5% ii) 28.6%
Vazquez-Barquero et al. (1985)	194	cardiology outpatients	Clinical Interview Schedule, & General Health Questionnaire-60	ICD-9 depressive neurosis ≥17	21.6% 28.4%
Carney et al. (1987)	50	coronary artery disease	Diagnostic Interview Schedule	DSM-III MDE	18.0%
Tarter et al. (1987)	53	i) Crohn's disease (n=26) ii) ulcerative colitis (n=27)	Diagnostic Interview Schedule	DSM-III MDE (lifetime)	i) 19.2% ii) 18.5%
Atkinson et al. (1988)	15	AIDS	Diagnostic Interview Schedule	DSM-III MDE (6 month) (lifetime)	6.7% 13.3%
"	13	AIDS-related complex (ARC)	Diagnostic Interview Schedule	(6 month) (lifetime)	7.7% 38.5%
"	17	HIV-positive	Diagnostic Interview Schedule	(6 month) (lifetime)	17.6% 35.3%
Frank et al. (1988)	137	rheumatoid arthritis	Diagnostic Interview Schedule	DSM-III MDE DD	16.8% 40.1%

Study	N	Sample	Interview	Criteria/Diagnosis	Prevalence
Malt (1988)	107	accidentally injured adults	semi-structured interview	DSM-III MDE	0.9%
				DD	2.8%
Maricle et al. (1989)	68	heart transplant candidates	semi-structured clinical interview	DSM-III MDE (current)	14.7%
				(past)	16.2%
				DD (current)	8.8%
				(past)	14.7%
				BAD (current)	1.5%
				(past)	1.5%
Beitman et al. (1990)	94	chest pain patients with normal angiography	structured clinical interview for DSM-III	DSM-III MDE (current)	28.1%
				MDE (lifetime)	37.5%

Several of the studies summarized in Table 1.7 were undertaken in the primary care setting. Three of these studies have reported similar point prevalence rates for major depressive episode, ranging from 5 percent (Von Korff et al., 1987) to 5.8 percent (Hoeper et al., 1979), to 7.1 percent (Coulehan et al., 1988) of patients. A single study found major depression in 12 percent of a combined sample of neurology and general medical patients (Koenig et al., 1988). The higher prevalence rate in this latter study could have been due to sample characteristics. Unlike studies undertaken in primary practice, most of the patients likely had at least one medical diagnosis. However, additional research is required to confirm the prevalence of major depression and other mood disorders in general medical patients.

A large number of studies of depressive disorders have been undertaken in patients with specific medical diagnoses (see Table 1.8). For some conditions, more than one investigation has been conducted, thereby allowing a comparison of results. Three studies have reported a prevalence rate of about 40 percent or more for major depression in oncology patients (Bukberg & Holland, 1980; Bukberg, Penman, & Holland, 1984; Morton et al., 1984). However, in one of these studies (Bukberg, Penman, & Holland, 1984), the authors reported that the prevalence of major depression decreased from 42 percent to 24 percent when somatic criteria were eliminated from consideration. Other studies have found that 6.0 percent (Derogatis et al., 1983), 9.7 percent (Dean, 1987), and 22.9 percent (Evans et al., 1986) of cancer patients experienced a major depressive episode. One group has also reported that the lifetime prevalence of this disorder in oncology patients was 24.2 percent (Weddington, Segraves, & Simon, 1986). Although the prevalence rates vary, these studies cumulatively support the contention that major depression is common in patients with cancer.

Three studies have been undertaken in patients with diabetes mellitus. Popkin et al. (1988) found that of diabetic patients applying for pancreatic transplantation, 10.7 percent demonstrated major depression at the time of interview and that 24 percent reported a lifetime history of this disorder. Lustman et al. (1986b) found that 32.5 percent of patients with diabetes mellitus had a lifetime history of MDE, whereas Robinson, Fuller, and Edmeades (1988) found a 5-year prevalence of 17.7 percent. Unfortunately, the reporting of various types of prevalence rates (i.e., point, lifetime, 5-year) makes comparison of these studies somewhat difficult. This problem could be resolved in the future if both the point and lifetime prevalence of depression were documented.

When lifetime prevalence is reported, knowing the proportion of cases in which depression occurred before the diagnosis of physical illness helps to determine the relationship of the illness to depression.

For some conditions, the prevalence rates reported are too diverse to allow any valid conclusions. For example, in patients with Parkinson's disease, Pfeiffer et al. (1986) found that 30.4 percent had a major depressive episode while Santamaria, Tolosa, and Valles (1986) found that only 2.9 percent had this diagnosis. Many clinical and methodological factors could account for this wide discrepancy. Because clinical rather than standardized interviews were used in each of these studies, differences in classifying somatic symptoms as due to depression or to physical illness, likely accounted for some of the difference in the results.

Four studies have reported prevalence rates for major depression in patients with endstage renal disease. Three of the studies found very similar results of 5.0 percent (Smith, Hong, & Robson, 1985), 8.1 percent (Craven et al., 1987), and 6.5 percent (Hinrichsen et al., 1989). The subjects in each of these three studies were administered standard diagnostic interviews, either the Diagnostic Interview Schedule (Craven et al., 1987) or the Schedule for Affective Disorders and Schizophrenia (Smith, Hong, & Robson, 1985; Hinrichsen et al., 1989). An earlier study found a higher prevalence of 22.4 percent in these patients (Lowry & Atcherson, 1979).

Associated Factors

Interestingly, many of the studies cited in Table 1.8 failed to find an association between major depression and increased severity of illness (e.g., Craven et al., 1987; Carney et al., 1987; Frank et al., 1988). The results of these studies are summarized in Table 1.9. This finding differs from the results of studies using depressive symptom inventories in which the association between depression and illness severity was both prominent and consistent. This discrepancy may be explained by several factors. As discussed previously, studies using depressive symptom inventories include a majority of patients with mild symptoms of depression whereas the studies summarized in this part of the chapter include only studies that identified depressive disorders as cases. Rodin and Voshart (1987) have previously suggested that depressive symptoms are directly associated with illness severity in the mild range of depression, but not necessarily with more severely depressed states. Depressive symptom measures are also more likely to include confounding somatic

TABLE 1.9. *Risk Factors for Major Depressive Episode (MDE) in Studies Using Structured Diagnostic Interviews and DSM-III Criteria*

Author(s) and Year	n	Illness	Prevalence of MDE	Risk Factors		
				Illness Severity	Female Sex	Past MDE
Carney et al. (1987)	50	coronary artery disease	18.0%	No	Yes	NST*
Craven et al. (1987)	99	endstage renal disease	8.1%	No	Yes	Yes
Minden, Orav, & Reich (1987)	50	multiple sclerosis	34.0%	No	No	Yes
Atkinson et al. (1988)	45	acquired immuno-deficiency syndrome, AIDS-related complex, HIV-infection	11.1%	No	---	Yes
Frank et al. (1988)	137	rheumatoid arthritis	16.8%	No	Yes	No
Popkin et al. (1988)	75	insulin-dependent diabetes mellitus	10.7%	No	Yes	---

* NST = non-significant trend

symptoms than are methods that utilize standardized criteria. Modern diagnostic criteria include both temporal and severity dimensions and, compared with depressive symptom inventories, minimize the likelihood that a transient physical symptom would count as a criterion for depression. Furthermore, when applied in the medically ill, most diagnostic systems incorporate at least some directive about whether to include confounding somatic symptoms. Nevertheless, the preliminary findings from these few studies indicate that illness severity may not be the most prominent factor in determining the occurrence of major depression in medical patients.

Several studies have examined the role of other etiological factors in the occurrence of major depression in medical patients. Compared with psychiatric depressives, physically ill patients with major depression are less likely to have a history of depression (Winokur, Black, & Nasrallah, 1988). However, compared with medical patients who are not depressed, those with major depression more often report symptoms suggesting a previous episode of major depression (Craven et al., 1987; Feldman et al., 1987; Carney et al., 1987). Whitlock and Siskind (1980) found that a history of depression prior to the onset of multiple sclerosis was a risk factor for the occurrence of depression following its onset. Similarly, Atkinson et al. (1988) found that a history of major depression and other psychiatric disorders was common in depressed patients with acquired immunodeficiency syndrome. These findings are compatible with the suggestion that major depression may occur in any patient secondary to the direct or indirect biopsychosocial stress of medical illness, but that patients with preexisting vulnerability (as evidenced by a history of depression) are most likely to become depressed again in the face of this stress. This vulnerability may result from genetic predisposition. Alternatively, a previous episode of major depression may itself increase the likelihood of recurrent depression during times of significant stress. This hypothesis is consistent with the findings of Paykel and Tanner (1976), who demonstrated that the occurrence of "undesirable" life events was associated with the relapse of depression. Other studies have found a preponderance of women in the depressed groups (Craven et al., 1987; Carney et al., 1987; Frank et al., 1988; Popkin et al., 1988). Further investigation is required into the epidemiology of major depression in the medically ill. However, these preliminary findings suggest that when standardized and strict diagnostic criteria are used, the risk factors for major depression in the medically ill are similar to those in the general population.

56 /   DEPRESSION IN THE MEDICALLY ILL

REFERENCES

Akiskal, H.S. & McKinney Jr., W.T. (1975). Overview of recent research in depression: Integration of ten conceptual models into a comprehensive clinical frame. *Archives of General Psychiatry, 32,* 285–305.

Akiskal, H.S., Rosenthal, R.H., Rosenthal, T.L., Kashgarian, M., Khani, M.K., & Puzantian, V.R. (1979). Differentiation of primary affective illness from situational, symptomatic, and secondary depressions. *Archives of General Psychiatry, 36,* 635–643.

American Psychiatric Association (1987). *Diagnostic and Statistical Manual of Mental Disorders (Third Edition—Revised).* Washington, D.C.: American Psychiatric Association.

Ananth, J. (1984). Physical illness and psychiatric disorders. *Comprehensive Psychiatry, 25,* 586–593.

Andreasen, N.C. & Winokur, G. (1979). Secondary depression: Familial, clinical, and research perspectives. *American Journal of Psychiatry, 136,* 62–66.

Atkinson Jr., J.H., Grant, I., Kennedy, C.J., Richman, D.D., Spector, S.A., & McCutchan, J.A. (1988). Prevalence of psychiatric disorders among men infected with human immunodeficiency virus: A controlled study. *Archives of General Psychiatry, 45,* 859–864.

Aylard, P.R., Gooding, J.H., McKenna, P.J., & Snaith, R.P. (1987). A validation study of three anxiety and depression self-assessment scales. *Journal of Psychosomatic Research, 31,* 261–268.

Barnes, G.E. & Prosen, H. (1984). Depression in Canadian general practice attenders. *Canadian Journal of Psychiatry, 29,* 2–10.

Beck, A.T., Steer, R.A., & Garbin, M.G. (1988). Psychometric properties of the Beck Depression Inventory: Twenty-five years of evaluation. *Clinical Psychology Review, 8,* 77–100.

Beck, A.T., Ward, C.H., Mendelson, M., Mock, J., & Erbaugh, J. (1961). An inventory for measuring depression. *Archives of General Psychiatry, 4,* 53–63.

Beitman, B.D., Mukerji, V., Lamberti, J.W., Schmid, L., & Kushner, M. (1990). Major depression and agoraphobia in patients with angiographically normal coronary arteries and panic disorder. *Canadian Journal of Psychiatry, 35,* 298–304.

Bergmann, K. & Eastham, E.J. (1974). Psychogeriatric ascertainment and assessment for treatment in an acute medical ward setting. *Age and Ageing, 3,* 174–188.

Bishop, D., Green, A., Cantor, S., & Torresin, W. (1987). Depression, anxiety and rheumatoid arthritis activity. *Clinical and Experimental Rheumatology, 5,* 147–150.

Bisno, B. & Richardson, J.L. (1987). The relationship between depression and reinforcing events in cancer patients. *Journal of Psychosocial Oncology, 5,* 63–71.

Blacker, C.V.R. & Clare, A.W. (1988). The prevalence and treatment of depression in general practice. *Psychopharmacology, 95,* S14–S17.

Blumenthal, M.D. (1975). Measuring depressive symptomatology in a general population. *Archives of General Psychiatry, 32,* 971–978.

Borson, S., Barnes, R.A., Kukull, W.A., Okimoto, J.T., Veith, R.C., Inui, T.S., Carter, W., & Raskind, M.A. (1986). Symptomatic depression in elderly medical outpatients. I: Prevalence, demography, and health service utilization. *Journal of the American Geriatrics Society, 34,* 341–347.

Boyd, J.H., Weissman, M.M., Thompson, D., & Myers, J.K. (1982). Screening for depression in a community sample: Understanding the discrepancies between depression symptoms and diagnostic scales. *Archives of General Psychiatry, 39,* 1195–1200.

Boyle, G.J. (1985). Self-report measures of depression: Some psychometric considerations. *British Journal of Clinical Psychology, 24,* 45–59.

Bridges, K.W. & Goldberg, D.P. (1984). Psychiatric illness in in-patients with neurological disorders: Patients' views on discussion of emotional problems with neurologists. *British Medical Journal, 289,* 656–658.

Brown, J.H. & Paraskevas, F. (1982). Cancer and depression: Cancer presenting with depressive illness: An autoimmune disease? *British Journal of Psychiatry, 141,* 227–232.

Brown, R.G. & MacCarthy, B. (1990). Psychiatric morbidity in patients with Parkinson's disease. *Psychological Medicine, 20,* 77–87.

Brown, R.G., MacCarthy, B., Gotham, A.M., Der, G.J., & Marsden, C.D. (1988). Depression and disability in Parkinson's disease: A follow-up of 132 cases. *Psychological Medicine, 18,* 49–55.

Bukberg, J., Penman, D., & Holland, J.C. (1984). Depression in hospitalized cancer patients. *Psychosomatic Medicine, 46,* 199–212.

Bukberg, J.B. & Holland, J.C. (1980). A prevalence study of depression in a cancer hospital population. *Proceedings of the American Association of Cancer Research, 21,* 382.

Burton, H.J., Kline, S.A., Lindsay, R.M., & Heidenheim, A.P. (1986). The relationship of depression to survival in chronic renal failure. *Psychosomatic Medicine, 48,* 261–268.

Byrne, P. (1984). Psychiatric morbidity in a gynaecology clinic: An epidemiological survey. *British Journal of Psychiatry, 144,* 28–34.

Cadoret, R.J., Widmer, R.B., & Troughton, E.P. (1980). Somatic complaints: Harbinger of depression in primary care. *Journal of Affective Disorders, 2,* 61–70.

Cain, E.N., Kohorn, E.I., Quinlan, D.M., Schwartz, P.E., Latimer, K., & Rogers, L. (1983). Psychosocial reactions to the diagnosis of gynecologic cancer. *Obstetrics and Gynecology, 62,* 635–641.

Carney, R.M., Rich, M.W., teVelde, A., Saini, J., Clark, K., & Jaffe, A.S. (1987). Major depressive disorder in coronary artery disease. *American Journal of Cardiology, 60,* 1273–1275.

Carroll, B.J. (1984). Problems with diagnostic criteria for depression. *Journal of Clinical Psychiatry, 45,* 14–18.

Cassidy, W.L., Flanagan, N.B., Spellman, M., & Cohen, M.E. (1957). Clinical observations in manic-depressive disease: A quantitative study of one hundred manic-depressive patients and fifty medically sick controls. *Journal of the American Medical Association, 164,* 1535–1546.

Cassileth, B.R., Lusk, E.J., Strouse, T.B., Miller, D.S., Brown, L.L., Cross, P.A., & Tenaglia, A.N. (1984). Psychosocial status in chronic illness: A comparative analysis of six diagnostic groups. *New England Journal of Medicine, 311,* 506–511.

Cavanaugh, S.V.A. (1983). The prevalence of emotional and cognitive dysfunction in a general medical population: Using the MMSE, GHQ, and BDI. *General Hospital Psychiatry, 5,* 15–24.

Celesia, G.G. & Wanamaker, W.M. (1972). Psychiatric disturbances in Parkinson's disease. *Diseases of the Nervous System, 33,* 577–583.

Chamberlain, B.B. & Chamberlain, K.R. (1985). Depression: A psychologic consideration in complete denture prosthodontics. *Journal of Prosthetic Dentistry, 53,* 673–675.

Cheah, K.C., Baldridge, J.A., & Beard, O.W. (1979). Geriatric evaluation unit of a medical service: Role of a geropsychiatrist. *Journal of Gerontology, 34,* 41–45.

Clark, D.C., Cavanaugh, S.V.A., & Gibbons, R.D. (1983). The core symptoms of depression in medical and psychiatric patients. *Journal of Nervous and Mental Disease, 171,* 705–713.

Comings, B.G. & Comings, D.E. (1987). A controlled study of Tourette syndrome. V. Depression and mania. *American Journal of Human Genetics, 41,* 804–821.

Comstock, G.W. & Helsing, K.J. (1976). Symptoms of depression in two communities. *Psychological Medicine, 6,* 551–563.

Coulehan, J.L., Schulberg, H.C., Block, M.R., & Zettler-Segal, M. (1988). Symptom patterns of depression in ambulatory medical and psychiatric patients. *Journal of Nervous and Mental Disease, 176,* 284–288.

Craig, T.J. & Abeloff, M.D. (1974). Psychiatric symptomatology among hospitalized cancer patients. *American Journal of Psychiatry, 131,* 1323–1327.

Craig, T.J. & Van Natta, P.A. (1976). Influence of demographic characteristics on two measures of depressive symptoms: The relation of prevalence and persistence of symptoms with sex, age, education, and marital status. *Archives of General Psychiatry, 36,* 149–154.

Craven, J., Littlefield, C., Rodin, G., & Murray, M. (1991). The Endstage Renal Disease Severity Index (ESRD-SI). *Psychological Medicine, 21 (2)* 237–244.

Craven, J.L. & Rodin, G. (1990). Somatic symptoms and the diagnosis of depression in medically ill patients (letter). *American Journal of Psychiatry, 147,* 814–815.

Craven, J.L., Rodin, G.M., Johnson, L., & Kennedy, S.H. (1987). The diagnosis of major depression in renal dialysis patients. *Psychosomatic Medicine, 49,* 482–492.

Craven, J.L., Rodin, G.M., & Littlefield, C.H. (1988). The Beck Depression Inventory as a screening device for major depression in renal dialysis patients. *International Journal of Psychiatry in Medicine, 18,* 373–382.

Craven, J.L., Rodin, G.M., & Littlefield, C. *Illness severity and depressive symptoms in dialysis patients.* (Unpublished data).

Culpan, R.H., Davies, B.M., & Oppenheim, A.N. (1960). Incidence of psychiatric illness among hospital outpatients and application of the Cornell Medical Index. *British Medical Journal, 1,* 855–857.

Davies, A.D.M., Davies, C., & Delpo, M.C. (1986). Depression and anxiety in patients undergoing diagnostic investigations for head and neck cancers. *British Journal of Psychiatry, 149,* 491–493.

Dean, C. (1987). Psychiatric morbidity following mastectomy: Preoperative predictors and types of illness. *Journal of Psychosomatic Research, 31,* 385–392.

Derogatis, L.R. (1983). *SCL-90-R: Administration, Scoring and Procedures Manual: II. For the Revised Version.* Towson, MD: Clinical Psychometric Research.

Derogatis, L.R., Morrow, G.R., Fetting, J., Penman, D., Piasetsky, S., Schmale, A.M., Henrichs, M., & Carnicke Jr., C.L.M. (1983). The prevalence of psychiatric disorders among cancer patients. *Journal of the American Medical Association, 249,* 751–757.

Dhadphale, M., Ellison, R.H., & Griffin, L. (1983). The frequency of psychiatric disorders among patients attending semi-urban and rural general outpatient clinics in Kenya. *British Journal of Psychiatry, 142,* 379–383.

Eastwood, M.R. (1975). *The Relation Between Physical and Mental Illness.* Toronto: University of Toronto Press.

Ebrahim, S., Barer, D., & Nouri, F. (1987). Affective illness after stroke. *British Journal of Psychiatry, 151,* 52–56.

Emmons, C.A., Fetting, J.H., & Zonderman, A.B. (1987). A comparison of the symptoms of medical and psychiatric patients matched on the Beck Depression Inventory. *General Hospital Psychiatry, 9,* 398–404.

Endicott, J. (1984). Measurement of depression in patients with cancer. *Cancer, 53,* 2243–2249.

Evans, D.L., McCartney, C.F., Nemeroff, C.B., Raft, D., Quade, D., Golden, R.N., Haggerty Jr., J.J., Holmes, V., Simon, J.S., Droba, M., Mason, G.Z., & Fowler, W.C. (1986). Depression in women treated for gynecological cancer: Clinical and neuroendocrine assessment. *American Journal of Psychiatry, 143,* 447–452.

Farmer, C.J., Bewick, M., Parsons, V., & Snowden, S.A. (1979). Survival on home haemodialysis: Its relationship with physical symptomatology, psychosocial background, and psychiatric morbidity. *Psychosomatic Medicine, 9,* 515–523.

Farmer, C.J., Snowden, S.A., & Parsons, V. (1979). The prevalence of psychiatric illness among patients on home haemodialysis. *Psychological Medicine, 9,* 509–514.

Fava, G.A., Pilowsky, I., Pierfederici, A., Bernardi, M., & Pathak, D. (1982a). Depression and illness behavior in a general hospital: A prevalence study. *Psychotherapy and Psychosomatics, 38,* 141–153.

Fava, G.A., Pilowsky, I., Pierfederici, A., Bernardi, M., & Pathak, D. (1982b). Depressive symptoms and abnormal illness behavior in general hospital patients. *General Hospital Psychiatry, 4,* 171–178.

Fava, G.A., Sonino, N., & Wise, T.N. (1988). Management of depression in medical patients. *Psychotherapy and Psychosomatics, 49,* 81–102.

Fava, G.A., Trombini, G., Barbara, L., Bernardi, M., Grandi, S., Callegari, C., & Miglioli, M. (1985). Depression and gastrointestinal illness: The joint use of biological and clinical criteria. *American Journal of Gastroenterology, 80,* 195–199.

Feighner, J.P., Robins, E., Guze, S.B., Woodruff Jr., R.A., Winokur, G., & Munoz, R. (1972). Diagnostic criteria for use in psychiatric research. *Archives of General Psychiatry, 26,* 57–63.

Feldman, E., Mayou, R., Hawton, K., Ardern, M., & Smith, E.B.O. (1987). Psychiatric disorder in medical in-patients. *Quarterly Journal of Medicine, 63,* 405–412.

Finklestein, S., Benowitz, L.I., Baldessarini, R.J., Arana, G.W., Levine, D., Woo, E., Bear, D., Moya, K., & Stoll, A.L. (1982). Mood, vegetative disturbance, and dexamethasone suppression test after stroke. *Annals of Neurology, 12,* 463–468.

Fogel, B.S. (1990). Major depression versus organic mood disorder: A questionable distinction. *Journal of Clinical Psychiatry, 51,* 53–56.

Folstein, S.E., Folstein, M.F., & McHugh, P.R. (1979). Psychiatric syndromes in Huntington's disease. In T.N. Chase, N.S. Wexler, & A. Barbeau (Eds.), *Advances in Neurology, Vol. 23.* (pp. 281–289). New York: Raven Press.

Foster, F.G., Cohn, G.L., & McKegney, F.P. (1973). Psychobiologic factors and individual survival on chronic renal hemodialysis: A two-year follow-up: Part 1. *Psychosomatic Medicine, 35,* 64–82.

Frank, R.G., Beck, N.C., Parker, J.C., Kashani, J.H., Elliott, T.R., Haut, A.E., Smith, E., Atwood, C., Brownlee-Duffeck, M., & Kay, D.R. (1988). Depression in rheumatoid arthritis. *Journal of Rheumatology, 15,* 920–925.

Frank, R.G., Kashani, J.H., Wonderlich, S.A., Lising, A., & Visot, L.R. (1985). Depression and adrenal function in spinal cord injury. *American Journal of Psychiatry, 142,* 252–253.

Frochtengarten, M.L., Villares, J.C.B., Maluf, E., & Carlini, E.A. (1987). Depressive symptoms and the Dexamethasone Suppression Test in parkinsonian patients. *Biological Psychiatry, 22,* 386–389.

Gibbons, R.D., Clark, D.C., Cavanaugh, S.V.A., & Davis, J.M. (1985). Application of modern psychometric theory in psychiatric research. *Journal of Psychiatric Research, 19,* 43–55.

Gillespie, L. (1929). The clinical differentiation of types of depression. *Guy's Hospital Reports, 79,* 231–233.

Glass, R.M. (1985). Situational and neurotic-reactive depression. *Archives of General Psychiatry, 42,* 1126–1127.

Glass, R.M., Allan, A.T., Uhlenhuth, E.H., Kimball, C.P., & Borinstein, D.I.

(1978). Psychiatric screening in a medical clinic: An evaluation of a self-report inventory. *Archives of General Psychiatry, 35,* 1189–1195.

Goldberg, D.P. (1972). *Detection of Psychiatric Illness by Questionnaire.* Oxford: Oxford University Press.

Gotham, A.M., Brown, R.G., & Marsden, C.D. (1986). Depression in Parkinson's disease: A quantitative and qualitative analysis. *Journal of Neurology, Neurosurgery, and Psychiatry, 49,* 381–389.

Gotlib, I.H. (1984). Depression and general psychopathology in university students. *Journal of Abnormal Psychology, 93,* 19–30.

Grossman, S. (1982). A psychoanalyst-liaison psychiatrist's overview of DSM-III. *General Hospital Psychiatry, 4,* 291–295.

Guze, S.B., Woodruff, R.A., & Clayton, P.J. (1971). 'Secondary' affective disorder: A study of 95 cases (preliminary communication). *Psychological Medicine, 1,* 426–428.

Hall, R.C., Gardner, E.R., Stickney, S.K., LeCann, A.F., & Popkin, M.K. (1980). Physical illness manifesting as psychiatric disease: II. Analysis of a state inpatient population. *Archives of General Psychiatry, 37,* 989–995.

Hankin, J.R. & Locke, B.Z. (1983). Extent of depressive symptomatology among patients seeking care in a prepaid group practice. *Psychological Medicine, 13,* 121–129.

Harding, T.W., de Arango, M.V., Baltazar, J., Climent, C.E., Ibrahim, H.H.A., Ladrido-Ignacio, L., Srinivasa-Murthy, R., & Wig, N.N. (1980). Mental disorders in primary health care: A study of their frequency and diagnosis in four developing countries. *Psychological Medicine, 10,* 231–241.

Harris, R.E., Mion, L.C., Patterson, M.B., & Frengley, J.D. (1988). Severe illness in older patients: The association between depressive disorders and functional dependency during the recovery phase. *Journal of the American Geriatrics Society, 36,* 890–896.

Hawley, D.J. & Wolfe, F. (1988). Anxiety and depression in patients with rheumatoid arthritis: A prospective study of 400 patients. *Journal of Rheumatology, 15,* 932–941.

Helzer, J.E., Chammas, S., Norland, C.C., Stillings, W.A., & Alpers, D.H. (1984). A study of the association between Crohn's disease and psychiatric illness. *Gastroenterology, 86,* 324–330.

Hengeveld, M.W., Ancion, F.A.J., & Rooijmans, H.G.M. (1987). Prevalence and recognition of depressive disorders in general medical inpatients. *International Journal of Psychiatry in Medicine, 17,* 341–349.

Henley, C.E. & Coussens, W.R. (1988). The ability of family practice residents to diagnose depression in outpatients. *Journal of the American Osteopathic Association, 88,* 118–122.

Hinrichsen, G.A., Lieberman, J.A., Pollack, S., & Steinberg, H. (1989). Depression in hemodialysis patients. *Psychosomatics, 30,* 284–289.

Hirschfeld, R.M.A., Klerman, G.L., Andreasen, N.C., Clayton, P.J., & Keller, M.B. (1985). Situational major depressive disorder. *Archives of General Psychiatry, 42,* 1109–1114.

Hoeper, E.W., Nycz, G.R., Cleary, P.D., Regier, D.A., & Goldberg, I.D. (1979). Estimated prevalence of RDC mental disorder in primary medical care. *International Journal of Mental Health, 8,* 6–15.

Holland, J. (1977). Psychological aspects of oncology. *Medical Clinics of North America, 61,* 737–748.

House, A. (1988). Mood disorders in the physically ill: Problems of definition and measurement. *Journal of Psychosomatic Research, 32,* 345–353.

Hughes, J.E., Barraclough, B.M., Hamblin, L.G., & White, J.E. (1983). Psychiatric symptoms in dermatology patients. *British Journal of Psychiatry, 143,* 51–54.

Jahanshahi, M. & Marsden, C.D. (1988). Depression in torticollis: A controlled study. *Psychological Medicine, 18,* 925–933.

Joffe, R.T., Lippert, G.P., Gray, T.A., Sawa, G., & Horvath, Z. (1987). Mood disorder and multiple sclerosis. *Archives of Neurology, 44,* 376–378.

Johnston, M., Wakeling, A., Graham, N., & Stokes, F. (1987). Cognitive impairment, emotional disorder and length of stay of elderly patients in a district general hospital. *British Journal of Medical Psychology, 60,* 133–139.

Judd, F.K., Stone, J., Webber, J.E., Brown, D.J., & Burrows, G.D. (1989). Depression following spinal cord injury: A prospective in-patient study. *British Journal of Psychiatry, 154,* 668–671.

Kashani, J.H., Frank, R.G., Kashani, S.R., Wonderlich, S.A., & Reid, J.C. (1983). Depression among amputees. *Journal of Clinical Psychiatry, 44,* 256–258.

Kathol, R.G. & Petty, F. (1981). Relationship of depression to medical illness: A critical review. *Journal of Affective Disorders, 3,* 111–121.

Katon, W. (1982). Depression: Somatic symptoms and medical disorders in primary care. *Comprehensive Psychiatry, 23,* 274–287.

Katon, W., Berg, A.O., Robins, A.J., & Risse, S. (1986). Depression—Medical utilization and somatization. *Western Journal of Medicine, 144,* 564–568.

Katon, W., Kleinman, A., & Rosen, G. (1982). Depression and somatization: A review: Part I. *American Journal of Medicine, 72,* 127–135.

Kirk, C.A., & Saunders, M. (1979). Psychiatric illness in a neurological out-patient department in North East England: Use of the General Health Questionnaire in the prospective study of neurological out-patients. *Acta Psychiatrica Scandinavica, 60,* 427–437.

Kleinman, A. (1988). *Rethinking Psychiatry: From Cultural Category to Personal Experience.* New York: Free Press (Macmillan).

Klerman, G.L. (1981). Depression in the medically ill. *Psychiatric Clinics of North America, 4,* 301–317.

Knights, E.B. & Folstein, M.F. (1977). Unsuspected emotional and cognitive disturbance in medical patients. *Annals of Internal Medicine, 87,* 723–724.

Koenig, H.G., Goli, V., Shelp, F., Cohen, H.J., Meador, K.G., & Blazer, D.G. (1989). Major depression and the NIMH Diagnostic Interview Schedule: Validation in medically ill hospitalized patients. *International Journal of Psychiatry in Medicine, 19,* 123–132.

Koenig, H.G., Meador, K.G., Cohen, H.J., & Blazer, D.G. (1988). Self-rated depression scales and screening for major depression in the older hospitalized patient with medical illness. *Journal of the American Geriatrics Society, 36,* 699–706.

Koenig, R., Levin, S.M., & Brennan, M.J. (1967). The emotional status of cancer patients as measured by a psychological test. *Journal of Chronic Diseases, 20,* 923–930.

Koranyi, E.K. (1980). Somatic illness in psychiatric patients. *Psychosomatics, 21,* 887–891.

Krupp, L.B., Alvarez, L.A., LaRocca, N.G., & Scheinberg, L.C. (1988). Fatigue in multiple sclerosis. *Archives of Neurology, 45,* 435–437.

Kupfer, D.J., Foster, F.G., & Coble, P.A. (1977). EEG sleep parameters for the classification and treatment of affective disorders. *Psychopharmacology Bulletin, 13,* 57–58.

Kutner, N.G., Fair, P.L., & Kutner, M.H. (1985). Assessing depression and anxiety in chronic dialysis patients. *Journal of Psychosomatic Research, 29,* 23–31.

Lalinec-Michaud, M., Engelsmann, F., & Marino, J. (1988). Depression after hysterectomy: A comparative study. *Psychosomatics, 29,* 307–314.

Lansky, S.B., List, M.A., Herrmann, C.A., Ets-Hokin, E.G., DasGupta, T.K., Wilbanks, G.D., & Hendrickson, F.R. (1985). Absence of major depressive disorder in female cancer patients. *Journal of Clinical Oncology, 3,* 1553–1560.

Lasry, J.C.M., Margolese, R.G., Poisson, R., Shibata, H., Fleischer, D., Lafleur, D., Legault, S., & Taillefer, S. (1987). Depression and body image following mastectomy and lumpectomy. *Journal of Chronic Diseases, 40,* 529–534.

Leigh, H., Price, L., Ciarcia, J., & Mirassou, M.M. (1982). DSM-III and consultation-liaison psychiatry: Toward a comprehensive medical model of the patient. *General Hospital Psychiatry, 4,* 283–289.

Levenson, J.L., Hamer, R., Silverman, J.J., & Rossiter, L.F. (1986). Psychopathology in medical inpatients and its relationship to length of hospital stay: A pilot study. *International Journal of Psychiatry in Medicine, 16,* 231–236.

Lewis, A. (1934). Melancholia: A clinical survey of depressive states. *Journal of Mental Science, 80,* 277–378.

Light, R.W., Merrill, E.J., Despars, J.A., Gordon, G.H., & Mutalipassi, L.R. (1985). Prevalence of depression and anxiety in patients with COPD: Relationship to functional capacity. *Chest, 87,* 35–38.

Lindemann, E. (1944). Symptomatology and the management of acute grief. *American Journal of Psychiatry, 101,* 141–148.

Linn, L.S. & Yager, J. (1980). The effect of screening, sensitization, and feedback on notation of depression. *Journal of Medical Education, 55,* 942–949.

Lipowski, Z.J. & Wolston, E.J. (1981). Liaison psychiatry: Referral patterns and their stability over time. *American Journal of Psychiatry, 138,* 1608–1611.

Lipsey, J.R., Spencer, W.C., Rabins, P.V., & Robinson, R.G. (1986). Phenomenological comparison of poststroke depression and functional depression. *American Journal of Psychiatry, 143,* 527–529.

Littlefield, C.H., Rodin, G.M., Murray, M.A., & Craven, J.L. (1990). The influence of functional impairment and social support on depressive symptoms in persons with diabetes. *Health Psychology 9,* 337–749.

Lloyd, G.G. & Cawley, R.H. (1978). Psychiatric morbidity in men one week after first acute myocardial infarction. *British Medical Journal, 2,* 1453–1454.

Louks, J., Hayne, C., & Smith, J. (1989). Replicated factor structure of the Beck Depression Inventory. *Journal of Nervous and Mental Disease, 177,* 473–479.

Lowry, M.R. & Atcherson, E. (1979). Characteristics of patients with depressive disorder on entry into home hemodialysis. *Journal of Nervous and Mental Disease, 167,* 748–751.

Lustman, P.J., Clouse, R.E., & Carney, R.M. (1988). Depression and the reporting of diabetes symptoms. *International Journal of Psychiatry in Medicine, 18,* 295–303.

Lustman, P.J., Griffith, L.S., Clouse, R.E., & Cryer, P.E. (1986a). Psychiatric illness in diabetes mellitus: Relationship to symptoms and glucose control. *Journal of Nervous and Mental Disease, 174,* 736–742.

Lustman, P.J., Harper, G.W., Griffith, L.S., & Clouse, R.E. (1986b). Use of the Diagnostic Interview Schedule in patients with diabetes mellitus. *Journal of Nervous and Mental Disease, 174,* 743–746.

Lyons, J.S., Strain, J.J., Hammer, J.S., Ackerman, A.D., & Fulop, G. (1989). Reliability, validity, and temporal stability of the Geriatric Depression Scale in hospitalized elderly. *International Journal of Psychiatry in Medicine, 19,* 203–209.

MacDonald, A.J. & Bouchier, I.A.D. (1980). Non-organic gastrointestinal illness: A medical and psychiatric study. *British Journal of Psychiatry, 136,* 276–283.

Mackenzie, T.B., Popkin, M.K., & Callies, A.L. (1983). Clinical applications of DSM-III in consultation-liaison psychiatry. *Hospital and Community Psychiatry, 34,* 628–631.

Magni, G., De Leo, D., & Schifano, F. (1985). Depression in geriatric and adult medical inpatients. *Journal of Clinical Psychology, 41,* 337–344.

Maguire, G.P. & Granville-Grossman, K.L. (1968). Physical illness in psychiatric patients. *British Journal of Psychiatry, 115,* 1365–1369.

Maguire, G.P., Julier, D.L., Hawton, K.E., & Bancroft, J.H.J. (1974). Psychiatric morbidity and referral on two general medical wards. *British Medical Journal, 1,* 268–270.

Malt, U. (1988). The long-term psychiatric consequences of accidental injury: A longitudinal study of 107 adults. *British Journal of Psychiatry, 153,* 810–818.

Maricle, R.A., Hosenpud, J.D., Norman, D.J., Woodbury, A., Pantley, G.A.,

Cobanoglu, A.M., & Starr, A. (1989). Depression in patients being evaluated for heart transplantation. *General Hospital Psychiatry, 11,* 418–424.

Massie, M.J., Grozynski, G., Mastrovito, R., Theis, D., & Holland, J. (1979). The diagnosis of depression in hospitalized patients with cancer. *Proceedings of the American Association of Cancer Research, 20,* 432.

Mayeux, R., Stern, Y., Rosen, J., & Leventhal, J. (1981). Depression, intellectual impairment, and Parkinson disease. *Neurology, 31,* 645–650.

Mayeux, R., Williams, J.B.W., Stern, Y., & Cote, L. (1984). Depression and Parkinson's disease. In R.G. Hassler & J.F. Christ (Eds.), *Advances in Neurology, Vol. 40.* (pp. 241–250). New York: Raven Press.

Mayou, R. (1975). Psychological morbidity in a clinic for sexually-transmitted disease. *British Journal of Venereal Disease, 51,* 57–60.

Mayou, R., & Hawton, K. (1986). Psychiatric disorder in the general hospital. *British Journal of Psychiatry, 149,* 172–190.

Mazure, C., Nelson, J.C., & Price, L.H. (1986). Reliability and validity of the symptoms of major depressive illness. *Archives of General Psychiatry, 43,* 451–456.

McSweeney, A.J., Grant, I., Heaton, R.K., Adams, K.M., & Timms, R.M. (1982). Life quality of patients with chronic obstructive pulmonary disease. *Archives of Internal Medicine, 142,* 473–478.

Millman, R.P., Fogel, B.S., McNamara, M.E., & Carlisle, C.C. (1989). Depression as a manifestation of obstructive sleep apnea: Reversal with nasal continuous positive airway pressure. *Journal of Clinical Psychiatry, 50,* 348–351.

Minden, S.L., Orav, J., & Reich, P. (1987). Depression in multiple sclerosis. *General Hospital Psychiatry, 9,* 426–434.

Moffic, H.S. & Paykel, E.S. (1975). Depression in medical inpatients. *British Journal of Psychiatry, 126,* 346–353.

Moore, J.T., Silimperi, D.R., & Bobula, J.A. (1978). Recognition of depression by family medicine residents: The impact of screening. *Journal of Family Practice, 7,* 509–513.

Morton, R.P., Davies, A.D.M., Baker, J., Baker, G.A., & Stell, P.M. (1984). Quality of life in treated head and neck cancer patients: A preliminary report. *Clinical Otolaryngology, 9,* 181–185.

Mossey, J.M., Mutran, E., Knott, K., & Craik, R. (1989). Determinants of recovery 12 months after hip fracture: The importance of psychosocial factors. *American Journal of Public Health, 79,* 279–286.

Myers, J.K. & Weissman, M.W. (1980). Use of a self-report symptom scale to detect depression in a community sample. *American Journal of Psychiatry, 137,* 1081–1084.

Nielsen, A.C. & Williams, T.A. (1980). Depression in ambulatory medical patients. *Archives of General Psychiatry, 37,* 999–1004.

Okimoto, J., Barnes, R.F., Veith, R.C., Raskind, M.A., Inui, T.S., & Carter, W.B. (1982). Screening for depression in geriatric medical patients. *American Journal of Psychiatry, 139,* 799–802.

66 / Depression in the Medically Ill

Parikh, R.M., Eden, D.T., Price, T.R., & Robinson, R.G. (1988). The sensitivity and specificity of the Center for Epidemiologic Studies Depression Scale in screening for post-stroke depression. *International Journal of Psychiatry in Medicine, 18,* 169–181.

Paykel, E.S. & Tanner, J. (1976). Life events, depressive relapse and maintenance treatment. *Psychological Medicine, 6,* 481–485.

Pfeiffer, R.F., Hsieh, H.H., Diercks, M.J., Glaeske, C., Jefferson, A., & Cheng, S.C. (1986). Dexamethasone suppression test in Parkinson's disease. In M.D. Yahr & K.J. Bergmann (Eds.), *Advances in Neurology, Vol. 45.* (pp. 439–442). New York: Raven Press.

Pincus, T., Callahan, L.F., Bradley, L.A., Vaughn, W.K., & Wolfe, F. (1986). Elevated MMPI scores for hypochondriasis, depression, and hysteria in patients with rheumatoid arthritis reflect disease rather than psychological status. *Arthritis and Rheumatism, 29,* 1456–1466.

Plumb, M.M. & Holland, J. (1977). Comparative studies of psychological function in patients with advanced cancer: I. Self-reported depressive symptoms. *Psychosomatic Medicine, 39,* 264–276.

Plumb, M.M. & Holland, J. (1981). Comparative studies of psychological function in patients with advanced cancer: II. Interviewer-rated current and past psychological symptoms. *Psychosomatic Medicine, 43,* 243–254.

Popkin, M.K., Callies, A.L., & Colon, E.A. (1987). A framework for the study of medical depression: A practical approach to classifying depression in the medically ill. *Psychosomatics, 28,* 27–33.

Popkin, M.K., Callies, A.L., Lentz, R.D., Colon, E.A., & Sutherland, D.E. (1988). Prevalence of major depression, simple phobia, and other psychiatric disorders in patients with long-standing Type I diabetes mellitus. *Archives of General Psychiatry, 45,* 64–68.

Porter, A.M.W. (1970). Depressive illness in a general practice: A demographic study and a controlled trial of imipramine. *British Medical Journal, 1,* 773–778.

Rabins, P.V. (1989). Depression and multiple sclerosis. In R.G. Robinson & P.V. Rabins (Eds.), *Depression and Coexisting Disease.* (pp. 226–233). New York: Igaku-Shoin.

Radloff, L. (1977). The CES-D scale: A self-report depression scale for research in the general population. *Applied Psychological Measurement, 1,* 385–401.

Rapp, S.R. & Vrana, S. (1989). Substituting nonsomatic for somatic symptoms in the diagnosis of depression in elderly male medical patients. *American Journal of Psychiatry, 146,* 1197–1200.

Robins, L.N., Helzer, J.E., Croughan, J., & Ratcliff, K.S. (1981). National Institute of Mental Health Diagnostic Interview Schedule: Its history, characteristics, and validity. *Archives of General Psychiatry, 38,* 381–389.

Robinson, N., Fuller, J.H., & Edmeades, S.P. (1988). Depression and diabetes. *Diabetic Medicine, 5,* 268–274.

Robinson, R.G., Lipsey, J.R., & Pearlson, G.D. (1984). The occurrence and treatment of poststroke mood disorders. *Comprehensive Therapy, 10,* 19–24.

Robinson, R.G. & Price, T.R. (1982). Post-stroke depressive disorders: A follow-up study of 103 patients. *Stroke, 13,* 635–641.

Robinson, R.G., Starr, L.B., Kubos, K.L., & Price, T.R. (1983). A two-year longitudinal study of post-stroke mood disorders: Findings during the initial evaluation. *Stroke, 14,* 736–741.

Rodin, G. & Voshart, K. (1987). Depressive symptoms and functional impairment in the medically ill. *General Hospital Psychiatry, 9,* 251–258.

Rodin, G.M., Voshart, K., Fenton, S.S.A., Cardella, C., Cattran, D.C., & Halloran, P.F. (1984). Depression and medical illness: A study of patients with end-stage renal disease. *Modern Medicine of Canada, 39,* 462–465.

Rose, J.D.R., Troughton, A.H., Harvey, J.S., & Smith, P.M. (1986). Depression and functional bowel disorders in gastrointestinal outpatients. *Gut, 27,* 1025–1028.

Rosen, D.H., Gregory, R.J., Pollock, D., & Schiffmann, A. (1987). Depression in patients referred for psychiatric consultation: A need for a new diagnosis. *General Hospital Psychiatry, 9,* 391–397.

Rosenberg, S.J., Peterson, R.A., Hayes, J.R., Hatcher, J., & Headen, S. (1988). Depression in medical in-patients. *British Journal of Medical Psychology, 61,* 245–254.

Rucker, L., Frye, E.B., & Cygan, R.W. (1986). Feasibility and usefulness of depression screening in medical outpatients. *Archives of Internal Medicine, 146,* 729–731.

Salkind, M.R. (1969). Beck Depression Inventory in general practice. *Journal of the Royal College of General Practitioners, 18,* 267–271.

Santamaria, J., Tolosa, E., & Valles, A. (1986). Parkinson's disease with depression: A possible subgroup of idiopathic parkinsonism. *Neurology, 36,* 1130–1133.

Schlesser, M.A., Winokur, G., & Sherman, B.M. (1980). Hypothalamic-pituitary-adrenal axis activity in depressive illness: Its relationship to classification. *Archives of General Psychiatry, 37,* 737–743.

Schmale, A.H. (1979). Psychological aspects of anorexia: Areas for study. *Cancer, 43,* 2087–2092.

Schulberg, H.C., Saul, M., McClelland, M., Ganguli, M., Christy, W., & Frank, R. (1985). Assessing depression in primary medical and psychiatric practices. *Archives of General Psychiatry, 42,* 1164–1170.

Schwab, J., Bialow, M., Clemmons, R., Martin, P., & Holzer, C. (1967a). The Beck Depression Inventory with medical inpatients. *Acta Psychiatrica Scandinavica, 43,* 255–266.

Schwab, J.J., Bialow, M., Brown, J.M., & Holzer, C.E. (1967b). Diagnosing depression in medical inpatients. *Annals of Internal Medicine, 67,* 695–707.

Schwab, J.J., Bialow, M.R., Clemmons, R.S., & Holzer, C.E. (1966). The affective symptomatology of depression in medical inpatients. *Psychosomatics, 7,* 214–217.

Seller, R.H., Blascovich, J., & Lenkei, E. (1981). Influence of stereotypes in the diagnosis of depression by family practice residents. *Journal of Family Practice, 12,* 849–854.

Shulman, R., Price, J.D.E., & Spinelli, J. (1989). Biopsychosocial aspects of long-term survival on endstage renal failure therapy. *Psychological Medicine, 19,* 945–954.

Silberfarb, P.M., Maurer, L.H., & Crouthamel, C.S. (1980). Psychosocial aspects of neoplastic disease: I. Functional status of breast cancer patients during different treatment regimens. *American Journal of Psychiatry, 137,* 450–455.

Sinyor, D., Amato, P., Kaloupek, D.G., Becker, R., Goldenberg, M., & Coopersmith, H. (1986). Post-stroke depression: Relationships to functional impairment, coping strategies, and rehabilitation outcome. *Stroke, 17,* 1102–1107.

Smith, M.D., Hong, B.A., & Robson, A.M. (1985). Diagnosis of depression in patients with end-stage renal disease: Comparative analysis. *American Journal of Medicine, 79,* 160–166.

Snaith, R.P. (1987). The concepts of mild depression. *British Journal of Psychiatry, 150,* 387–393.

Spitzer, R.L., Endicott, J., & Robins, E. (1978). Research Diagnostic Criteria: Rationale and reliability. *Archives of General Psychiatry, 35,* 773–782.

Stancer, H.C., Persaud, E., Jorna, T., Flood, C., & Wagener, D.K. (1984). The occurrence of secondary affective disorder in an in-patient population with severe and recurrent affective disorder. *British Journal of Psychiatry, 144,* 630–635.

Starkstein, S.E., Preziosi, T.J., Bolduc, P.L., & Robinson, R.G. (1990). Depression in Parkinson's disease. *Journal of Nervous and Mental Disease, 178,* 27–31.

Starkstein, S.E. & Robinson, R.G. (1989). Depression and Parkinson's disease. In R.G. Robinson & P.V. Rabins (Eds.), *Depression and Coexisting Disease.* (pp. 213–225). New York: Igaku-Shoin.

Steer, R.A., Beck, A.T., & Garrison, B. (1986). Applications of the Beck Depression Inventory. In N. Sartorius & T.A. Ban (Eds.), *Assessment of Depression.* (pp. 123–142). Berlin: Springer-Verlag.

Stein, R.E., Gortmaker, S.L., Perrin, E.C., Perrin, J.M., Pless, I.B., Walker, D.K., & Weitzman, M. (1987). Severity of illness: Concepts and measurements. *Lancet, 2,* 1506–1509.

Stern, M.J., Pascale, L., & Ackerman, A. (1977). Life adjustment postmyocardial infarction: Determining predictive variables. *Archives of Internal Medicine, 137,* 1680–1685.

Stewart, M.A., Drake, F., & Winokur, G. (1965). Depression among medically ill patients. *Diseases of the Nervous System, 26,* 479–485.

Tarter, R.E., Switala, J., Carra, J., Edwards, K.L., & Van Thiel, D.H. (1987). Inflammatory bowel disease: Psychiatric status of patients before and after disease onset. *International Journal of Psychiatry in Medicine, 17,* 173–181.

Teiramaa, E. (1979). Asthma, psychic disturbances and family history of atopic disorders. *Journal of Psychosomatic Research, 23,* 209–217.

Vazquez-Barquero, J.L., Padierna Acero, J.A., Pena Martin, C., & Ochoteco,

A. (1985). The psychiatric correlates of coronary pathology: Validity of the GHQ-60 as a screening instrument. *Psychological Medicine, 15,* 589-596.

Von Korff, M., Shapiro, S., Burke, J.D., Teitlebaum, M., Skinner, E.A., German, P., Turner, R.W., Klein, L., & Burns, B. (1987). Anxiety and depression in a primary care clinic: Comparison of Diagnostic Interview Schedule, General Health Questionnaire, and practitioner assessments. *Archives of General Psychiatry, 44,* 152-156.

Wade, D.T., Legh-Smith, J., & Hewer, R.A. (1987). Depressed mood after stroke: A community study of its frequency. *British Journal of Psychiatry, 151,* 200-205.

Wai, L., Richmond, J., Burton, H., & Lindsay, R.M. (1981). Influence of psychosocial factors on survival of home-dialysis patients. *Lancet, 2,* 1155-1156.

Warburton, J.W. (1967). Depressive symptoms in Parkinson patients referred for thalamotomy. *Journal of Neurology, Neurosurgery, and Psychiatry, 30,* 368-370.

Ward, H.W., Moss, R.L., Darko, D.F., Berry, C.C., Anderson, J., Kolman, P., Green, A., Nielsen, J., Klauber, M., Wachtel, T.L., & Frank, H. (1987). Prevalence of postburn depression following burn injury. *Journal of Burn Care and Rehabilitation, 8,* 294-298.

Weddington, W.W., Segraves, K.B., & Simon, M.A. (1986). Current and lifetime incidence of psychiatric disorders among a group of extremity sarcoma survivors. *Journal of Psychosomatic Research, 30,* 121-125.

Whitlock, F.A. & Siskind, M.M. (1980). Depression as a major symptom of multiple sclerosis. *Journal of Neurology, Neurosurgery, and Psychiatry, 43,* 861-865.

Williamson, M.T. (1987). Sex differences in depression symptoms among adult family medicine patients. *Journal of Family Practice, 25,* 591-594.

Williamson, P.S. & Yates, W.R. (1989). The initial presentation of depression in family practice and psychiatric outpatients. *General Hospital Psychiatry, 11,* 188-193.

Winokur, G., Black, D.W., & Nasrallah, A. (1988). Depressions secondary to other psychiatric disorders and medical illnesses. *American Journal of Psychiatry, 145,* 233-237.

Wood, D., Othmer, S., Reich, T., Viesselman, J., & Rutt, C. (1977). Primary and secondary affective disorder: I. Past social history and current episodes in 92 depressed inpatients. *Comprehensive Psychiatry, 18,* 201-210.

Wright, J.H., Bell, R.A., Kuhn, C.C., Rush, E.A., Patel, N., & Redmon Jr., J.E. (1980). Depression in family practice patients. *Southern Medical Journal, 73,* 1031-1034.

Wulsin, L.R., Hillard, J.R., Geier, P., Hissa, D., & Rouan, G.W. (1988). Screening emergency room patients with atypical chest pain for depression and panic disorders. *International Journal of Psychiatry in Medicine, 18,* 315-323.

Yang, L., Zuo, C., Su, L., & Eaton, M.T. (1987). Depression in Chinese medical inpatients. *American Journal of Psychiatry, 144,* 226–228.

Zaphiropoulos, G. & Burry, H.C. (1974). Depression in rheumatoid disease. *Annals of the Rheumatic Diseases, 33,* 132–135.

Zigmond, A.S. & Snaith, R.P. (1983). The Hospital Anxiety and Depression Scale. *Acta Psychiatrica Scandinavica, 67,* 361–370.

Zung, W.W.K. (1965). A self-rating depression scale. *Archives of General Psychiatry, 12,* 63–70.

Zung, W.W.K. (1986). Zung Self-Rating Depression Scale and Depression Status Inventory. In N. Sartorius & T.A. Ban (Eds.), *Assessment of Depression.* (pp. 221–231). Berlin: Springer-Verlag.

Zung, W.W.K., Magill, M., Moore, J.T., & George, D.T. (1983). Recognition and treatment of depression in a family medicine practice. *Journal of Clinical Psychiatry, 44,* 3–6.

2

Assessment and Diagnosis: II

In the previous chapter, we examined the prevalence of depression in the medically ill and discussed various diagnostic approaches. This chapter addresses additional selected issues relevant to the diagnosis of depression in medical settings. It begins with a review of studies regarding the detection of depression by nonpsychiatric clinicians. Not surprisingly, the failure to recognize depression is a major impediment to the institution of appropriate treatment in the medical setting. Our discussion here highlights factors that may interfere with detection. Some potential solutions to the problems of underdiagnosis and undertreatment are examined in a discussion of the role of screening techniques and laboratory tests to detect and diagnose depressive disorders in medical settings.

PHYSICIAN RECOGNITION OF DEPRESSION IN THE MEDICALLY ILL

Before primary care patients can be properly investigated and treated for depression, the disturbance in mood must first come to the attention of their physicians. Nonpsychiatric medical staff with the primary responsibility for routine patient care are best situated to identify medical patients who are suffering from depression. However, as early as 1967, Wynn found that although depression contributed to functional disability in 40 percent of 400 patients with ischemic heart disease, it was largely unrecognized by the treating physicians. He concluded that an important source of unwarranted suffering and invalidism was the failure to recognize or treat depression in these patients. Since that time, physician recognition of depression has been examined by others.

A common research design has been to compare the rate of physician recognition of depression with the proportion of patients who score highly on self-report inventories of depressive symptoms.

Based on BDI scores of ≥14, Moffic and Paykel (1975) found that 24 percent of 150 general medical inpatients were at least mildly depressed. However, the medical residents responsible for their care had identified depression in just 14 percent of the depressed cases and had treated only 9 percent with antidepressants. Similar studies undertaken in general medical inpatients (Feldman et al., 1987) and general practice outpatients (Shepherd et al., 1966; Marks, Goldberg, & Hillier, 1979; Nielsen & Williams, 1980; Borus et al., 1988; Henley & Coussens, 1988) have shown that medical physicians with responsibility for primary care recognized depressive symptoms in no more than one-half, and often less than one-third, of the patients who reported significant depressive symptoms on self-report surveys.

Other studies have examined physicians' detection of depression in patients with specific medical illnesses. With coronary artery disease, depressive symptoms are rarely recognized either by the cardiologist or by the general practitioner (Wynn, 1967; Mayou, Foster, & Williamson, 1979; Kurosawa et al., 1983). Derogatis, Abeloff, and McBeth (1976) found in a sample of oncology patients that the treating physicians usually rated depression in their patients as less severe than did the patients themselves. Similarly, DePaulo and Folstein (1978) found that depression and other manifestations of emotional distress in neurology patients were frequently undetected by neurologists.

Although many investigators have concluded from such findings that medically oriented physicians are poor at detecting depression in their patients, self-report measures are relatively nonspecific indicators of depressive disorders (see Chapter 1). In fact, many of the patients included as "cases" of depression in the above surveys reported only mild symptoms of depression. These patients may not have suffered from clinical depression and their symptoms may have been the most likely to diminish either spontaneously or following remission of the associated medical state. Although it may be of value for physicians to recognize mild to moderate symptoms of depression, it is more important that they detect and treat patients with more severe depressive symptoms or disorders. Although Hankin and Locke (1983) found that more severe self-reported depressive symptoms were more likely to be detected by practitioners, it is unclear from many of the studies using self-report depression measures whether physicians are better able to recognize clinical depression in its more severe forms.

A small number of studies have addressed this issue by comparing physicians' detection of actual cases of depressive disorders with those identified using structured diagnostic interviews and/or standardized diagnostic criteria. Sireling et al. (1985) interviewed 167 patients who had been flagged for depression during preliminary screening, and they examined the rate of detection by the patients' general practitioners. They found that even major depression based on RDC criteria had often been undiagnosed by the physicians. Similarly, Kessler, Cleary, and Burke (1985) found that although major depression could be diagnosed in one-third of primary care patients using a self-report questionnaire and clinical interview, few cases were detected by the primary care physicians. The morbidity may have been significant, since depression persisted in many of the patients at a follow-up assessment six months later. Moreover, a study of 126 consecutively admitted oncology patients (Hardman, Maguire, & Crowther, 1989) showed that other health care practitioners performed little better than physicians in detecting depression. The rate of agreement with the diagnosis of depression in this study was 40 percent for physicians, 40 percent for specialized nurse practitioners, and, interestingly, 63 percent for other nurses.

Investigators conducting each of the above studies have concluded that there is a substantial risk that mood disorders will be under-diagnosed by the treating physicians of patients who have a physical illness or who attend medical clinics. This is worrisome, in view of the prevalence of depression in the physically ill, and the sizable proportion of patients with such mental disorders who initially present to primary care services and to medically oriented physicians, rather than to mental health practitioners (Hankin et al., 1982; Schurman, Kramer, & Mitchell, 1985). In fact, Regier, Goldberg, and Taube (1978) estimated that 60 percent of persons with mental disorders are seen in the primary care/outpatient sector, and approximately one-half of these people may suffer from depression (Casey, Dillon, & Tyrer, 1984).

Undertreatment of depression has been suspected for some time in oncology, where rates of major depression have been reported as high as 42 percent (Bukberg, Penman, & Holland, 1984). Such undertreatment is suggested by a study of psychotropic drug prescriptions for 1,579 oncology inpatients (Derogatis et al., 1979). Although psychotropic medications were prescribed for 51 percent of this sample, antidepressants accounted for only 1 percent of the psychotropic drug prescriptions. Furthermore, Levine, Silberfarb, and Lipowski (1978) reported that far fewer cancer patients are referred for psychiatric consultation than are known to be depressed. Low rates of referral and/or treatment are extremely unfortunate considering that treatment studies of antidepressant pharmacotherapy in oncology patients have shown beneficial effects for major depression (see Chapter 10).

Several additional studies suggest that depression is undertreated in the medically ill. In a study of 220 general medical patients, Hengeveld, Ancion, and Rooijmans (1987) interviewed the 35 percent who scored in the range of at least mild depression on the Beck Depression Inventory. Although these authors diagnosed major depression in 9.5 percent of this selected group, only one-third of those patients with MDE had previously been referred for psychiatric consultation. Carney et al. (1987) interviewed 50 consecutive patients undergoing elective cardiac catheterization. They found that only two of nine patients with a current major depressive episode were being treated for depression. Similar findings have emerged from studies of poststroke patients. Feibel, Berk, and Joynt (1979) found that although 37 percent of a sample of 85 poststroke patients demonstrated moderate to severe depressive disorders, few had been diagnosed or treated. In a later study of 103 poststroke patients, none of the 30 patients with mood disorders were receiving any type of antidepressant treatment (Robinson & Price, 1982). Similarly, Wade, Legh-Smith, and Hewer (1987) found that few poststroke patients in their sample had been treated with antidepressants, even though depression persisted for one year or more in many cases.

Our group (Craven et al., 1987) administered the Diagnostic Interview Schedule to 99 renal dialysis patients and found that 8.1 percent of the sample had a current major depressive episode and 6.1 percent had a dysthymic disorder. However, only one patient was receiving pharmacological treatment for depression at the time of the study. We later conducted a clinical trial of desipramine in renal dialysis patients with major depression, including most of the patients with this diagnosis who had been identified in the previous study. We found that five out of the six patients who completed a six-week trial of antidepressant therapy recovered from the depressive episode (Kennedy, Craven, & Rodin, 1989).

The successful treatment of depression may significantly reduce psychological morbidity in patients with a medical illness. However, several other factors underscore the importance of recognizing and treating depression in these people. When depression is missed, somatic complaints related to the mood disturbance may be needlessly investigated with unnecessary procedures. In this regard, a study by Katon et al. (1986) showed that patients with depression visited and telephoned their physicians more frequently and had more medical evaluations than did a non-depressed control group. Studies have shown that recognition and appropriate treatment of depression in primary care settings dramatically reduces the use of laboratory tests and patient visits to medically oriented physicians (Goldberg, Krantz, & Locke, 1970; Linn & Yager, 1982). In addition, it may also not be appreciated that depressive symptoms can represent an organic feature of the illness. For example, DiGiovanni (1987) stated that in patients with HIV infection, the automatic dismissal of depressive symptoms as an "understandable" reaction to severe illness may mean that an early manifestation of AIDS dementia complex is missed, and that treatment is delayed unnecessarily. Finally, untreated depression in the physically ill patient is more likely to run a protracted or recurrent course (Keller et al., 1983), with impaired quality of life, and increased likelihood of suicide or medical deterioration. At least one study has found that the frequency of nonsuicidal deaths and myocardial infarction is significantly greater in a group with untreated depression compared with a group treated adequately for depression (Avery & Winokur, 1976). Thus, the low rate of diagnosis and treatment of depression in the medically ill may have significant adverse implications.

Reasons for Underdiagnosis

The studies cited above suggest that depression is often missed by physicians working with the medically ill. It has also been shown (Marks, Goldberg, & Hillier, 1979) that physicians vary widely in their rates of detection. A series of interrelated explanations have been proposed by various authors to explain why depression is under-recognized in the physically ill (Salkind, 1969; Raft et al., 1975; Hankin & Locke, 1983; Massie & Holland, 1984; Goldberg, 1985; Schulberg et al., 1986). These explanations involve factors that are both physician-related and situational (see Table 2.1).

An important patient characteristic that determines the rate of detection of depression is the ability and capacity to communicate emotional symptoms. Goldberg (1985) has suggested that unless specifically requested to do so, many patients do not provide verbal, or even nonverbal clues, about psychological distress. Prusoff, Klerman, and Paykel (1972) also noted that physically ill patients are particularly hesitant to report symptoms of depression. Similarly, Comaroff and Maguire (1981) found that of cancer patients who developed psychiatric problems, less than 25 percent spontaneously discussed their symptoms with anyone involved in their health care. These findings suggest that there may be a general under-reporting of emotional symptoms by medical patients to their physicians.

TABLE 2.1.   *Factors Contributing to the Underdiagnosis of Depression by Physicians*

Physician-Related Factors

Limitations in clinical experience and training

Concern about adverse social consequences of a psychiatric diagnosis

Fear of a negative reaction to the diagnosis of depression

Uncertainty regarding management

Reluctance to address emotional issues

Misunderstanding of diagnosis and classification of clinical depression

Misattribution of somatic symptoms of depression to physical illness

Minimization of clinical signs which are assumed to be an "expected and understandable" reaction to illness

Ignorance about treatment potential

Subspecialist focus on particular organ system with neglect of psychosocial factors

Structural Factors

Time and/or financial restraints

Lack of privacy for interview

Patient Factors

Somatization and diminished affective awareness

Fear of stigma of reporting emotional illness

Lack of knowledge about available assistance and/or treatment

Depressed patients who do not spontaneously report their symptoms to their physicians are unlikely to have a mood disorder diagnosed. For example, Maguire (1984) found that general practitioners caring for oncology patients erroneously assumed that any patient who developed psychological problems serious enough to warrant help would consult them and request treatment. Katon, Kleinman, and Rosen (1982) found that primary care physicians tended to consider the diagnosis of depression only when cognitive-affective symptoms were prominent. In fact, in patients with an active medical illness, physicians may be too ready to attribute many depressive symptoms (e.g., anorexia, insomnia) to the physical illness, rather than to consider the possibility of an associated depressive syndrome (Katon, 1984).

The under-reporting of symptoms of depression may reflect a relative deficiency in the capacity of some patients to identify and interpret emotional distress. This may be due to denial of emotional experience, a common means of coping with medical illness and diminishing potentially overwhelming affective reactions. Also, for developmental or other reasons, some patients may have less ability to recognize emotional states (Lane & Schwartz, 1987). Rather than recognizing or identifying depressive affect, some individuals experience it instead as vague or undifferentiated somatic discomfort. Patients and their physicians might attribute such discomfort to a physical disturbance or illness, thereby delaying or missing the diagnosis of mood disorder. This may help to explain why depression is typically missed when patients with somatization disorder present to medical facilities, even though 48 percent of these patients meet DSM-III criteria for a major depressive disorder (Katon, Ries, & Kleinman, 1984). The presentation of depression as a somatization syndrome is discussed more fully in Chapter 3.

Katon, Ries, and Kleinman (1984) have suggested that depressed patients who attend a medical facility may be more likely to complain of somatic rather than psychological symptoms of depression. Using the DIS, Coulehan et al. (1988) compared the symptom profile of 294 patients with major depression who presented to one of three primary care medical settings, to 269 patients with major depression who presented to one of three community mental health centers. They found major depression based on DSM-III criteria in 7.1 percent of the patients presenting to the medical setting met DSM-III criteria for current major depressive episode, and in 25 percent of patients presenting to the mental health setting. Although the patients in the medical setting were significantly more likely to present with functional somatic symptoms, the symptom profile of depression in both settings was virtually identical. In particular, DSM-III somatic criteria for depression were reported with equal frequency in the two depressed groups. The authors concluded that patients with MDE who present to a medical setting are more likely to present with multiple somatic complaints compared with depressed patients presenting to a mental health facility. However, since the symptom profile of MDE is almost identical in both groups, a simple functional enquiry based on standard DSM-III criteria would have led to a diagnosis of depression in all of the patients.

Some patients may be aware of depression or other emotional distress, but are hesitant to report their feelings. The physically ill patient may already feel stigmatized and reluctant to admit to additional problems coping with the psychological or emotional aspects of their illness. At times, patients may deny symptoms of depression, feeling that a "positive" attitude is necessary for optimal medical outcome. Reluctance to report recognized symptoms of depression may also occur if patients assume that such feelings are abnormal, are a sign of personal weakness, or represent an additional and unwanted onus on the family or health care staff. Men may be particularly hesitant to report symptoms of depression (Warren, 1983) unless they are first made aware that depressive symptoms are often part of a normal process of adjustment. In addition, such individuals can also be helped to understand that acknowledgment and subsequent treatment of a mood disorder may improve not only mental health but also physical well-being.

Particular clinical circumstances may inhibit patients from disclosing emotional symptoms. For example, patients may be more reluctant to report depressive symptoms if medical interviews are conducted in public areas, or in a manner that suggests that the physician is either short of time or disinterested. Bridges and Goldberg (1984) asked neurological inpatients their opinion about discussing emotional problems with their neurologists. Many of these patients believed that it was the neurologist's role to investigate only physical causes for their symptoms. Several respondents said that their doctors were very busy and did not wish to burden them further with their emotional problems. Others expressed dissatisfaction, criticizing the lack of privacy to discuss emotional issues, and the evasiveness of some doctors when these issues were raised.

The perceptions that physicians are hesitant to discuss emotional problems is often accurate. Maguire (1984) found that physicians treating oncology patients were reluctant to ask their patients routinely about the psychological impact of cancer and its treatment, and believed that such questions might lead to uncomfortable affective experiences. The doctors feared they would be unable to help patients contain or deal with the distress that might be provoked by such questions. However, there is little or no evidence to suggest that tactful questioning about emotional distress is harmful. In fact, routine enquiry about feeling states such as depression and anxiety can deliver an important message to patients, namely that it is appropriate to discuss emotional experiences in the doctor's office. Without the routine inclusion of depressive symptoms in the functional enquiry, many physicians simply fail to consider a diagnosis of depression (Schulberg & McClelland, 1987). Goldberg (1985) also reported that many physicians lack confidence in their ability to recognize, diagnose, and treat psychiatric conditions. He stated that physicians often feel incompetent to deal with patients' questions about the etiology, treatment, and prognosis of depression and other mental disorders. Zung et al. (1983) have suggested that physicians may avoid diagnosing or treating depression because of exaggerated concerns about the potential harmfulness of antidepressant medication.

Hankin and Locke (1983) specifically studied the factors that might account for the varying ability of individual physicians to detect depression. In a survey of 1,921 medical outpatients, they identified characteristics of both patients and of nonpsychiatric physicians that correlated with recognition of depression. Depression was most likely to be recognized in patients with more severe depressive symptoms, more frequent clinic visits, and in patients who were female and Caucasian. Recognition also depended upon the department and special interests of the physician. Shepherd et al. (1966) reported that the primary care physicians most likely to detect depression in their patients were those who had an interest in providing counselling and psychotherapy. Goldberg and Huxley (1980) found that the physicians most likely to make accurate diagnoses were those who were sensitive to their patients' cues about emotional distress, confident in their assessment and interview skills, and aware of their own needs and feelings. These two studies suggest that physicians with more personal and interpersonal awareness are more likely to diagnose depression in their patients.

It has been suggested that depression is diagnosed more often in female patients in medical settings because of sex stereotyping. Seller, Blascovich, and Lenkei (1981) found no significant difference in the proportion of male and female family medicine patients who scored over 20 on the Beck Depression Inventory. Yet, women were significantly more likely to be given a diagnosis of depression by resident physicians. It may be that gender differences in the presentation of symptoms make depression more difficult to recognize in men (Warren, 1983). Williamson (1987) has found evidence to support this hypothesis in patients attending an adult family medicine clinic. She found that men were less likely than women to report dysphoric mood when depressed, but were more likely to report irritability, social withdrawal, and interpersonal behavior changes at these times.

Finally, the relationship of demographic characteristics of patients to the recognition of depression by physicians is equivocal. Whereas Salkind (1969) and Raft et al. (1975) found that the race and social class of the patients were influential, Hankin and Locke (1983) and Sireling et al. (1985) found no differences in the demographic characteristics of depressed primary care patients who were or were not diagnosed with depression by their physicians.

Physicians' beliefs about the association of medical illness and depression may also influence whether they will question patients about emotional symptoms. Massie and Holland (1984) described three beliefs that can interfere with the diagnosis and management of depression in cancer patients: the belief that all cancer patients are depressed; that it is "understandable" and therefore nonpathological for a patient with cancer to be depressed; and that treatment for depression in cancer patients is either ineffective or intolerable because of side effects. These beliefs do not reflect current knowledge about the relationship of depression to cancer and its potential response to treatment. A more accurate set of statements which reflect present knowledge would be that: depression occurs in some but not all cancer patients; depression in cancer patients may or may not result from a realistic response to the condition, but that this difference does not necessarily determine the need for treatment; and that, with a careful and systematic approach, depression in cancer patients is a potentially treatable condition.

To assess doctors' perception and interpretation of depressive symptoms in their patients, Zung et al. (1984) administered a questionnaire to 89 physicians, mostly general practitioners, attending a medical conference. Almost all of the respondents stated that depression had an important impact on their patients' well-being. However, when presented with lists of depressive symptoms, the majority of physicians recognized the psychological manifestations of depression but believed that no follow-up management was required. The investigators concluded that the psychological symptoms of depression were regarded by these physicians as a reasonable or natural result of illness. In particular, the tendency to ignore the somatic manifestations of depression interfered with the recognition of depressive disorders that might require biologic or other specific management. Similarly, in a study of patients who had committed suicide, Murphy (1975) found that a psychosocial "explanation" of a patient's depressed mood prior to suicide had frequently preempted careful diagnostic enquiry. We would suggest that although an understanding of the psychological determinants of depression may guide the nature of treatment provided, this understanding should not preclude specific antidepressant treatment.

Kamerow (1988) suggested four additional explanations for the failure of physicians to detect depression in the physically ill. First, many physicians think of depression and anxiety as problems that can be solved through an act of will or volition. This belief of some physicians leads them to disregard emotional distress as an indicator of the need for professional assistance. Second, physicians have often received their psychiatric training on inpatient psychiatric units, where there is insufficient experience with depression in the medically ill. Third, the frequent coexistence of depression and other medical or mixed psychiatric symptoms contributes to the difficulty diagnosing mood disorders in the medical setting. Finally, third party reimbursement plans may subtly interfere with the diagnostic process by providing more financial incentive for physical procedures than for the thoughtful assessment of psychological distress or for ambulatory treatment of mental disorders. In addition, Reifler (1988) has suggested that the time constraints of general practice often do not allow for the extended verbal assessment required to make a firm diagnosis of a depressive disorder. He suggested further research to improve screening techniques for use during the physician's routine interview.

We hope that highlighting the problem of depression in the medically ill will foster a greater awareness of depression in these patients. However, as Kamerow (1988) noted, the diagnosis and treatment of depression in the physically ill continues to challenge even experienced clinicians and researchers in the field. We discussed the measures and techniques currently being used to diagnose depression in the physically ill in the previous chapter. Continuous refinement of this methodology is needed to improve its reliability and validity. Further, physicians require ongoing education to increase their cognizance of depression and their ability to detect this and other psychiatric disorders in the medical setting (Schulberg & McClelland, 1987). Patients also need to be educated about the symptoms of depression and encouraged to seek help when they need it.

AIDS IN THE DETECTION AND DIAGNOSIS OF DEPRESSION IN THE MEDICALLY ILL

Screening Instruments

In the previous chapter, we examined the use of self-report measures to document depressive symptoms in medical patients. We noted that self-report measures alone are inadequate to diagnose depressive disorders in medical or nonmedical patients. In this section we discuss the use of self-report, paper-and-pencil measures as screening devices for depression in the clinical setting. We review here some aspects of these measures, including practical issues specifically involved in screening for depression.

Interest in the use of self-report measures to screen for depression was stimulated both by the difficulty recognizing depression in medical patients, and by the relative ease of administration of these measures. However, a major challenge for researchers in this area has been to establish the validity of these instruments for use as screening devices. It is necessary to answer two principal questions before a self-report measure can be considered adequate to screen medical patients for depression. First, what is the "hit" rate of the instrument (i.e., the proportion of cases correctly identified), and second, what cutoff should be used to optimize its usefulness. To answer both questions, results with screening devices should be compared with a "gold standard" of diagnosis, namely a structured diagnostic interview (e.g., the Diagnostic Interview Schedule) in conjunction with standardized diagnostic criteria (e.g., DSM-III-R). Different calculations can then be used to determine the sensitivity, specificity, and positive and negative predictive values of the self-report measure. Sensitivity refers to the proportion of individuals with depression who have a positive score on the self-report measure. Specificity refers to the proportion of persons without depression who have a negative score. The positive predictive value is the proportion of persons with a positive self-report score who have a depressive disorder, and the negative predictive value is the proportion of individuals with a negative score who do not have a depressive disorder. Because positive and negative predictive values are highly influenced by the proportion of depressive disorders in the sample, validity studies should report not only data on sensitivity, specificity, and positive and negative predictive values, but also the prevalence rate of depression. Unfortunately, few studies in this area have satisfied these minimal criteria.

To determine the appropriate cutoff score on a self-report measure used for screening purposes, the investigator must weigh the disadvantages of missing cases of depression (i.e., low sensitivity) against the cost of increasing the rate of false positives (i.e., low specificity) (Ford, 1988). A higher cutoff will contribute to a lowered sensitivity and possibly a higher specificity, whereas a lower cutoff will result in a higher sensitivity and lower specificity. Thus, although a lower threshold is more likely to include the greatest proportion of depressed cases in the sample, it will also identify more false positives. Further assessment of these individuals is then needed to rule out the presence of a depressive disorder. On the other hand, a higher threshold will identify fewer false positives, but is more likely to miss cases of depressive disorders. Mathematical methods exist to identify an optimal cutoff (Feinstein, 1977). However, the clinical demands of the situation must take priority over mathematical methods in determining the optimal cutoff to be used. In the medically ill, cutoff scores low enough to identify the greatest proportion of depressive disorders are usually sought.

The Beck Depression Inventory (BDI) has been studied by several groups to determine its usefulness as a screen for depression in the medical setting. Nielsen and Williams (1980) administered the BDI to 526 medical outpatients. They calibrated the results according to the findings from psychiatric interviews in a subset of 41 patients with diagnoses of primary and secondary depression based on Feighner criteria. They determined that a cutoff of >9 on the BDI provided an optimal combination of sensitivity (0.92) and specificity (0.35) for its use as a screening device for primary and secondary depression. Even with a higher cutoff of >12, the BDI still performed much better than medical physicians in detecting depression. However, the optimal cutoff score in this sample cannot be determined because the predictive values or diagnostic accuracy were not reported, and the base rate of mood disorders in this sample is unknown.

Other studies have examined the use of the BDI to screen for mood disorders in patients with specific medical illnesses. For example, Carney et al. (1987) administered the Diagnostic Interview Schedule and the BDI to 50 patients undergoing elective cardiac catheterization for coronary artery disease. Using a cutoff of >10, they found a sensitivity of 0.78 and a specificity of 0.90 for MDE, the base prevalence of which was 18 percent. They concluded that this instrument would be a suitable screening device for major depression in these patients. However, since the positive predictive value was not reported, the total number of patients who must undergo further assessment to identify those patients with MDE cannot be determined.

Our group (Craven, Rodin, & Littlefield, 1988) administered the BDI and the Diagnostic Interview Schedule to a sample of 99 renal dialysis subjects. We reported the sensitivity, specificity, predictive values, and Youden's Index of Validity for all cutoffs of the BDI ranging from >9 through to >21. We found that a cutoff of >14 was optimal for use of the BDI as a screening device both for major depressive disorder (MDE) and for dysthymic disorder (DD) in this sample. Using this cutoff, the sensitivity was 0.92, the specificity 0.80, the negative predictive value 0.99, and the positive predictive value 0.39. With this cutoff on the BDI, one-third of the total sample required further assessment to diagnose most cases of MDE and DD. Following screening, it would be necessary for approximately 30 patients to undergo additional assessment in order to identify the 12 patients with a major mood disorder.

Other measures that have been assessed as screening instruments include the Center for Epidemiologic Studies Depression Scale (CES-D) and various forms of the General Health Questionnaire (GHQ). Schulberg et al. (1985) compared the results of the CES-D with diagnoses of DSM-III disorders derived from the Diagnostic Interview Schedule in 563 primary care medical outpatients. They found that the usual CES-D cutoff of >15 provided excellent sensitivity (>0.96), but poor specificity (<0.39). They also found that raising the cutoff to >26 continued to provide adequate sensitivity (0.89) for a screening device, but increased the specificity substantially (0.70). However, the positive predictive level of the test at the cutoff of >26 was only 0.35. They concluded that the CES-D is highly sensitive and adequate as a screening device for depression in the medically ill, but that it is relatively nonspecific for diagnosable depressive disorders.

Parikh et al. (1988) examined the sensitivity and specificity of the CES-D as a screening device for poststroke depression. Administering the CES-D to a sample of 80 poststroke patients, they found that a cutoff of >15 correlated with DSM-III diagnoses of depression, and had a sensitivity of 0.86, a specificity of 0.90, and a positive predictive value of 0.80. Raising the cutoff to >20 raised the specificity to 0.94 and the positive predictive value to 0.85, but decreased the sensitivity to 0.72. In addition, they found that a CES-D score of >15 had good predictive validity for depressive scores at 3-, 6-, and 12-month follow-up assessments. These authors concluded that with a cutoff of >15, the CES-D was adequate as a screening device for depression in poststroke patients.

Mayou and Hawton (1986) extensively reviewed the use of the General Health Questionnaire (GHQ) as a screening device for psychiatric disorders in medical patients. This questionnaire has various forms including the GHQ-60, the GHQ-30, and the GHQ-28. Summarizing work from a number of studies, these authors concluded that a cutoff of >11 for the GHQ-60 and >4 for the GHQ-30 provided adequate sensitivity and specificity for use as a screening device in medical inpatients. This measure has most commonly been validated against the Clinical Interview Schedule and the Present State Examination. Mayou and Hawton (1986) correctly noted that the validity of the Clinical Interview Schedule itself is suspect as it does not define a single procedure for case definition. Instead, "caseness" may be based on an arbitrary total score, on psychiatric judgment, or on a combination of both methods. Furthermore, the validation of the GHQ is further compromised as the majority of the studies they reviewed did not specify the prevalence of depression as opposed to other DSM-III disorders.

Razavi et al. (1990) examined the utility of the Hospital Anxiety and Depression Scale (HADS) as a screen for major depression in a sample of 210 oncology patients. DSM-III diagnoses of major depression were obtained by clinical psychiatric interview and compared to the results of the HADS. When using the HADS to screen for major depression, receiving operating characteristic analysis demonstrated an optimal cutoff of greater than or equal to 19. This threshold resulted in a sensitivity of 0.70, a specificity of 0.75, and a positive predictive value of 0.50. A threshold of 13 was considered optimal to screen for both major depression and adjustment disorders. When used in this manner, the HADS demonstrated a sensitivity of 0.70, a specificity of 0.75 and a positive predictive value of 0.90. The prevalence of mood disorders in the sample was not reported. This group suggested that the HADS was useful as a simple and sensitive screen for depression in inpatients with cancer.

A small number of studies have attempted to validate screening instruments for major depression in elderly medical patients. Kitchell et al. (1982) examined the utility of the Zung Self-Rating Depression Scale (SDS) in a sample of geriatric patients hospitalized for medical illness. Compared with diagnoses of MDE obtained by blind clinical interview, they found that the SDS had a sensitivity of 0.58, a specificity of 0.87, and a diagnostic accuracy of 0.74. Forty-five percent of this sample were diagnosed with MDE. These authors concluded that the SDS seemed useful to screen for depression in elderly medical patients, but less so than in younger groups of physically ill patients. In another study, Koenig et al. (1988) administered the Geriatric Depression Scale (GDS) and the Brief Carroll Depression Rating Scale (BCDRS) to a sample of 128 elderly male inpatients. The optimal cutoff for the GDS was >10, a threshold which provided a sensitivity of 0.92, a specificity of 0.89, a negative predictive value of 0.99, and a positive predictive value of 53 percent, compared with the diagnosis of major depression using structured interviews. The optimal cutoff for the BCDRS was >5, providing a sensitivity of 1.0, a specificity of 0.93, a negative predictive value of 0.93, and a positive predictive value of 0.66. The prevalence of major depression determined by structured psychiatric interview was 12 percent. These authors concluded that both the GDS and the BCDRS would be useful as screening devices for major depression in elderly medical inpatients.

The findings of screening studies have been interpreted somewhat inconsistently in the literature. For example, several investigators concluded that the BDI is an adequate screening device for depression (Salkind, 1969; Nielsen & Williams, 1980; Craven et al., 1987), whereas others have suggested that it is unacceptable for this use (Kathol & Petty, 1981; Kearns et al., 1982; Zigmond & Snaith, 1983; Hengeveld, Ancion, & Rooijmans, 1987). However, the validity of such interpretations depends not only on the psychometric properties of the instrument, but on other factors as well. Some of these factors, which have also been reviewed by Ford (1988), are discussed in the remainder of this section.

Both the setting in which a screening instrument is administered and its purposes can influence its usefulness. In general practice settings, it may be practical for patients to fill out a screening instrument in the waiting room, with the results available immediately, followed by brief questioning during the clinical examination. It was for this type of setting that Salkind (1969) concluded that the Beck Depression Inventory was most useful in detecting and assessing depression in general practice. Used in this way, the screen may alert the physician to the presence of emotional distress. Even with patients not suffering from major depression, it may be valuable for the primary practitioner to be aware of other forms of emotional distress. Because the follow-up examination for depression in this setting is immediate, relatively brief, and nonintrusive, a screening instrument that is sensitive for depression is desirable even if it produces a substantial number of false positives. However, in a busy consulting practice for cardiological or neurological disorders, this same test may be less suitable due to insufficient time available for follow-up assessment.

A small number of studies have evaluated how primary care physicians utilize information from screening instruments for depressive symptoms. Moore, Silimperi, and Bobula (1978) examined the impact of screening on the recognition of depression by physicians. The Zung Self-Rating Depression Scale (SDS) was administered to 212 patients attending a general medical outpatient practice. Feedback to the physicians as to which patients scored above the cutoff for mild depression increased physician recognition from 22 percent to 56 percent. A similar study by Linn and Yager (1980) found that feedback of screening results increased the detection of depression from 8 percent to 25 percent. However, it should be noted that the group scoring above the screening cutoff almost certainly included false positives.

Rucker, Frye, and Cygan (1986) found that the short form of the BDI (BDI-SF) (Beck & Beck, 1972) was well accepted by general practice patients, and was completed by 375 out of 500 patients who were asked to do so. By examining the results of the BDI-SF, physicians found that 17 percent of patients were more depressed than initially recognized, and that management plans were altered in 21 percent of patient visits due to the results of the BDI-SF. Ninety-four percent of the physicians who used the BDI-SF as part of their clinical assessment found the measure useful, and none found it to be harmful. The latter finding is important, as a screening test should rate high in acceptability to both patients and medical staff.

Zung et al. (1983) examined the effect of the screening procedure on treatment and outcome of general practice patients. They administered the SDS to 1,086 patients and found that 143 scored above the cutoff of 55, indicating the presence of at least mild depression. The patients were then randomized into two groups, one in which physicians were told which patients scored high on the screening instrument and one in which physicians were not given this information. Fifty percent of the high scorers in the identified group were subsequently treated with an antidepressant by their physician. In this identified group, 28 percent of untreated patients and 64 percent of treated patients had improved. By contrast, at four weeks follow-up, only 18 percent of the unidentified patients had improved. These authors concluded that screening increased the likelihood of detection and successful treatment of depression.

Although the benefits of screening in general practice settings appear encouraging, some caution is warranted. For example, House (1988) notes that current findings do not offer convincing evidence that the failure of medically oriented physicians to detect depression is best addressed by introducing self-report measures of depressive symptoms. The introduction of screening measures might simply add another set of variables with which clinicians may not be familiar. Also, self-report instruments do not detect all cases of depression because some patients lack emotional awareness and/or are secretive about personal feelings. Thus, clinicians must maintain a high index of suspicion for depression, even with patients who do not score above the screening threshold. It should also be noted that the instruments available are nonspecific, and therefore should not be given undue weight compared with clinical assessment and verbal functional enquiry. In addition, false positive identifications may have some negative implications. They may produce an unmanageable need for follow-up assessments of patients who are identified as at risk. Individuals who are transiently depressed may feel stigmatized or demoralized by inappropriate labelling as "cases." Also, Ford (1988) has suggested that such patients are at risk of being inappropriately streamed into the mental health system. To reduce the problems of overdiagnosis, it may be helpful to require that patients score positively on two consecutive administrations of the screening instrument before being referred for further assessment.

The burden of follow-up when screening for depression in the medically ill should not be underestimated. The instruments presently in use are relatively nonspecific indicators of major depression, especially in patients with symptomatic physical illness. Therefore, even if a screening test detects a sizable proportion of the patients with major depression (i.e., high sensitivity), the predictive value is often low so that only one out of every three or four patients identified by the screening test will actually receive the diagnosis of major depression when subsequently assessed. Indeed, the greatest disadvantage to current screening instruments may be the low predictive value, particularly when a cutoff that is sensitive enough to detect most cases of depressive disorder is used. As House (1988) notes, screening tests may identify more depression in the medical setting than there is either the understanding or the resources to treat. Post-screening evaluation may be practical in primary care settings where follow-up examinations are routine and brief, but more problematic to arrange in most hospital settings in which facilities are directed primarily toward treating the physical aspects of medical disease.

It may be, as Mayou & Hawton (1986) suggested, that there is no simple, generally acceptable screening instrument to detect depression in medical inpatients, and that simple questions relevant to mood disorder are better included in the routine functional enquiry conducted by physicians and nurses. Ford (1988) was similarly unable to recommend a single preferred instrument for this use. We agree that ideal measures may not exist, and that any screening instrument may be inferior to clinical screening for depression during physicians' interviews. However, we believe that there are clinical circumstances in which screening tests can be useful. Further, the valid criticisms of current research in this area may be overcome or circumvented with improved methodology. For example, revision of screening tests for the medically ill may result in greater predictive ability.

An additional method to optimize the predictive validity of screening measures that has received little attention is the selective administration of the measure to the subject group known to be at greatest risk. It is well recognized that the positive predictive value of an instrument is highly dependent upon the frequency of the disorder in the sample tested. For example, even with the same sensitivity and specificity, the predictive value of a measure will be much lower in a setting in which the prevalence of depressive disorder is 5 percent compared to one in which the prevalence is 25 percent (Ford, 1988). Parikh et al. (1988) found that the CES-D provided a very high positive predictive value of 0.80 for DSM-III diagnosis of depression in a sample of poststroke patients. Although these authors did not report the prevalence of depression in their sample, their data suggest that it was more than 25 percent. This relatively high prevalence of depression may, in part, account for the rather high positive predictive value obtained in this study. However, Wulsin et al. (1988) administered the CES-D to 49 patients presenting to emergency with atypical chest pain. In this sample, 30 patients scored >15 on the CES-D but only one of these received any psychiatric diagnosis at all, and this diagnosis was not depression. Thus, two studies using the same screening device and the same cutoff had strikingly different predictive values, most likely because of widely different base prevalence rates of major depression in the respective samples. The CES-D performs well with an acceptable positive predictive value during the first two years following stroke (i.e., when the base prevalence rate of depressive disorders is high), but it performs poorly as a screen for depressive disorders in emergency patients with atypical chest pain (i.e., when the base prevalence rate is apparently low).

Screening a preselected subgroup of patients at highest risk for depressive disorders could substantially improve the utility of the screen by decreasing the number of patients who would require further assessment. However, the practicality of this recommendation depends on whether accurate information regarding risk factors for depression in that sample is available. We found that following BDI screening of 99 randomly selected renal dialysis patients, 28 patients required further assessment to diagnose the 10 patients in the sample with major depression or dysthymic disorder (Craven, Rodin, & Littlefield, 1988). However, in another report on the same sample of 99 patients, we showed that almost all of the patients with major depression had been on dialysis for two years or less (Craven et al., 1987). A recommendation that might follow from these findings would be to administer the screening device during the first two years following initiation of dialysis. This more selective use of a screening test would increase the base rate of mood disorder from 12 percent to 26 percent in the sample to be screened, and would thereby increase the positive predictive value of the test from 39 percent to 80 percent in this same sample (Craven,

Rodin, & Littlefield, unpublished data). This approach may be of value with other medical groups at high risk for depressive disorders.

In summary, presently available screening methods are likely most appropriate for use in general practice settings, where follow-up assessments are easily undertaken and minimally intrusive. When screening for depression is carried out in hospitalized patients or in specialized medical clinics, it may be desirable to minimize the number of false positives, the intrusiveness, and the stigma of follow-up assessments, and to optimize the positive predictive value of the screen. Administering screening instruments only to those medical patients at highest risk for depressive disorders would optimize the utility of the available instruments and facilitate the efficient utilization of follow-up resources. Finally, further empirical validation of the instruments used for screening for depressive disorders in medical samples is required. In this regard, studies in the literature would be more comparable if research reports included the following information: the sensitivity, specificity, positive predictive values, negative predictive values, description of the medical illness and setting, and the prevalence of depressive disorders in the setting in which the screening device is being administered. In addition, screening devices are most beneficial in medical practice when used as aids to the recognition and diagnosis of depression, rather than as replacements for thorough clinical assessments and sound clinical judgment.

THE DEXAMETHASONE SUPPRESSION TEST (DST) IN MEDICAL SETTINGS

The identification of consistent biological alterations in depression would contribute enormously not only to the validation of a case of major depression, but also to the development of diagnostic laboratory tests. This objective is not unrealistic since major depression has demonstrable validity as a psychobehavioral syndrome, in terms of its course, family and personal history, and response to treatment. In addition, major depression is associated with physiological, biochemical, and hormonal alterations. The latter findings have led to the search for biologic markers of depressive disorders. Considering how difficult it is to diagnose depression in the medically ill, a reliable and valid laboratory test would be a tremendous addition to the clinician's diagnostic armamentarium. To date, the only laboratory test that has been seriously considered for the clinical diagnosis of major depression in the medically ill is the dexamethasone suppression test (DST) (Carroll et al., 1981; Carroll, 1985).

The development of the DST was based on the finding of hyper-responsivity of the hypothalamic-pituitary-adrenal axis in major depression. However, although numerous investigators continue to study these disturbances, it is not yet known whether they are related etiologically to depression or are simply a manifestation or complication of depression (Stokes, 1987). The administration of the DST usually involves giving 1 mg of dexamethasone at 2300 hours and determining plasma cortisol levels either once (1600 hours), twice (1600 and 2300 hours) or three times (0800, 1600 and 2300 hours) on the day following dexamethasone administration. An abnormal DST (i.e., nonsuppression of endogenous cortisol production by administration of dexamethasone) is defined by at least one plasma cortisol level above 5 mg/dl after dexamethasone administration. When two levels are examined, a procedure that increases the sensitivity of the test somewhat, approximately 50 percent of patients with unipolar depression show nonsuppression (Davis, 1987).

The above findings suggest that although the DST may prove useful to define a subgroup of depressed patients, the test is of no value for screening purposes in view of its low sensitivity. At present, no meaningful clinical conclusion can be drawn from the finding of a single negative DST. In fact, approximately 4 percent of normal adults are DST nonsuppressors (Carroll et al., 1981). Also, a number of factors may cause false positive DST results. Specific factors that may account for DST nonsuppression include medical illness, weight loss, pregnancy, extreme stress, and withdrawal from sedative agents. Fogel and Satel (1985) found that age and concurrent medical illness were associated with higher rates of nonsuppression in 89 general hospital inpatients assessed for depression. Due to the large number of false positives, the routine application of the test to patients who might be depressed is unlikely to assist with diagnosis. However, it has been suggested that the test may be of clinical value when applied to preselected patients with the lowest risk of being false positives. Also, for some depressed patients who are nonsuppressors, the test shows some promise for monitoring treatment response (Davis, 1987).

In view of the limitations noted above, patients with physical illness have often been excluded from studies examining the utility of the DST. However, a small number of investigators have specifically examined the use of the DST in the medical setting. The available reports include both case studies, and a few empirical studies with larger samples. The case reports do little to substantiate the utility of the test, and therefore, are not discussed here. The systematic studies in this area are briefly reviewed in the remainder of this chapter. As with psychological screening tests, the sensitivity, specificity, positive predictive value, and negative predictive value of a biologic test should be determined in the sample in which it is applied. To assess these parameters, a diagnostic test that is considered the "gold standard" of diagnosis for the disorder must also be administered.

Studies Using the DST in Medical Samples

Thase et al. (1985) routinely administered the DST to medical or surgical inpatients referred for psychiatric consultation because a major depressive disorder was suspected. They selected subjects who were not likely to show a false positive result for medical reasons (Carroll et al., 1981). Compared with a clinical psychiatric evaluation using diagnoses of major depression based on DSM-III criteria, the test showed a sensitivity of 0.63, a specificity of 0.75, and diagnostic confidence of 0.75. The diagnostic confidence indicates that 75 percent of subjects were correctly classified as depressed or not depressed on the basis of the DST. However, the positive and negative predictive values were not reported in this study. Major depressive disorder was diagnosed in 14 (44 percent) of the 32 subjects tested. In addition, more severe depression or more severe medical illness were each associated with higher rates of DST nonsuppression. Although the authors concluded that the diagnostic utility of the DST in this medical sample was similar to that in inpatient psychiatric samples, they acknowledged that their sample did not include the most difficult diagnostic cases (i.e., those with an active medical illness). Thus, the benefit of the test was not, in fact, demonstrated with regard to the complexities of diagnosis in the general hospital setting.

Evans et al. (1986) examined both the DST and the Thyrotropine Releasing Hormone (TRH) Test in 83 women with gynecological cancer. The patients were screened prior to administration of the biologic tests and 19 (23 percent) were excluded due to the presence of obviously recognizable medical conditions that would create false positive results. They found a sensitivity of 0.40 and a specificity of 0.80 for the DST in this group of patients. The prevalence of major depressive episodes was approximately 23 percent. The TRH test was positive in 29 percent of patients with MDE, and in 8 percent of patients with no affective disorder. They concluded that depression in these cancer patients involved hypothalamic-pituitary changes and that antidepressant medication may be warranted. However, they were cautious about recommending the clinical use of the DST, the TRH, or the two tests combined in cancer patients. These authors noted that, with the exception of ovarian tumors, gynecological cancers are not known to synthesize peptide hormones or steroid metabolites which would invalidate the neuroendocrine tests used. Nevertheless, the possibility remains that neuroendocrine changes with cancer may confound results with the DST. In this regard, Werk, MacGee, and Sholiton (1964) have previously demonstrated increased and abnormal cortisol secretion with various malignancies, suggesting that oncology patients are particularly likely to show false positive nonsuppression on the DST.

Fava et al. (1985) administered a clinical interview, devised by Paykel, Klerman, and Prusoff (1970), to diagnose DSM-III major depression in a consecutive series of 40 gastroenterology outpatients. Their sample included 23 patients with organic digestive disease and 17 patients with functional bowel disorders. In the organic group, the sensitivity of the DST was 0.40, the specificity 0.86, and the positive and negative predictive values 0.66. In the functional group, the sensitivity was higher (0.75), although the test was much less specific (0.50) and had a lower positive predictive value (0.38). These authors concluded that the DST is not clinically useful to screen for major depression in patients suffering from gastrointestinal disorders.

Two studies have examined the use of the DST in poststroke patients. Finklestein et al. (1982) administered the DST to 25 randomly selected elderly stroke patients, and 13 nonstroke control patients who were hospitalized in a rehabilitation center. All patients included in the study had an average of four medical diagnoses. The patients were also administered three separate, brief psychiatric interviews. At least moderate symptoms of depression were found in 48 percent of stroke patients compared with 0 percent of nonstroke controls. Abnormal DST results were associated with moderate to severe depressed mood, and with appetite and sleep disturbances. These findings were all more common in patients with left hemispheric than right hemispheric strokes, occurring in 69 percent of the former and 25 percent of the latter.

In a study that attempted to replicate and extend these findings, Reding et al. (1985) administered the DST on a routine clinical basis to 78 poststroke patients during their second week at an inpatient rehabilitative center. In addition, the patients were administered the Zung Self-Rating Depression Scale (SDS), a version of the Hamilton Rating Scale for Depression (HRS-D) that had been modified for use in poststroke patients, and the Barthel Activities of Daily Living Scale. DST nonsuppression was found in 49 percent of the patients, and was associated with more extensive strokes but not with age, sex, or the time interval between the stroke or diagnostic testing. Patients with positive DST results scored significantly higher on the SDS and the

HRS-D, but the clinical utility of this finding is minimal since the actual difference between the mean scores of the two groups was small and both were within the range of mild depression. When the results of the DST were compared with clinical diagnoses of major depression based on DSM-III criteria, the specificity was more than 80 percent, but the sensitivity was less than 55 percent. However, these results are difficult to interpret because inadequate information was provided regarding the method of diagnosis for mood disorders. No association among the DST and laterality of the stroke, functional status, or rehabilitative outcome was found.

In a study of patients with Parkinson's disease, Pfeiffer et al. (1986) found DST nonsuppression in 43 percent of those who were depressed and 16 percent of those nondepressed. This group concluded, as have other investigators with other medical conditions, that the low sensitivity (0.43) limits the value of the DST to rule out depression, but that the specificity of 0.86 provides increased confidence in the diagnosis of MDE. Frochtengarten et al. (1987) reported similar findings in patients with Parkinson's disease. Frank et al. (1985) found that the DST had both low sensitivity (0.60) and specificity (0.50) for major depression based on DSM-III criteria in a sample of 32 patients with spinal cord injury. These authors postulated that the high rate of DST false positives resulted from alteration of the normal rhythm of 17-hydroxy-corticosteroid excretion caused by deafferentation of the central nervous system. They concluded, therefore, that the test was not useful for the diagnosis of depression in patients with spinal cord injury.

Several recent studies have examined the use of the DST in patients with chronic pain. Major depression has been reported in a sizable proportion of these patients, although the identification and diagnosis of depression remains problematic in this context (see Chapter 3). DST nonsuppression may be more frequent in chronic pain patients with major depression compared with euthymic pain patients (Atkinson et al., 1983; France & Krishnan, 1985; France et al., 1984; Syvalahti, Hyyppa, & Salminen, 1985), but the clinical utility of this difference is not evident.

Syvalahti, Hyyppa, and Salminen (1985) administered the DST to a sample of 115 chronic pain patients who were referred to psychiatrists consulting at a rehabilitation research center and a university hospital setting. They hypothesized that the DST might assist in the diagnosis of depression in these patients, and might be useful as a screening device for patients with "masked" depression who present primarily with somatic symptoms. All referred patients were interviewed clinically and diagnosed using Research Diagnostic Criteria. The rate of nonsuppression in the entire sample was 24 percent, but the prevalence of depressive disorders in the sample was not reported. The authors concluded that the test was "rather good as a diagnostic aid" for the diagnosis of depression in these patients based on a positive predictive value of 0.78. However, almost two-thirds of the depressed patients in the sample had a negative DST (sensitivity = 0.36), and the test was of no value in detecting masked depression in somatizing patients.

In a study of 73 consecutive admissions to an assessment center for chronic low back pain, France et al. (1987) found that the DST was relatively insensitive (0.42) to major depression, but was highly specific for major depression when positive. They concluded that the DST showed promise in discriminating patients with chronic pain from those with primary major depression. Rihmer, Szadoczky, and Arato (1983) administered the DST to 16 female patients diagnosed with masked depression who had presented to medical internists with somatic complaints. Of the 16 patients, 12 were DST positive, and 10 of the 12 responded well to treatment with a tricyclic antidepressant. However, only one of the four patients with a normal DST result showed a positive response to treatment. These authors concluded that a positive DST result in masked depression may indicate treatment responsiveness.

Two reports have discussed the utility of the DST for the diagnosis of organic mood disorders. In a single case study, Kronfol et al. (1982) monitored with serial DSTs, a woman with delusional depression secondary to thyrotoxicosis. Although the patient showed markedly elevated nocturnal plasma cortisol concentration before dexamethasone administration, the results of the DST were consistently negative. These authors suggested that the negative result indicated an absence of the limbic-adrenocortical dysfunction characteristic of melancholia, and was consistent with depression secondary to some factor and/or mechanism that was different from that in primary depression. It has since been clarified that the DST is not a sensitive indicator of major depression and that a negative result has little clinical utility. The second study in this area arrived at different conclusions. Evans and Nemeroff (1984) found DST nonsuppression in four of six patients with organic affective disorder (DSM-III criteria). These authors suggested that the DST nonsuppression in depression secondary to organic etiologies, at a similar frequency to that found in primary depression, indicated that hypothalamic-pituitary-adrenal axis hyperactivity may be present in depression of both types. Thus, these findings suggest that the DST does not distinguish between these two categories of depression. Clinically, the DST appears to be no more or less useful in the diagnosis of organic mood disorder than it is in the diagnosis of primary major depression.

In summary, laboratory aids for the diagnosis of major depression may eventually become a substantial asset to the clinician in a medical setting. However, although DST results may be different in medical patients with depression than in medical patients who are euthymic, there is no consistent evidence that the DST is a practical diagnostic tool. Because a large proportion of medical patients with severe or active physical illness tend to show false positive DST nonsuppression, they have been excluded from many studies assessing its use, thereby limiting the generalizability of these findings. The test may have some promise for confirming major depression in patients with chronic pain, but there is no evidence that the DST is useful to detect depression in patients who present primarily with somatic symptoms. In addition, systematic studies have not fully demonstrated the usefulness of the DST for predicting antidepressant response in medical patients with major depression.

REFERENCES

American Psychiatric Association (1987). *Diagnostic and Statistical Manual of Mental Disorders (Third Edition—Revised)*. Washington, D.C.: American Psychiatric Association.

Atkinson, J.H., Kremer, E.F., Risch, S.C., & Bloom, F.E. (1983). Neuroendocrine function and endogenous opioid peptide systems in chronic pain. *Psychosomatics, 24*, 899–913.

Avery, D. & Winokur, G. (1976). Mortality in depressed patients treated with electroconvulsive therapy and antidepressants. *Archives of General Psychiatry, 33*, 1029–1037.

Beck, A.T. & Beck, R.W. (1972). Screening depressed patients in family practice: A rapid technique. *Postgraduate Medicine, 52*, 81–85.

Borus, J.F., Howes, M.J., Devins, N.P., Rosenberg, R., & Livingston, W.W. (1988). Primary health care providers' recognition and diagnosis of mental disorders in their patients. *General Hospital Psychiatry, 10*, 317–321.

Bridges, D.W. & Goldberg, D.P. (1984). Psychiatric illness in inpatients with neurological disorder: Patients' views on discussion of emotional problems with neurologists. *British Medical Journal, 389*, 656–658.

Bukberg, J., Penman, D., & Holland, J.C. (1984). Depression in hospitalized cancer patients. *Psychosomatic Medicine, 46*, 199–212.

Carney, R.M., Rich, M.W., teVelde, A., Saini, J., Clark, K., & Jaffe, A.S. (1987). Major depressive disorder in coronary artery disease. *American Journal of Cardiology, 60*, 1273–1275.

Carroll, B.J. (1985). Dexamethasone Suppression Test: A review of temporary confusion. *Journal of Clinical Psychiatry, 46,* 13–24.

Carroll, B.J., Feinberg, M., Greden, J.F., Tarika, J., Abala, A.A., Haskett, R.F., Steiner, M., de Vigne, J.P., & Young, E. (1981). A specific laboratory test for the diagnosis of melancholia: Standardization, validation, and clinical utility. *Archives of General Psychiatry, 38,* 15–22.

Casey, P.R., Dillon, S., & Tyrer, P.J. (1984). The diagnostic status of patients with conspicuous psychiatric morbidity in primary care. *Psychological Medicine, 14,* 673–681.

Comaroff, J. & Maguire, P. (1981). Ambiguity and the search for meaning: Childhood leukemia in the modern clinical context. *Social Science and Medicine, 15B,* 115–123.

Coulehan, J.L., Schulberg, H.C., Block, M.R., & Zettler-Segal, M. (1988). Symptom patterns of depression in ambulatory medical and psychiatric patients. *Journal of Nervous and Mental Disease, 176,* 284–288.

Craven, J.L., Rodin, G.M., Johnson, L., & Kennedy, S.H. (1987). The diagnosis of major depression in renal dialysis patients. *Psychosomatic Medicine, 49,* 482–492.

Craven, J.L., Rodin, G.M., & Littlefield, C.H. (1988). The Beck Depression Inventory as a screening device for major depression in renal dialysis patients. *International Journal of Psychiatry in Medicine, 18,* 373–382.

Craven, J.L., Rodin, G.M., & Littlefield, C.H. *Optimizing the utility of the Beck Depression Inventory as a screen for mood disorders in dialysis patients.* (Unpublished data).

Davis, J.M. (1987). Clinical utility of biochemical assays in psychiatry. *Annual Review of Medicine, 38,* 149–156.

DePaulo Jr., J.R. & Folstein, M.F. (1978). Psychiatric disturbances in neurological patients: Detection, recognition, and hospital course. *Annals of Neurology, 4,* 225–228.

Derogatis, L.R., Abeloff, M.D., & McBeth, C.D. (1976). Cancer patients and their physicians in the perception of psychological symptoms. *Psychosomatics, 17,* 197–201.

Derogatis, L.R., Feldstein, M., Morrow, G., Schmale, A., Schmitt, M., Gates, C., Murawski, B., Holland, J., Penman, D., Melisaratos, N., Enelow, A.J., & Adler, L.M. (1979). A survey of psychotropic drug prescriptions in an oncology population. *Cancer, 44,* 1919–1929.

DiGiovanni, C. (1987). Psychiatric aspects. *Maryland Medical Journal, 36,* 35–36.

Evans, D.L., McCartney, C.F., Nemeroff, C.B., Raft, D., Quade, D., Golden, R.N., Haggerty Jr., J.J., Holmes, V., Simon, J.S., Droba, M., Mason, G.Z., & Fowler, W.C. (1986). Depression in women treated for gynecological cancer: Clinical and neuroendocrine assessment. *American Journal of Psychiatry, 143,* 447–452.

Evans, D.L. & Nemeroff, C.B. (1984). The dexamethasone suppression test in organic affective syndrome. *American Journal of Psychiatry, 141,* 1465–1467.

Fava, G.A., Trombini, G., Barbara, L., Bernardi, M., Grandi, S., Callegari, C., & Miglioli, M. (1985). Depression and gastrointestinal illness: The joint use of biological and clinical criteria. *American Journal of Gastroenterology, 80,* 195-199.

Feibel, J.G., Berk, S., & Joynt, R.J. (1979). The unmet needs of stroke survivors. *Neurology, 29,* 592.

Feinstein, A.R. (1977). Clinical biostatistics. XL. Stochastic significance, consistency, apposite data, and some other remedies for the intellectual pollutants of statistical vocabulary. *Clinical Pharmacology and Therapeutics, 22,* 113-123.

Feldman, E., Mayou, R., Hawton, K., Ardern, M., & Smith, E.B. (1987). Psychiatric disorder in medical inpatients. *Quarterly Journal of Medicine, 63,* 405-412.

Finklestein, S., Benowitz, L.I., Baldessarini, R.J., Arana, G.W., Levine, D., Woo, E., Bear, D., Moya, K., & Stoll, A.L. (1982). Mood, vegetative disturbance, and Dexamethasone Suppression Test after stroke. *Annals of Neurology, 12,* 463-468.

Fogel, B.S. & Satel, S.L. (1985). Age, medical illness, and the DST in depressed general hospital inpatients. *Journal of Clinical Psychiatry, 46,* 95-97.

Ford, D.E. (1988). Principles of screening applied to psychiatric disorders. *General Hospital Psychiatry, 10,* 177-188.

France, R.D. & Krishnan, K.R. (1985). The Dexamethasone Suppression Test as a biological marker of depression in chronic pain. *Pain, 21,* 49-55.

France, R.D., Krishnan, K.R.R., Houpt, J.L., & Maltbie, A.A. (1984). Differentiation of depression from chronic pain using a comparison of DST and diagnostic criteria. *American Journal of Psychiatry, 141,* 1577-1579.

France, R.D., Krishnan, K.R.R., Trainor, M., & Pelton, S. (1987). Chronic pain and depression. IV. DST as a discriminator between chronic pain and depression. *Pain, 28,* 39-44.

Frank, R.G., Kashani, J.H., Wonderlich, S.A., Lising, A., & Visot, L.R. (1985). Depression and adrenal function in spinal cord injury. *American Journal of Psychiatry, 142,* 252-253.

Frochtengarten, M.L., Villares, J.C.B., Maluf, E., & Carlini, E.A. (1987). Depressive symptoms and the Dexamethasone Suppression Test in parkinsonian patients. *Biological Psychiatry, 22,* 386-389.

Goldberg, D. (1985). Identifying psychiatric illness among general medical patients. *British Medical Journal, 291,* 161-162.

Goldberg, D. & Huxley, P. (1980). *Mental Illness in the Community.* London: Tavistock Publications.

Goldberg, I.D., Krantz, G., & Locke, Z. (1970). Effect of a short-term outpatient psychiatric therapy benefit on the utilization of medical services in a prepaid group practice medical program. *Medical Care, 8,* 419-426.

Hankin, J.R. & Locke, B.Z. (1983). Extent of depressive symptomatology among patients seeking care in a prepaid group practice. *Psychological Medicine, 13,* 121-129.

Hankin, J.R., Steinwachs, D.M., Regier, D.A., Burns, B.J., Goldberg, I.D., & Hoeper, E.W. (1982). Use of general medical care services by persons with mental disorders. *Archives of General Psychiatry, 39,* 225–231.

Hardman, A., Maguire, P., & Crowther, D. (1989). The recognition of psychiatric morbidity on a medical oncology ward. *Journal of Psychosomatic Research, 33,* 235–239.

Hengeveld, M.W., Ancion, F.A.J., & Rooijmans, H.G.M. (1987). Prevalence and recognition of depressive disorders in general medical inpatients. *International Journal of Psychiatry in Medicine, 17,* 341–349.

Henley, C.E. & Coussens, W.R. (1988). The ability of family practice residents to diagnose depression in outpatients. *Journal of the American Osteopathic Association, 88,* 118–122.

House, A. (1988). Mood disorders in the physically ill: Problems of definition and measurement. *Journal of Psychosomatic Research, 32,* 345–353.

Kamerow, D.B. (1988). Anxiety and depression in the medical setting: An overview. *Medical Clinics of North America, 72,* 745–751.

Kathol, R.G. & Petty, F. (1981). Relationship of depression to medical illness: A critical review. *Journal of Affective Disorders, 3,* 111–121.

Katon, W. (1984). Panic disorder and somatization: Review of 55 cases. *American Journal of Medicine, 77,* 101–106.

Katon, W., Berg, A.O., Robins, A.J., & Risse, S. (1986). Depression—medical utilization and somatization. *Western Journal of Medicine, 144,* 564–568.

Katon, W., Kleinman, A., & Rosen, G. (1982). Depression and somatization: A review: Part I. *American Journal of Medicine, 72,* 127–135.

Katon, W., Ries, R.K., & Kleinman, A. (1984). Part II: A prospective DSM-III study of 100 consecutive somatization patients. *Comprehensive Psychiatry, 25,* 305–314.

Kearns, N.P., Cruickshank, C.A., McGuigan, K.J., Riley, S.A., Shaw, S.P., & Snaith, R.P. (1982). A comparison of depression rating scales. *British Journal of Psychiatry, 141,* 45–49.

Keller, M.B., Lavori, P.W., Lewis, C.E., & Klerman, L.G. (1983). Predictors of relapse in major depressive disorder. *Journal of the American Medical Association, 250,* 3295–3304.

Kennedy, S.H., Craven, J.L., & Rodin, G.M. (1989). Major depression in renal dialysis patients: An open trial of antidepressant therapy. *Journal of Clinical Psychiatry, 50,* 60–63.

Kessler, L.G., Cleary, P.D., & Burke Jr., J.D. (1985). Psychiatric disorders in primary care: Results of a follow-up study. *Archives of General Psychiatry, 42,* 583–587.

Kitchell, M.A., Barnes, R.F., Veith, R.C., Okimoto, J.T., & Raskind, M.A. (1982). Screening for depression in hospitalized geriatric medical patients. *Journal of the American Geriatrics Society, 30,* 174–177.

Koenig, H.G., Meador, K.G., Cohen, H.J., & Blazer, D.G. (1988). Self rated depression scales and screening for major depression in the older hospitalized patient with medical illness. *Journal of the American Geriatrics Society, 36,* 699–706.

Kronfol, Z., Greden, J.F., Condon, M., Feiberg, M., & Carroll, B.J. (1982). Application of biological markers in depression secondary to thyrotoxicosis. *American Journal of Psychiatry, 139,* 1319–1322.

Kurosawa, H., Shimizu, Y., Nishimatsu, Y., Hirose, S., & Takano, T. (1983). The relationship between mental disorders and physical severities in patients with acute myocardial infarction. *Japanese Circulation Journal, 47,* 723–728.

Lane, R.D. & Schwartz, G.E. (1987). Levels of emotional awareness: A cognitive-developmental theory and its application to psychopathology. *American Journal of Psychiatry, 144,* 133–143.

Levine, P.M., Silberfarb, P.M., & Lipowski, Z.J. (1978). Mental disorders in cancer patients: A study of 100 psychiatric referrals. *Cancer, 42,* 1385–1391.

Linn, L.S. & Yager, J. (1980). The effect of screening, sensitization, and feedback on notation of depression. *Journal of Medical Education, 55,* 942–949.

Linn, L.S. & Yager, J. (1982). Screening of depression in relationship to subsequent patient and physician behavior. *Medical Care, 20,* 1233–1240.

Maguire, P. (1984). The recognition and treatment of affective disorders in cancer patients. *International Review of Applied Psychology, 33,* 479–491.

Marks, J.N., Goldberg, D.P., & Hillier, V.F. (1979). Determinants of the ability of general practitioners to detect psychiatric illness. *Psychological Medicine, 9,* 337–353.

Massie, M.J. & Holland, J.C. (1984). Diagnosis and treatment of depression in the cancer patient. *Journal of Clinical Psychiatry, 45,* 25–28.

Mayou, R., Foster, A., & Williamson, B. (1979). Medical care after myocardial infarction. *Journal of Psychosomatic Research, 23,* 23–26.

Mayou, R. & Hawton, K. (1986). Psychiatric disorder in the general hospital. *British Journal of Psychiatry, 149,* 172–190.

Moffic, H.S. & Paykel, E.S. (1975). Depression in medical inpatients. *British Journal of Psychiatry, 126,* 346–353.

Moore, J.T., Silimperi, D.R., & Bobula, J.A. (1978). Recognition of depression by family medicine residents: The impact of screening. *Journal of Family Practice, 7,* 509–513.

Murphy, G.E. (1975). The physicians' responsibility for suicide: II. Errors of omission. *Annals of Internal Medicine, 82,* 305–309.

Nielsen, A.C. & Williams, T.A. (1980). Depression in ambulatory medical patients. *Archives of General Psychiatry, 37,* 999–1004.

Parikh, R.M., Eden, D.T., Price, T.R., & Robinson, R.G. (1988). The sensitivity and specificity of the Center for Epidemiologic Studies Depression Scale in screening for poststroke depression. *International Journal of Psychiatry in Medicine, 18,* 169–181.

Paykel, E.S., Klerman, G.L., & Prusoff, B.A. (1970). Treatment setting and clinical depression. *Archives of General Psychiatry, 22,* 11–21.

Pfeiffer, R.F., Hsieh, H.H., Diercks, M.J., Glaeske, C., & Jefferson, A. (1986). Dexamethasone Suppression Test in Parkinson's disease. In M.D. Yahr & K.J. Bergmann (Eds.), *Advances in Neurology, Vol. 45.* (pp. 439–442). New York: Raven Press.

Prusoff, B.A., Klerman, G.L., & Paykel, E.S. (1972). Concordance between clinical assessments and patients' self-report in depression. *Archives of General Psychiatry, 26,* 546–552.

Raft, D., Davidson, J., Toomey, T.C., Spencer, R.F., & Lewis, B.F. (1975). Inpatient and outpatient patterns of psychotropic drug prescribing by nonpsychiatrist physicians. *American Journal of Psychiatry, 132,* 1309–1312.

Razavi, D., Delvaux, N., Farvacquez, C., & Robaye, E. (1990). Screening for adjustment disorders and major depressive disorders in cancer inpatients. *British Journal of Psychiatry, 156,* 79–83.

Reding, M., Orto, L., Willensky, P., Fortuna, I., Day, N., Steiner, S.F., Gehr, L., & McDowell, F. (1985). The Dexamethasone Suppression Test: An indicator of depression in stroke but not a predictor of rehabilitation outcome. *Archives of Neurology, 42,* 209–212.

Regier, D.A., Goldberg, I.D., & Taube, C.A. (1978). The de facto U.S. mental health services system: A public health perspective. *Archives of General Psychiatry, 35,* 685–696.

Reifler, B.V. (1988). Physical illness and depression. *Journal of Family Practice, 27,* 27–28.

Rihmer, Z., Szadoczky, E., & Arato, M. (1983). Dexamethasone Suppression Test in masked depression. *Journal of Affective Disorders, 5,* 293–296.

Robinson, R.G. & Price, T.R. (1982). Post-stroke depressive disorders: A follow-up study of 103 patients. *Stroke, 13,* 635–641.

Rucker, L., Frye, E.B., & Cygan, R.W. (1986). Feasibility and usefulness of depression screening in medical outpatients. *Archives of Internal Medicine, 146,* 729–731.

Salkind, M.R. (1969). Beck Depression Inventory in general practice. *Journal of the Royal College of General Practitioners, 18,* 267–271.

Schulberg, H.C. & McClelland, M. (1987). A conceptual model for educating primary care providers in the diagnosis and treatment of depression. *General Hospital Psychiatry, 9,* 1–10.

Schulberg, H.C., McClelland, M., Coulehan, J.L., Block, M., & Werner, G. (1986). Psychiatric decision making in family practices: Future research directions. *General Hospital Psychiatry, 8,* 1–6.

Schulberg, H.C., Saul, M., McClelland, M., Ganguli, M., Christy, W., & Frank, R. (1985). Assessing depression in primary medical and psychiatric practices. *Archives of General Psychiatry, 42,* 1164–1170.

Schurman, R.A., Kramer, P.D., & Mitchell, J.B. (1985). The hidden mental health network: Treatment of mental illness by nonpsychiatrist physicians. *Archives of General Psychiatry, 42,* 89–94.

Seller, R.H., Blascovich, J., & Lenkei, E. (1981). Influence of stereotypes in the diagnosis of depression by family practice residents. *Journal of Family Practice, 12,* 849–854.

Shepherd, M., Cooper, B., Brown, A.C., & Kalton, G.W. (1966). *Psychiatric Illness In General Practice.* London: Oxford University Press.

Sireling, L.I., Paykel, E.S., Freeling, P., Rao, B.M., & Patel, S.P. (1985). Depression in general practice: Case thresholds and diagnosis. *British Journal of Psychiatry, 147,* 113–119.

Stokes, P.E. (1987). DST update: The hypothalamic-pituitary-adrenocortical axis and affective illness. *Biological Psychiatry, 22,* 245–248.

Syvalahti, E., Hyyppa, M.T., & Salminen, J.K. (1985). Depression and the Dexamethasone Suppression Test (DST) in patients with non-specific somatic complaints: Atypical depression and DST. *Annals of Clinical Research, 17,* 148–151.

Thase, M.E., Brent, D.A., Neil, J.F., & Horn, T.L. (1985). Evaluation of depression in a general hospital: Utility and limitations of the Dexamethasone Suppression Test. *General Hospital Psychiatry, 7,* 43–48.

Wade, D.T., Legh-Smith, J., & Hewer, R.A. (1987). Depressed mood after stroke: A community study of its frequency. *British Journal of Psychiatry, 151,* 200–205.

Warren, L.W. (1983). Male intolerance of depression: A review with implications for psychotherapy. *Clinical Psychology Review, 3,* 147–156.

Werk, E.E., MacGee, J., & Sholiton, L.J. (1964). Altered cortisol metabolism in advanced cancer and other terminal illnesses: Excretion of 6-hydroxycortisol. *Metabolism, 13,* 1425–1438.

Williamson, M.T. (1987). Sex differences in depression symptoms among adult family medicine patients. *Journal of Family Practice, 25,* 591–594.

Wulsin, L.R., Hillard, J.R., Geier, P., Hissa, D., & Rouan, G.W. (1988). Screening emergency room patients with atypical chest pain for depression and panic disorder. *International Journal of Psychiatry in Medicine, 18,* 315–323.

Wynn, A. (1967). Unwarranted emotional distress in men with ischaemic heart disease (IHD). *Medical Journal of Australia, 2,* 847–851.

Zigmond, A.S. & Snaith, R.P. (1983). The Hospital Anxiety and Depression Scale. *Acta Psychiatrica Scandinavica, 67,* 361–370.

Zung, W.W.K., George, D.T., Woodruff III, W.W., & Mahorney, S.L. (1984). Symptom perception by nonpsychiatric physicians in evaluating for depression. *Journal of Clinical Psychiatry, 45,* 26–29.

Zung, W.W.K., Magill, M., Moore, J., & George, D.T. (1983). Recognition and treatment of depression in a family medicine practice. *Journal of Clinical Psychiatry, 44,* 3–6.

3

Ambiguous Presentations of Depression

It has long been observed that depression is sometimes manifest in forms that are not immediately recognizable as a mood disorder (Lesse, 1967). Certain patients typically deny emotional distress altogether, or else selectively complain of the somatic rather than the cognitive-affective symptoms of depression (Katon, Kleinman, & Rosen, 1982). These patients have been labelled "somatizers." Somatization is defined as the presence of somatic symptoms in the absence of organic disease (Kellner, 1986), or alternatively, as the expression of emotional discomfort and psychosocial distress in the language of physical or bodily symptoms (Barsky, Wyshak, & Klerman, 1986). This phenomenon deserves attention here because it is possible that the rate of detection of mood disorders in the medical setting (see Chapter 2) is reduced because somatic presentations of depression are often assumed to be manifestations of physical illness. Primary care physicians tend to consider the diagnosis of depression only when cognitive-affective symptoms are prominent (Katon, Kleinman, & Rosen, 1982).

Somatic complaints are the most common presentation of depression in certain cultures (Kleinman, 1977), and in the primary care setting (Cadoret, Widmer, & Troughton, 1980; Williamson & Yates, 1989). Approximately one-quarter of persons in psychiatric settings with major depression have presented initially with somatic complaints (Jones & Hall, 1963; Hagnell & Rorsman, 1978). This proportion increases to one-half for depressed patients who were referred from medical or surgical settings (Jones & Hall, 1963). These patients often present difficult diagnostic problems. In that regard, Stoudemire et al. (1985)

found that "masked" depression was a common reason for patients to be admitted for investigation to a combined medical-psychiatric treatment unit. Unfortunately, practitioners in the medical or primary care setting often do not consider psychiatric disorders in the differential diagnosis of unexplained somatic complaints. When cognitive-affective depressive symptoms are absent, clinicians may erroneously conclude that a medical condition, rather than a mood disorder, is directly responsible for the presenting somatic symptoms. Such patients with "masked" depression may be subjected to extensive medical investigations and then dismissed when no physical basis for their complaints can be found. As Barsky (1981) noted, psychosocial factors are often among the "hidden reasons" for a medical visit. This failure to consider psychological and psychiatric factors in medical patients may be costly since somatization is often associated with the preferential use of medical services (Escobar et al., 1989), persistent psychiatric morbidity, and excessive overall health care utilization. This cost is further highlighted by Akiskal's (1983) assertion that somatic presentations are likely the most predominant forms of mood disorder in the community.

It is understandable that medically oriented physicians are most concerned about the physical manifestations of disease. However, awareness of the role of emotional factors in disease presentation is necessary to detect potentially treatable psychiatric disorders in somatizing patients. It must be appreciated that a variety of psychiatric disorders are known to be associated with and to contribute to somatization (Rodin, 1984). Depression is particularly important to detect among patients who are unable or unwilling to communicate distress in psychological terms because such patients may respond well to psychiatric treatment (House, 1988).

The present chapter begins with a selective discussion of somatization and depression, and of related phenomena that contribute to the preferential reporting of physical, rather than emotional complaints. The relationship among depression, somatization, and organic disease is explored further through the examination of some specific and perplexing syndromes. These are characterized by prominent somatic complaints that are not entirely explained on either a psychological or a physical basis. The syndromes that are discussed in this chapter are chronic fatigue, chronic pain, fibrositis, and irritable bowel syndrome. We have included a discussion of these conditions in this text because they pose substantial dilemmas in the differential diagnosis of both depression and medical illness. Depression has often been thought to be a common underlying or coexisting disorder in these conditions. These and other similar conditions highlight diagnostic problems related to somatization, depression, and the differential diagnosis of organic versus functional conditions.

It is not known whether the ill-defined conditions noted above represent medical disorders aggravated by psychological factors, psychological disturbances manifest with prominent somatic symptoms, or coexisting medical and psychiatric disorders. Thus, although depression has been associated, to a greater or lesser extent, with each of these syndromes, it is unclear whether the mood disturbance r` presents a primary aspect of the condition, a complication of it, or a coincidental occurrence. To confuse matters even further, individual patients differ in the way in which physical abnormality, depression, and somatization of related (Lipowski, 1990).

SOMATIZATION AND DEPRESSION

To recognize and communicate depression in other than somatic terms requires some capacity to identify the cognitive-affective aspects of emotional experience. Lane and Schwartz (1987) suggested that the cognitive-affective dimensions are involved in the more differentiated, attenuated aspects of emotional experience, whereas less differentiated emotional experience tends to be experienced as bodily sensations and action tendencies. The term alexithymia, coined by Sifneos in 1972, refers to an extreme end of the continuum in which patients are limited in their awareness of emotional experience and have great difficulty discriminating between emotional states and bodily sensations (Taylor, 1984). The tendency toward alexithymia may be increased as patients experience the severe and chronic stress associated with a medical illness (Freyberger et al., 1985). Indeed, the presence of a physical illness may heighten bodily anxieties and contribute to a selective focus on the physical manifestations of emotional disturbances.

It has been suggested (Sifneos, 1973; Martin & Pihl, 1985) that alexithymic individuals are unable to respond adequately to emotionally stressful situations. Such individuals may be prone to develop withdrawn, "frozen," depression-like states in response to severe stress (Horowitz et al., 1984). Engel (1962) regarded these states as manifestations of "conservation-withdrawal" or "depression-withdrawal," which he considered a response to the need to conserve energy. Engel (1962) further suggested that these clinical states might be variants of depression associated with feelings of helplessness, hopelessness, and resignation. However, the diagnosis of depression is problematic when there is an associated severe medical illness. It is unclear whether the so-called states of "depression-withdrawal" in response to severe stress represent a physical or psychological disturbance, or both. Further, it is unclear whether either of these possibilities may be equated with a depressive disorder.

Controversy persists concerning the link between depression and the somatizing disorders. Lipowski (1990) has recently noted that prior to the eighteenth century, the terms melancholia and hypochondriasis were synonymous. Orenstein (1989) recently proposed that the psychiatric comorbidity of major depression, panic disorder and agoraphobia, and the somatoform disorders reflects a shared diathesis causing these conditions to aggregate together. Several studies have found a high frequency of major depression in patients with somatization disorder (Fabrega et al., 1988; Morrison & Herbstein, 1988; Orenstein, 1989). However, a unique association does not exist between depression and a particular somatoform disorder, namely hypochondriasis. In this regard, Kellner et al. (1989) found that although depression was more common in hypochondriacal patients than in normal controls, it was not more common than in other psychiatric patients. Similarly, Barsky, Wyshak, and Klerman (1986) reported that although depression and hypochondriacal attitudes are strongly related, an appreciable proportion of hypochondriacal patients are not depressed. Together, these findings suggest that depression and somatization are overlapping but distinct phenomena.

The relationship of functional somatic complaints to depression may be stronger in some physical conditions than in others. For example, depression may be the most common psychiatric diagnosis in patients with chronic pain (Magni, 1987) or chronic fatigue (Kruesi, Dale, & Straus, 1989). However, with a more specific condition such as functional chest pain, depression is less common than anxiety disorders (Katon et al., 1988; Wulsin et al., 1988).

Some of the common clinical situations in which it is difficult to distinguish among depression, physical illness, and somatization are discussed next.

Depression Presenting with Somatic Features

Factors within the family and the culture may lead to somatization. In developing countries, somatic complaints are the most common presentation of psychiatric illness (Kirkmayer, 1984). Studies from Africa (Makanjuola & Olaifa, 1987), Asia (Kleinman, 1977), and the Mediterranean (Ierodiakonou & Iacovides, 1987) have confirmed this tendency. However, the relationship between somatization and cultural factors is complex and multidetermined.

Cultural factors may influence the development of emotional awareness, and the subsequent tendency toward somatization, through their
impact on child-rearing practices and the nature of early child-parent
relationships. The extent to which parents become attuned to and value
the emotional life of the child, and are able or willing to assist in the
identification, validation, and expression of feelings, may be significant
determinants of the child's capacity for emotional awareness and his
or her ability to express feelings in more than physical terms (Greenspan,
1981; Stolorow, Brandchaft, & Atwood, 1987). In the absence of parental
responsiveness of this kind, children may learn to respond somatically
to situations in which it might be more appropriate or adaptive to
respond emotionally (Greenspan, 1981). Physical illness during childhood may also affect parent-child relationships and the subsequent
tendency of individuals to focus on somatic symptoms (Burns & Nichols, 1972).

The following case illustrates how family and personality factors may
contribute to the masked, or somatic presentation of major depression
in association with medical illness.

Case Example

■ Mrs. L. was a 55-year-old married woman referred by her cardiovascular surgeon for psychiatric assessment. She suffered from a mild
but progressive abnormality of her mitral valve, but her surgeon believed
that the degree of her disability far exceeded what might have been
expected based on the physical findings alone.

When she arrived for the psychiatric interview, Mrs. L. presented as
a well-groomed, middle-aged woman who was mildly agitated and
appeared moderately depressed. However, she did not initially report
symptoms of depression. She commented on how difficult it was for
her to attend the appointment due to her physical condition. She warned
the psychiatrist that she might have to leave the office should her heart
"act up." She proceeded to describe a progressive deterioration in her
physical health such that she had felt forced to quit work one year
previously and now felt unable to perform daily household duties.
Although Mrs. L. admitted to some undifferentiated emotional distress
secondary to forced inactivity, she maintained a strained smile throughout the medical history and was adamant that she had adjusted well
to her situation and was not "crazy." She added that she had never
had any emotional problems, had never seen herself as someone who
would require psychiatric help, and was quite surprised when her
surgeon had referred her to a psychiatrist.

Soon after the description of her medical history, Mrs. L. began to cry profusely. She reported that her 20-year-old son had "dropped dead" of a brain aneurysm a few years before, that her stepfather had died six months prior to the interview, and that she now felt unable to continue to care for her partially disabled mother. Even while crying, Mrs. L. continued to smile and repeatedly tried to reassure the interviewer that she did not suffer from an emotional problem. However, with specific but gentle questioning, she acknowledged that she had felt depressed for about a year, had withdrawn socially, was no longer interested in activities that she has previously enjoyed, and uncharacteristically, now had little interest in her physical exercise program. She also reported feeling hopeless about her future health and the benefits of surgery, having recurrent passive wishes for death, and marked feelings of guilt and self-recrimination regarding her inability to care for her mother. She denied having previously recognized any emotional difficulty, but now stated that her depressed feelings made sense to her in the light of her predicament.

Factors that may have contributed to this patient's tendency to suppress and deny distressing affect were apparent in her developmental history. Her father had been killed at an early age, and she remembered her mother was often absent, working long hours to support the family. She recalled her mother as being a stoical individual who never complained and would not tolerate complaining by her children. At the age of 19, Mrs. L. married a sailor who was away from home for extended periods of time. They had three children and Mrs. L.'s life was focused on caring for them. She adopted this life style with the same self-denial and stoicism that was evident in her mother. Depressive feelings represented for her, a kind of self-indulgence to which she did not feel entitled.

The psychiatric diagnosis in this case was that of a major depressive episode in an individual with obsessional personality traits. Treatment involved both individual and marital interventions. With some assistance, Mrs. L. and her husband were able to reconceptualize her difficulties in terms of a depressive illness that had occurred as a result of multiple stressors. A combination of antidepressant pharmacotherapy and focal psychotherapy was used to help resolve her grief and to improve her functional adjustment. ■

This case illustrates how multiple stressors, in combination with particular personality features, may lead to a depression that is unacknowledged or unrecognized by the patient. An important role for the therapist in such cases is to identify, acknowledge, and legitimize depressive feelings. Also of note in this case, is that although the depression was initially masked, gentle but direct questioning easily elicited the characteristic history of major depression. The failure to enquire into her emotional disturbance might have led to a missed diagnosis, persistent disability, and unnecessary medical investigations and treatment.

Whereas somatization is usually considered a characteristic of the patient, it may also arise out of the physician-patient relationship. Many aspects of the medical setting may suggest to patients that physicians are too busy or too preoccupied with other matters to attend to emotional distress. When physicians seem insensitive to their emotional state, patients may come to believe that they need somatic complaints to justify their wish for emotional support. This perception may contribute to the tendency of some patients in the medical setting to report depression in somatic terms. Changes in the structure of the medical setting and in the attitude of medical staff may be necessary to convey a more permissive message to patients regarding emotional expression. Indeed, as Kleinman (1988) has suggested, legitimizing the patient's illness experience is a key task in the care of the physically ill.

Depression Producing or Amplifying Somatic Symptoms

Considerable evidence suggests that depression may not only produce a wide variety of physical complaints directly, but also that it may amplify or increase the patient's general awareness of physical symptoms. For instance, Widmer and Cadoret (1978) and Cadoret, Widmer, and Troughton (1980) found, in primary care patients, that a tendency to report somatic complaints was an early manifestation of depression which appeared before other features of depression were present; these complaints diminished after the depressive symptoms resolved. Similarly, Kellner (1986) reported that hypochondriacal beliefs and fears were common in patients who had major depression with melancholia, but that these symptoms tended to disappear after treatment with amitriptyline. Waxman et al. (1985) observed that individuals in the community who reported more depressive symptoms also tended to report more somatic complaints and more chronic medical illness. However, the increased somatic complaints in the depressed individuals were not necessarily accounted for by an increased number of chronic medical illnesses. They suggested, instead, that depression amplified the perceived discomfort associated with physical illness. Finally, Lustman, Clouse, and Carney (1988) examined the relationship of physical symptoms to current mood and metabolic control in 114 patients with diabetes mellitus. They found that the severity of depression, as measured by the Beck Depression Inventory, contributed more strongly to the reporting of physical symptoms than did the degree of metabolic dyscontrol. They concluded that many symptoms often attributed to diabetes are related more to depressive mood than to the true physical state of the patient.

Physical Illness with Both Somatic and Depressive Features

Depression and somatic complaints can coexist in medical patients not because of somatization but because both arise independently consequent to the medical illness. It is prudent for clinicians to keep an open mind about the underlying cause of the symptoms they observe. The tendency of some primary care physicians to focus on organic disease and to underdiagnose depression in patients with physical conditions has been previously discussed. Equally problematic, particularly with patients who have frequent functional somatic symptoms or a past psychiatric history, is the tendency of physicians to assume that unexplained somatic complaints are a manifestation of psychopathology. In such cases, coexisting or underlying organic disease may go undetected. For example, Chandler and Gerndt (1988) found, in a psychiatric setting, that somatic complaints with major depression were not always a manifestation of depression, but at times were due to associated medical problems in these patients. They cautioned against automatically attributing a psychiatric origin to somatic complaints in individuals with major depression.

We turn now to a discussion of several specific conditions with ill-defined characteristics and etiology in which there is particular difficulty differentiating organically based symptoms from those of depression.

SPECIFIC CONDITIONS WITH FUNCTIONAL SOMATIC COMPLAINTS

Chronic Fatigue

The symptom of fatigue refers both to the failure to maintain expected or required muscular force and to the subjective experience of excessive weakness or decreased energy. Fatigue is a common complaint of medical patients, and when persistent, it is frequently associated with significant impairment in the quality of life (Nelson et al., 1987). Fatigue is also a well-recognized symptom of depression and is included as one of the DSM-III-R criteria both for dysthymic disorder and for major depressive episode.

Fatigue may arise through any one of a variety of mechanisms (Swartz, 1988). In the physically ill, fatigue may arise from impairment at any site from cerebral cortex to spinal cord to peripheral nerve to muscle cell membrane. For example, myasthenia gravis may produce muscle weakness and generalized fatigue due to disruption of synaptic transmission. Systemic factors may also produce fatigue. For instance, fatigue secondary to cachexia may occur when there is diversion of nutrients to a large or rapidly growing tumor. Fatigue is also commonly reported by renal dialysis patients, and is likely due, in part, to a chronic sleep disturbance associated with their medical illness (Moldofsky et al., 1985). Although fatigue is also commonly associated with depression, it may be difficult in some medical patients to determine whether this symptom is due to depression or to the physical condition. Fatigue has not been found to be a reliable indicator of depression in dialysis patients (Craven et al., 1987), oncology patients (Bukberg, Penman, & Holland, 1984), patients with rheumatoid arthritis (Frank et al., 1988), and those with multiple sclerosis (Krupp et al., 1988). However, it may still be useful in the diagnosis of major depression in other medical conditions in which fatigue is not a prominent feature (e.g., mild coronary artery disease).

The search for organic causes of ill-defined symptoms such as fatigue has longstanding roots in both medicine and psychiatry. During the 19th century, George Beard (1880) described the syndrome of nervous exhaustion or neurasthenia, which he believed to be due both to the demands of life in North America and to nervous irritability. He advocated treatment of this condition with electricity. During the past few decades, other explanations have been advanced for the syndrome of chronic fatigue. These include viral infections and psychiatric disorders, particularly depression.

Chronic fatigue syndrome is associated with weakness, myalgia, memory loss, and depression. Investigators who regard chronic fatigue as a postviral syndrome have referred to it variously in the literature as benign myalgic encephalomyelitis (Acheson, 1959), Royal Free disease (The Medical Staff of the Royal Free Hospital, 1957), Iceland disease (Sigurdsson et al., 1950), epidemic neuromyasthenia (Henderson & Shelokov, 1959), and postviral fatigue syndrome (Behan, Behan, & Bell, 1985). So-called postviral asthenia has been attributed by Swartz (1988) to a variety of organic factors including deconditioning because of bed rest or limited activity, and muscle proteolysis due to the presence of interleukin-1 and prostaglandin E2. More specifically, it has been suggested that persistent fatigue might arise as a long-term sequela of Epstein-Barr virus (EBV) infection (Cadie, Nye, & Storey, 1976; Tobi et al., 1982; Jones et al., 1985; Straus et al., 1985), although other viruses including enterovirus (Yousef et al., 1988) and Coxsackie B virus (Wilson et al., 1989) have also been implicated. The clinical syndrome of infectious mononucleosis, known to be caused by Epstein-Barr virus (EBV), is typically characterized by a variety of nonspecific symptoms including severe fatigue, malaise, weakness, subjective fever, sore throat, painful lymph nodes, decreased memory, confusion, and decreased concentration (Holmes et al., 1988). Depression and constitutional symptoms have been reported to occur for months and even years after the acute physical symptoms subside (Straus et al., 1985).

Although EBV antibodies have been found in patients with a postviral syndrome of chronic fatigue, the diagnostic value of Epstein-Barr virus serologic tests, and the proposed causal relationship between infection with this virus and the syndrome of chronic fatigue remains doubtful (Holmes et al., 1987; Buchwald, Sullivan, & Komaroff, 1987; Holmes et al., 1988). To date, controlled studies (Hellinger et al., 1988; Holmes et al., 1987) have shown that patients with the chronic fatigue syndrome and antibody to the Epstein-Barr virus cannot be distinguished from age and sex-matched controls with chronic fatigue and no EBV antibodies. Indeed, although more than 20 percent of patients in a general medical practice suffered from a chronic fatigue syndrome not due to documented organic disease or to chronic psychiatric disease, EBV antibody titers in these patients did not differ from those of age and sex-matched controls (Buchwald, Sullivan, & Komaroff, 1987). One study did show increased EBV antibody titers in 15 patients with severe chronic fatigue of undetermined etiology compared to controls (Holmes et al., 1987). However, this association with EBV antibodies was not unique. The chronic fatigue patients also had increased titers of antibodies to cytomegalovirus, herpes simplex, and measles viruses, so that any one or a combination of all of these viruses were just as likely to have caused the chronic fatigue.

The observation that psychological or psychiatric factors may be involved in chronic postviral fatigue is not new. It was noted that persistent fatigue during the 1957 Asian influenza epidemic (Imboden, Canter, & Cluff, 1961) and in cases of so-called chronic brucellosis (Imboden et al., 1959) tended to occur in individuals with premorbid depression and difficulties in emotional adjustment. Others suggested that recovery from infectious mononucleosis is delayed in individuals with "low ego strength" (Greenfield, Roessler, & Crosley, 1959). More recent studies suggest that depression is associated with postviral fatigue syndrome. Cadie, Nye, and Storey (1976) suggested that women with serologically positive infectious mononucleosis were more likely than controls to report depressive symptoms one year after the onset of this infection. Taerk et al. (1987) reported that major depression based on the Diagnostic Interview Schedule could be diagnosed in 15 out of 24 patients referred for complaints of subjective weakness of at least three months duration in the absence of significant physical findings and following an apparent infective episode. Evidence of some preexisting vulnerability is suggested by the finding that chronic fatigue patients in this study reported a higher frequency of previous major depression than did controls. Kruesi, Dale, and Straus (1989) similarly found that 13 of 28 patients with chronic fatigue syndrome had a history of major depression. Although the idea of identifying a specific relationship between viral infection and depression in these patients is appealing, current evidence does not support it. In fact, Amsterdam et al. (1986) reported that antibodies to EBV were not more common among patients with major depression than among controls. Indeed, by middle age, more than 90 percent of the general population will have been infected by and possess antibodies to the EB virus (Straus et al., 1988).

It has been suggested (Holmes et al., 1988) that the term chronic fatigue syndrome be used to indicate the uncertain etiology of this condition, and that standardized working case definitions be used in systematic research. Holmes et al. (1988) suggested the following criteria for the diagnosis of chronic fatigue: (1) new onset of persistent debilitating fatigue that reduces average daily activity below 50 percent of the premorbid level for at least six months; (2) absence of diagnosed physical or psychiatric disease that can account for the symptoms; and (3) a specified number of physical signs or symptoms. Patients with the chronic fatigue syndrome should not be presumed a priori to be suffering from depression or from the specific after effects of a viral syndrome. It is likely that the chronic fatigue syndrome is heterogeneous and includes individuals with masked depression, those in whom a viral or other medical illness has acted as a biologic and/or psychologic stressor that triggers prolonged somatization and/or depression, those in whom the medical illness is coincidental, and others in whom the prolonged somatic symptoms are indeed the direct biological consequences of a medical condition. Somatization is likely to be an important process that contributes to this symptom complex and to other functional syndromes with somatic complaints. In this regard, Manu et al. (1989) found the prevalence of somatization disorder in a chronic fatigue population to be similar to that found in other common functional medical syndromes including chronic pain and irritable bowel.

Some of the relationships between fatigue and depression may be illustrated in the following case:

Case Example

■ Mrs. A. was a 65-year-old married woman who had been treated by a gastroenterologist for gastric acid hypersecretory pain associated with the Zollinger-Ellison syndrome. The specialist noted that medical treatment resulted in a reduction in both her pain symptoms and in gastric secretion. However, she continued over the course of one year to complain of persistent fatigue, which did not seem to be explained by her physical condition. Eventually, the referring physician wondered if emotional factors might be contributing to her chronic fatigue syndrome.

She presented to psychiatric assessment as a well-groomed woman who appeared moderately depressed and tended to be vague and circumstantial. Her major complaint was of feeling "absolutely dead-tired" from the time her pain began. This fatigue persisted even when her pain subsided. She felt unable to resume any of her normal activities including light housework and socializing with friends. She also reported marked difficulty in falling asleep, early morning awakening, concentration difficulties, and loss of appetite with minimal weight loss. She was preoccupied with her physical symptoms and worried that she was suffering from the chronic fatigue syndrome about which she had read in a popular magazine. She became tearful when she reported that the article said that the syndrome could persist for several years.

This patient reported having been a "shy and sensitive" child who felt disturbed by her alcoholic father's frequent and prolonged absences and eventual departure from the home when she was six years old. However, as a child, she was able to make friends, enjoy school, and later marry a successful businessperson to whom she felt very attracted. His work involved frequent travel and entertaining, and, at his request, they remained childless. Mrs. A. had suffered a series of losses over the past decade, including the death of her father as a result of alcoholic liver disease, the death of her only sibling following an injury that seemed alcohol-related, and the death of her mother due to Parkinson's disease. She commented that she seemed not to have grieved any of these losses when they occurred. She felt unable to share her feelings with her husband who seemed uncomfortable with emotions.

A diagnosis of major depression was made in this patient, although she initially presented with symptoms consistent with chronic fatigue syndrome. She was readily able to identify profound feelings of depression and grief when her feelings were explored. Her recent depressive symptoms seemed to have been triggered by the onset of a medical condition that responded favorably to medication, but which nevertheless aroused fears of dependency and disability. The illness also activated feelings of helplessness and abandonment related to previous significant unmourned losses. A marital assessment was carried out that confirmed both the patient's symptoms and her husband's unwillingness to be more involved with her emotional distress. She was started on antidepressant medication and within two to three weeks reported an alleviation of her symptoms and a gradual resumption of her social engagements. ■

This case illustrates major depression triggered by a physical illness but subsequently manifest with somatic complaints, particularly fatigue. This patient had emphasized her fatigue both to herself and to her physician. However, although she presented with somatic symptoms, she was able, upon direct enquiry, to identify a depressed mood. As this case demonstrates, the ability of patients to report emotional symptoms relates not only to their capacity for emotional awareness but also to the extent to which caregivers are attuned to emotional distress. Psychiatric referral permitted the diagnosis of major depression to be made and appropriate treatment to be instituted. For many other patients, the symptom of chronic fatigue is experienced in the absence of other features of major depression and antidepressants appear to be of little help. This may be true even for chronic fatigue patients with a history of major depressive episode.

Chronic Pain

Chronic pain not explained by organic factors has been variously regarded as a cause of depression, a metaphor for it, or a coexisting disturbance. Chronic pain of obscure origin has been referred to in the past as chronic pain syndrome (Black, 1975), idiopathic pain disorder (Williams & Spitzer, 1982), pain prone-disorder (Blumer & Heilbronn, 1981), depression-pain syndrome (Lindsay & Wyckoff, 1981), and dysthymic pain disorder (Blumer & Heilbronn, 1987). The last two terms are based upon a postulated relationship between chronic pain and a disturbance in mood, although controversy persists regarding the presence and nature of such a relationship. The multiple diagnostic labels that have been assigned to patients with chronic pain reflects, to some extent, differing perspectives on this condition.

No assumption is made in the DSM-III-R about the relationship of depression to chronic pain. Chronic pain unrelated to a medical disorder is grouped not with the affective disorders, but with the somatoform disorders under the diagnosis of somatoform pain disorder. The term somatoform pain disorder is used in the DSM-III-R to refer to a condition in which there is a preoccupation with pain in the absence of organic pathology adequate enough to account either for the pain or for the associated social or occupational impairment. No judgment as to the apparent or presumed presence of depression is required for this diagnosis.

Most studies have found that the diagnosis of major depression can be made in about one-half of patients with chronic pain (France et al., 1986; Kramlinger, Swanson, & Maruta, 1983; Schaffer, Donlon, & Bittle, 1980). Blumer and Heilbronn (1987) suggested, based upon features such as the chronicity, the lack of psychotic features, and the relative absence of biological markers for depression, that chronic pain may be more closely related to dysthymic disorder than to major depression. It was for these reasons that they proposed the term dysthymic pain disorder. However, other evidence suggests that pain symptoms are not specific for depression. Slocumb et al. (1989) reported that patients with the abdominal pelvic pain syndrome reported not only more symptoms of depression but also more anxiety and hostility than matched gynecologic controls. Romano and Turner (1985) suggested that without adequately controlled studies, it is impossible to conclude that syndromal depression is higher in pain patients than in other groups. Also, although headaches and other pain symptoms are common in depressed patients, it is not known whether such symptoms are as frequent in other psychiatric populations. Controlled studies are needed to document the association between various pain syndromes and psychiatric illnesses.

Three major points of view have been espoused in the recent literature regarding the association between depression and chronic pain:

1. *Pain is analogous to depression or is a depressive equivalent.* Blumer and Heilbronn (1982) favor this hypothesis, viewing the pain-prone patient as alexithymic with emotions tending to be poorly differentiated, poorly verbalized, and experienced mostly in the somatic sphere. Similarly, Postone (1986) reported that chronic pain patients were significantly more alexithymic than an outpatient psychotherapy control group although not more alexithymic than their spouses. Pilowsky, Chapman, and Bonica (1977) reported that, compared to a general medical control group, 100 chronic pain patients were less willing to consider their problems in psychological terms and tended to deny current life problems. Although a subgroup of the pain patients did

suffer from significant depression, they suggested that, in general, the chronic pain symptoms in these patients should be regarded as a form of abnormal illness behavior.

The response of pain symptoms to antidepressant medication has suggested to some, that pain and depression are analogous. In a review of the literature on the use of antidepressants in chronic pain, France, Houpt, and Ellinwood (1984) concluded that current evidence supported their efficacy, but often at lower doses and with more rapid onset of action than is usual with depression. However, they concluded that it remains unclear whether antidepressants act in such patients through the potentiation of analgesic effects or through a mood-activating property. The mechanism most widely accepted is that, when used in the manner described, antidepressants likely alleviate chronic pain symptoms by the potentiation of analgesic activity.

2. *Depression arises secondary to chronic pain.* This point of view is well represented in the literature (Hendler, 1984; Turk & Salovey, 1984). Hendler (1984) supported this perspective with the observation that chronic pain almost always leads to depression but that depression is rarely manifested by chronic pain. Turk and Salovey (1984) suggested that the most parsimonious explanation for the association of chronic pain and depression is that depressive symptoms are secondary to the experience of having distressing chronic symptoms that are poorly understood and ineffectively treated. This certainly may be the case with a variety of diagnosed and undiagnosed medical disorders and is supported by the findings of Maruta, Vatterot, and McHardy (1989) who found that depressive symptoms resolved in almost all chronic pain patients following admission to a pain management program.

3. *Chronic pain and depression are coincidental.* It may be that some cases of depression in individuals with chronic pain are coincidental or that both are related to an underlying medical disorder and/or psychological vulnerability. In the latter case, the coexistence of depressive and pain syndromes might be expected without there being a direct causal relationship.

In some patients, the diagnosis of chronic pain is complicated by the presence of a serious medical illness. In these cases, the pain may be secondary to an underlying medical disorder and appropriate analgesia may be the most effective therapeutic measure. In other cases, even when a medical illness is present, the degree of pain may not be fully explainable on an organic basis. In such cases, the pain may reflect a tendency to experience psychological distress in physical terms or to amplify somatic symptoms (Barsky et al., 1988). The clinician should consider the possibility that clinical or subclinical depression is present in patients with chronic pain, although current evidence does not support the view that chronic pain and depression are necessarily synonymous. At present, a therapeutic trial of antidepressant medication is often indicated for patients with chronic pain although a positive response does not necessarily confirm the diagnosis of depression. Further, the possibility of undetected or untreated organic disease must not be neglected in any chronic pain patient.

Fibrositis

A subgroup of patients who are perplexing with regard to both the presence of organic illness and of depression are those with so-called fibrositis. The multiple diagnostic labels applied to this syndrome again reflect the uncertainty that has existed in the literature regarding its nature and pathogenesis. Terms that have been used synonymously include fibrositis, fibromyalgia, fibromyositis, myofibrositis, myofascitis, myofascial pain syndrome, rheumatic pain modulation disorder, and chronic pain syndrome.

Gowers (1904) coined the term fibrositis to refer to a form of muscular rheumatism affecting the fibrous tissue of muscle. At the same time, Stockman (1904) identified tender nodules associated with this condition. Fibrositis has subsequently been described as "a poorly defined painful disorder of presumably rheumatic origin in which specially skilled examiners might appreciate tender, nodular abnormalities in muscle and other associated soft tissues" (Rice, 1986, p. 456). A number of authors have suggested that there are not enough consistent or specific findings to support the view that fibrositis is a discrete pathological disorder, and that many patients with this diagnosis have other associated syndromes including irritable bowel, headaches, anxiety, and pain syndromes (Hadler, 1986; Rice, 1986). Rice (1986) noted that fibrositis is a misnomer that persists in spite of the lack of evidence for any structural disorder of fibrous or soft tissue. The term fibromyalgia is preferred by some for this reason (Yunus, 1983).

Whereas the original descriptions of this syndrome referred to musculoskeletal pain, fatigue and sleep disturbance were subsequently included in the clinical description (Traut, 1968). It was not until 1981 that a controlled study of the condition was reported (Yunus et al., 1981). Rice (1986) suggested that the following criteria be used to identify fibrositis in clinical practice: musculoskeletal pain or tenderness in characteristic locations that is unexplained by associated structural or systemic disease; symptoms of three or more months duration; and associated sleep disturbance or chronic fatigue.

Depression has not been regarded as an essential component of fibrositis. However, as with almost all conditions in which there are prominent physical symptoms not fully explained by organic factors, some have postulated that it represents some form of depression. In support of this hypothesis is the observation that sleep disorder and fatigue, central features of fibrositis, are commonly associated with major depression. Hudson et al. (1985) studied a sample of patients with fibrositis referred to a rheumatologist at a university arthritis clinic. Based on the DIS, they found a current or past major affective disorder in 71 percent of the fibromyalgia patients, a prevalence rate significantly greater than the 14 percent found in rheumatoid arthritis patients, and the 12 percent in a control group without affective illness. Also, the family history of major depression was significantly stronger in the fibromyalgia patients than in the rheumatoid arthritis patients. Because the major depression occurred at least one year before the development of the fibromyalgia in the majority of cases, the authors concluded that the depression likely represented a preexisting condition or vulnerability. However, in another study, no significant difference in the prevalence of depression or other psychological symptoms was found in patients with fibrositis selected from a general medical population compared to control patients (Clark et al., 1985). Similarly, Ahles, Yunus, and Masi (1987) found no difference in the frequency of depressive symptoms between patients with the primary fibromyalgia syndrome (PFS) and those with rheumatoid arthritis, although both were more depressed than normal controls. These authors concluded that their data do not support the concept that PFS is a variant of "depressive disease," although a subgroup may well be clinically depressed.

It would appear that depression is common but not synonymous with fibrositis. This condition still remains enigmatic with regard to its functional and organic components. Depression cannot be assumed to be present nor is this condition a clearly defined medical illness. Finally, studies of depressive symptoms in fibrositis patients must take into account the nature of the population studied and the relationship of depressive symptoms to help-seeking behavior.

Irritable Bowel Syndrome (IBS)

The irritable bowel syndrome (IBS) has been defined as the persistence of abdominal pain or discomfort, and/or an alteration of bowel habit lasting for longer than three months in the absence of any demonstrable underlying organic disease (Ford, 1986). The symptoms that may help distinguish IBS from organic gastrointestinal disease include abdominal pain relieved by defecation, abdominal distension, and a change in bowel habit at the onset of abdominal pain (Manning et al., 1978). Although a variety of organic factors including GI motility disorders, dietary fiber deficiency, food intolerance, and bile acid malabsorption have been postulated or observed in some cases, consistent findings have not been evident in IBS patients compared to control groups (Ford, 1986).

Psychiatric disorders were diagnosed in the majority of patients with IBS in some early studies (Liss, Alpers, & Woodruff, 1973). However, in subsequent research, specific psychiatric or psychological disturbances have not been identified and the findings are even more inconsistent when nonreferred cases are studied. Walker, Roy-Byrne, and Katon (1990) reported, based on a prospective study using structured diagnostic interviews, that major depression was no more common in patients with irritable bowel syndrome than in those with inflammatory bowel disease. Studying selected patients with severe symptoms, many of whom had undergone surgery, Kingham and Dawson (1985) found that 64 percent were significantly depressed according to the Hamilton Rating Scale for Depression. However, using strict criteria for IBS, Whitehead et al. (1988) found that females with IBS who had not sought medical treatment reported no more psychological distress than asymptomatic controls, whereas those who had attended a medical clinic reported more psychological distress than asymptomatic controls or nonconsulters with the same diagnoses. When broader and more conventional criteria for IBS were used, individuals with IBS reported more psychological distress than controls, whether or not they had consulted a physician. Whitehead et al. (1988) concluded that the core symptoms of IBS are related to altered GI motility and not necessarily to psychological distress. They suggest that the association between bowel symptoms and psychological distress in many studies of medical clinic patients may be accounted for by patients with psychological distress who seek treatment of bowel symptoms that other people either ignore or treat themselves. Others believe that patients with IBS may have hypersensitive bowels such that symptoms are easily produced in response to both physiological and emotional stimuli (Toner, Garfinkel, & Jeejeebhoy, 1990; Read, 1987).

In summary, it would appear that patients with IBS who seek medical help often are emotionally distressed, and that some of these individuals suffer from depression of varying degrees of severity. However, there is little evidence to suggest that there is a causal relationship between depression and IBS.

CONCLUSIONS

Chronic pain and other syndromes such as irritable bowel, chronic fatigue, and fibrositis represent difficult clinical problems because of the discrepancy between subjective complaints and objective physical findings. At different points in time, these conditions have been regarded by various investigators as being predominantly organic or psychological in origin. Depression and other psychological symptoms have been identified in many studies of these patients, especially with samples derived from help-seeking populations. Such individuals are often psychologically distressed and may report somatic symptoms because of their tendency toward somatization and symptom amplification. Depression may be associated with any of these syndromes but cannot be considered to be synonymous with or to be a universal accompaniment of any of them. Goldberg and Bridges (1988) recently suggested that somatization may require no particular explanation and that psychologization may be a phenomenon that is peculiar to Western cultures where introspection is highly valued. However, even if this point of view is accepted, it cannot be denied that somatic symptoms complicate the differential diagnosis of medical and psychiatric illness. The problem of diagnosing depression is considerable when there is an obvious medical condition that produces somatic symptoms that mimic depression. The difficulty is further complicated when a poorly defined condition with physical symptoms is also present.

REFERENCES

Acheson, E.D. (1959). The clinical syndrome variously called benign myalgic encephalomyelitis, Iceland disease, and epidemic neuromyasthenia. *American Journal of Medicine, 26,* 569–595.
Ahles, T.A., Yunus, M.B., & Masi, A.T. (1987). Is chronic pain a variant of depressive disease? The case of primary fibromyalgia syndrome. *Pain, 29,* 105–111.
Akiskal, H.S. (1983). Diagnosis and classification of affective disorders: New insights from clinical and laboratory approaches. *Psychiatric Developments, 2,* 123–160.
Amsterdam, J.D., Henle, W., Winokur, A., Wolkowitz, O.M., Pickar, D., & Paul, S.M. (1986). Serum antibodies to Epstein-Barr virus in patients with major depressive disorder. *American Journal of Psychiatry, 143,* 1593–1596.

Barsky, A.J. (1981). Hidden reasons some patients visit doctors. *Annals of Internal Medicine, 94,* 492–498.

Barsky, A.J., Goodson, J.D., Lane, R.S., & Cleary, P.D. (1988). The amplification of somatic symptoms. *Psychosomatic Medicine, 50,* 510–519.

Barsky, A.J., Wyshak, G., & Klerman, G.L. (1986). Hypochondriasis: An evaluation of the DSM-III criteria in medical outpatients. *Archives of General Psychiatry, 43,* 493–500.

Beard, G. (1880). *Nervous Exhaustion (Neurasthenia): Its Nature, Symptoms, and Treatment.* New York: G.P. Putnam's Sons.

Behan, P.O., Behan, W.M.H., & Bell, E.J. (1985). The postviral fatigue syndrome—an analysis of the findings in 50 cases. *Journal of Infection, 10,* 211–222.

Black, R.G. (1975). The chronic pain syndrome. *Surgical Clinics of North America, 55,* 999–1011.

Blumer, D. & Heilbronn, M. (1981). The pain-prone disorder: A clinical and psychological profile. *Psychosomatics, 22,* 395–402.

Blumer, D. & Heilbronn, M. (1982). Chronic pain as a variant of depressive disease: The pain-prone disorder. *Journal of Nervous and Mental Disease, 170,* 381–406.

Blumer, D. & Heilbronn, M. (1987). Depression and chronic pain. In O.E. Cameron (Ed.), *Presentations of Depression: Depressive Symptoms in Medical and Psychiatric Disease.* (pp. 215–235). New York: John Wiley & Sons.

Buchwald, D., Sullivan, J.L., & Komaroff, A.L. (1987). Frequency of "chronic active Epstein-Barr virus infection" in a general medical practice. *Journal of the American Medical Association, 257,* 2303–2307.

Bukberg, J., Penman, D., & Holland, J.C. (1984). Depression in hospitalized cancer patients. *Psychosomatic Medicine, 46,* 199–212.

Burns, B.H. & Nichols, M.A. (1972). Factors related to localization of symptoms to the chest in depression. *British Journal of Psychiatry, 121,* 405–409.

Cadie, M., Nye, F.J., & Storey, P. (1976). Anxiety and depression after infectious mononucleosis. *British Journal of Psychiatry, 128,* 559–561.

Cadoret, R.J., Widmer, R.B., & Troughton, E.P. (1980). Somatic complaints: Harbinger of depression in primary care. *Journal of Affective Disorders, 2,* 61–70.

Chandler, J.D. & Gerndt, J. (1988). Somatization, depression, and medical illness in psychiatric inpatients. *Acta Psychiatrica Scandinavica, 77,* 67–73.

Clark, S., Campbell, S.M., Forehand, M.E., Tindall, E.A., & Bennett, R.M. (1985). Clinical characteristics of fibrositis: II. A "blinded," controlled study using standard psychological tests. *Arthritis and Rheumatism, 28,* 132–137.

Craven, J.L., Rodin, G.M., Johnson, L., & Kennedy, S.H. (1987). The diagnosis of major depression in renal dialysis patients. *Psychosomatic Medicine, 49,* 482–492.

Engel, G.L. (1962). Anxiety and depression-withdrawal: The primary effects of unpleasure. *International Journal of Psychoanalysis, 43,* 89–97.

Escobar, J.I., Rubio-Stipec, M., Canino, G., & Karno, M. (1989). Somatic Symptom Index (SSI): A new and abridged somatization construct: Prevalence and epidemiological correlates in two large community samples. *Journal of Nervous and Mental Disease, 177,* 140–146.

Fabrega Jr., H., Mezzich, J., Jacob, R., & Ulrich, R. (1988). Somatoform disorder in a psychiatric setting: Systematic comparisons with depression and anxiety disorders. *Journal of Nervous and Mental Disease, 176,* 431–439.

Ford, M.J. (1986). The irritable bowel syndrome. *Journal of Psychosomatic Research, 30,* 399–410.

France, R.D., Houpt, J.L., & Ellinwood, E.H. (1984). Therapeutic effects of antidepressants in chronic pain. *General Hospital Psychiatry, 6,* 55–63.

France, R.D., Houpt, J.L., Skott, A., Krishnan, K.R.R., & Varia, I.M. (1986). Depression as a psychopathological disorder in chronic low back pain patients. *Journal of Psychosomatic Research, 30,* 127–133.

Frank, R.G., Beck, N.C., Parker, J.C., Kashani, J.H., Elliott, T.R., Haut, A.E., Smith, E., Atwood, C., Brownlee-Duffeck, M., & Kay, D.R. (1988). Depression in rheumatoid arthritis. *Journal of Rheumatology, 15,* 920–925.

Freyberger, H., Kunsebeck, H.W., Lempa, W., Wellmann, W., & Avenarius, H.J. (1985). Psychotherapeutic interventions in alexithymic patients: With special regard to ulcerative colitis and Crohn patients. *Psychotherapy and Psychosomatics, 44,* 72–81.

Goldberg, D.P. & Bridges, K. (1988). Somatic presentations of psychiatric illness in primary care setting. *Journal of Psychosomatic Research, 32,* 137–144.

Gowers, W.R. (1904). Lumbago: Its lessons and analogues. *British Medical Journal, 1,* 117–121.

Greenfield, N.S., Roessler, R., & Crosley Jr., A.P. (1959). Ego strength and length of recovery from infectious mononucleosis. *Journal of Nervous and Mental Disease, 128,* 125–128.

Greenspan, S.I. (1981). *Psychopathology and Adaptation in Infancy and Early Childhood: Principles of Clinical Diagnosis and Preventive Intervention.* New York: International Universities Press.

Hadler, H.M. (1986). A critical reappraisal of the fibrositis concept. *American Journal of Medicine, 81,* 26–32.

Hagnell, O. & Rorsman, B. (1978). Suicide and endogenous depression with somatic symptoms in the Lundby study. *Neuropsychobiology, 4,* 180–187.

Hellinger, W.C., Smith, T.F., Van Scoy, R.E., Spitzer, P.G., Forgacs, P., & Edson, R.S. (1988). Chronic fatigue syndrome and the diagnostic utility of antibody to Epstein-Barr virus early antigen. *Journal of the American Medical Association, 260,* 971–973.

Henderson, D.A. & Shelokov, A. (1959). Epidemic neuromyasthenia: Clinical syndrome. *New England Journal of Medicine, 260,* 757–764.

Hendler, N. (1984). Depression caused by chronic pain. *Journal of Clinical Psychiatry, 45,* 30–38.

Holmes, G.P., Kaplan, J.E., Gantz, N.M., Komaroff, A.L., Schonberger, L.B.,

124 /   DEPRESSION IN THE MEDICALLY ILL

Straus, S.E., Jones, J.F., Dubois, R.E., Cunninghan-Rundles, C., Pahwa, S., Tosato, G., Zegans, L.S., Purtilo, D.T., Brown, N., Schooley, R.T., & Brus, I. (1988). Chronic fatigue syndrome: A working case definition. *Annals of Internal Medicine, 108,* 387–389.

Holmes, G.P., Kaplan, J.E., Stewart, J.A., Hunt, B., Pinsky, P.F., & Schonberger, L.B. (1987). A cluster of patients with a chronic mononucleosis-like syndrome: Is Epstein-Barr virus the cause? *Journal of the American Medical Association, 257,* 2297–2302.

Horowitz, M., Marmar, C., Krupnick, J., Wilner, N., Kaltreider, N., & Wallerstein, R. (1984). *Personality Styles and Brief Psychotherapy.* New York: Basic Books, Inc.

House, A. (1988). Mood disorders in the physically ill: Problems of definition and measurement. *Journal of Psychosomatic Research, 32,* 345–353.

Hudson, J.I., Hudson, M.S., Pliner, L.F., Goldenberg, D.L., & Pope Jr., H.G. (1985). Fibromyalgia and major affective disorder: A controlled phenomenology and family history study. *American Journal of Psychiatry, 142,* 441–446.

Ierodiakonou, C.S. & Iacovides, A. (1987). Somatic manifestations of depressive patients in different psychiatric settings. *Psychopathology, 20,* 136–143.

Imboden, J.B., Canter, A., & Cluff, L.E. (1961). Convalescence from influenza: A study of the psychological and clinical determinants. *Archives of Internal Medicine, 108,* 393–399.

Imboden, J.B., Canter, A., Cluff, L.E., & Trever, R.W. (1959). Psychological aspects of delayed convalescence. *Archives of Internal Medicine, 103,* 406–414.

Jones, D. & Hall, S.B. (1963). Significance of somatic complaints in patients suffering from psychotic depression. *Acta Psychotherapeutica, 11,* 193–199.

Jones, J.F., Ray, C.G., Minnich, L.L., Hicks, M.J., Kibler, R., & Lucas, D.O. (1985). Evidence for active Epstein-Barr virus infection in patients with persistent, unexplained illnesses: Elevated anti-early antigen antibodies. *Annals of Internal Medicine, 102,* 1–7.

Katon, W., Hall, M.L., Russo, J., Cormier, L., Hollifield, M., Vitaliano, P.P., & Beitman, B.D. (1988). Chest pain: Relationship of psychiatric illness to coronary arteriographic results. *American Journal of Medicine, 84,* 1–9.

Katon, W., Kleinman, A., & Rosen, G. (1982). Depression and somatization: A review: Part I. *American Journal of Medicine, 72,* 127–135.

Kellner, R. (1986). *Somatization and Hypochondriasis.* New York: Praeger Publishers.

Kellner, R., Abbott, P., Winslow, W.W., & Pathak, D. (1989). Anxiety, depression, and somatization in DSM-III hypochondriasis. *Psychosomatics, 30,* 57–64.

Kingham, J.G.C. & Dawson, A.M. (1985). Origin of chronic right upper quadrant pain. *Gut, 26,* 783–788.

Kirkmayer, L. (1984). Culture, affect, and somatization. *Transcultural Psychiatry Research Review, 21,* 159–188.

Kleinman, A. (1988). *The Illness Narratives: Suffering, Healing and the Human Condition.* New York: Basic Books, Inc.

Kleinman, A.M. (1977). Depression, somatization, and the "new cross-cultural psychiatry." *Social Science and Medicine, 11,* 3–10.

Kramlinger, K.G., Swanson, D.W., & Maruta, T. (1983). Are patients with chronic pain depressed. *American Journal of Psychiatry, 140,* 747–749.

Kruesi, M.J.P., Dale, J., & Straus, F.E. (1989). Psychiatric diagnoses in patients who have chronic fatigue syndrome. *Journal of Clinical Psychiatry, 50,* 53–56.

Krupp, L.B., Alvarez, L.A., LaRocca, N.G., & Scheinberg, L.C. (1988). Fatigue in multiple sclerosis. *Archives of Neurology, 45,* 435–437.

Lane, R.D. & Schwartz, G.E. (1987). Levels of emotional awareness: A cognitive-developmental theory and its application to psychopathology. *American Journal of Psychiatry, 144,* 133–143.

Lesse, S. (1967). Hypochondriasis and psychosomatic disorders masking depression. *American Journal of Psychotherapy, 21,* 607–620.

Lindsay, P. & Wyckoff, M. (1981). The depression-pain syndrome and its response to antidepressants. *Psychosomatics, 22,* 511–577.

Lipowski, Z.J. (1990). Somatization and depression. *Psychosomatics, 31,* 13–21.

Liss, J.L., Alpers, D., & Woodruff Jr., R.A. (1973). The irritable colon syndrome and psychiatric illness. *Diseases of the Nervous System, 34,* 151–157.

Lustman, P.J., Clouse, R.E., & Carney, R.M. (1988). Depression and the reporting of diabetes symptoms. *International Journal of Psychiatry in Medicine, 18,* 295–303.

Magni, G. (1987). On the relationship between chronic pain and depression when there is no organic lesion. *Pain, 31,* 1–21.

Makanjuola, J.D.A. & Olaifa, E.A. (1987). Masked depression in Nigerians treated at the Neuro-Psychiatric Hospital Aro, Abeokuta. *Acta Psychiatrica Scandinavica, 76,* 480–485.

Manning, A.P., Thompson, W.G., Heaton, K.W., & Morris, A.F. (1978). Towards positive diagnosis of the irritable bowel. *British Medical Journal, 2,* 653–654.

Manu, P., Lane, T.J., Matthews, K.A., & Escobar, J.I. (1989). Screening for somatization disorder in patients with chronic fatigue. *General Hospital Psychiatry, 11,* 294–297.

Martin, J.B. & Pihl, R.O. (1985). The stress-alexithymia hypothesis: Theoretical and empirical considerations. *Psychotherapy and Psychosomatics, 43,* 169–176.

Maruta, T., Vatterot, M.D., & McHardy, M.J. (1989). Pain management as an antidepressant: Long-term resolution of pain-associated depression. *Pain, 36,* 335–337.

The Medical Staff of the Royal Free Hospital (1957). An outbreak of encephalomyelitis in the Royal Free Hospital Group, London, in 1955. *British Medical Journal, 2,* 895–904.

Moldofsky, H., Krueger, J.M., Walter, J., Dinarello, C.A., Lue, F.A., Quance,

126 /   DEPRESSION IN THE MEDICALLY ILL

G., & Oreopoulos, D.G. (1985). Sleep-promoting material extracted from peritoneal dialysate of patients with end-stage renal disease and insomnia. *Peritoneal Dialysis Bulletin, 5,* 189–193.

Morrison, J. & Herbstein, J. (1988). Secondary affective disorder in women with somatization disorder. *Comprehensive Psychiatry, 29,* 433–440.

Nelson, E., Kirk, J., McHugo, G., Douglass, R., Ohler, J., Wasson, J., & Zubkoff, M. (1987). Chief complaint fatigue: A longitudinal study from the patient's perspective. *Family Practice Research Journal, 6,* 175–188.

Orenstein, H. (1989). Briquet's syndrome in association with depression and panic: A reconceptualization of Briquet's syndrome. *American Journal of Psychiatry, 146,* 334–338.

Pilowsky, I., Chapman, C.R., & Bonica, J.J. (1977). Pain, depression, and illness behavior in a pain clinic population. *Pain, 4,* 183–192.

Postone, N. (1986). Alexithymia in chronic pain patients. *General Hospital Psychiatry, 8,* 163–167.

Read, N.W. (1987). Irritable Bowel Syndrome (IBS): Definition and pathophysiology. *Scandinavian Journal of Gastroenterology, 130,* 7–13.

Rice, J.R. (1986). "Fibrositis" syndrome. *Medical Clinics of North America, 70,* 455–468.

Rodin, G. (1984). Somatization and the self: Psychotherapeutic issues. *American Journal of Psychotherapy, 38,* 257–263.

Romano, J.M. & Turner, J.A. (1985). Chronic pain and depression: Does the evidence support a relationship? *Psychological Bulletin, 97,* 18–34.

Schaffer, C.B., Donlon, P.T., & Bittle, R.M. (1980). Chronic pain and depression: A clinical and family history survey. *American Journal of Psychiatry, 137,* 118–120.

Sifneos, P. (1972). *Short-Term Psychotherapy and Emotional Crisis.* Boston: Harvard University Press.

Sifneos, P.E. (1973). The prevalence of "alexithymic" characteristics in psychosomatic patients. *Psychotherapy and Psychosomatics, 22,* 255–262.

Sigurdsson, B., Sigurjonsson, J., Sigurdsson, J.H.J., Thorkelsson, J., & Gudmundsson, K.R. (1950). A disease epidemic in Iceland simulating poliomyelitis. *American Journal of Hygiene, 52,* 222–238.

Slocumb, J.C., Kellner, R., Rosenfeld, R.C., & Pathak, D. (1989). Anxiety and depression in patients with the abdominal pelvic pain syndrome. *General Hospital Psychiatry, 11,* 48–53.

Stockman, R. (1904). The causes, pathology, and treatment of chronic rheumatism. *Edinburgh Medical Journal, 15,* 107–116.

Stolorow, R.D., Brandchaft, B., & Atwood, G.E. (1987). *Psychoanalytic Treatment: An Intersubjective Approach.* New Jersey: The Analytic Press.

Stoudemire, A., Kahn, M., Brown, J.T., Linfors, E., & Houpt, J.L. (1985). Masked depression in a combined medical-psychiatric unit. *Psychosomatics, 26,* 221–228.

Straus, S.E., Dale, J.K., Tobi, M., Lawley, T., Preble, O., Blaese, R.M., Hallahan, C., & Henle, W. (1988). Acyclovir treatment of the chronic fatigue syndrome: Lack of efficacy in a placebo-controlled trial. *New England Journal of Medicine, 319,* 1692–1698.

Straus, S.E., Tosato, G., Armstrong, G., Lawley, T., Preble, O.T., Henle, W., Davey, R., Pearson, G., Epstein, J., Brus, I., & Blaese, R.M. (1985). Persisting illness and fatigue in adults with evidence of Epstein-Barr virus infection. *Annals of Internal Medicine, 102,* 7–16.

Swartz, M.N. (1988). The chronic fatigue syndrome: One entity or many? *New England Journal of Medicine, 319,* 1726–1728.

Taerk, G.S., Toner, B.B., Salit, I.E., Garfinkel, P.E., & Ozersky, S. (1987). Depression in patients with neuromyasthenia (benign myalgic encephalomyelitis). *International Journal of Psychiatry in Medicine, 17,* 49–56.

Taylor, G.J. (1984). Alexithymia: Concept, measurement, and implications for treatment. *American Journal of Psychiatry, 141,* 725–732.

Tobi, M., Ravid, Z., Feldman-Weiss, V., Ben-Chetrit, E., Morag, A., Chowers, I., Michaeli, Y., Shalit, M., & Knobler, H. (1982). Prolonged atypical illness associated with serological evidence of persistent Epstein-Barr virus infection. *Lancet, 1,* 61–64.

Toner, B.B., Garfinkel, P.E., & Jeejeebhoy, K.N. (1990). Psychological factors in Irritable Bowel Syndrome. *Canadian Journal of Psychiatry, 35,* 158–161.

Traut, E.F. (1968). Fibrositis. *Journal of the American Geriatrics Society, 16,* 531–538.

Turk, D.C. & Salovey, P. (1984). 'Chronic pain as a variant of depressive disease': A critical reappraisal. *Journal of Nervous and Mental Disease, 172,* 398–404.

Walker, E.A., Roy-Byrne, P.P., & Katon, W.J. (1990). Irritable bowel syndrome and psychiatric illness. *American Journal of Psychiatry, 147,* 565–572.

Waxman, H.M., McCreary, G., Weinrit, R.M., & Carner, E.A. (1985). A comparison of somatic complaints among depressed and non-depressed older persons. *Gerontologist, 25,* 501–507.

Whitehead, W.E., Bosmajian, L., Zonderman, A.B., Costa Jr., P.T., & Schuster, M.M. (1988). Symptoms of psychologic distress associated with irritable bowel syndrome: Comparison of community and medical clinic samples. *Gastroenterology, 95,* 709–714.

Widmer, R.B. & Cadoret, R.J. (1978). Depression in primary care: Changes in pattern of patient visits and complaints during a developing depression. *Journal of Family Practice, 7,* 293–302.

Williams, J.B.W. & Spitzer, R.L. (1982). Idiopathic Pain Disorder: A critique of Pain-Prone Disorder and a proposal for a revision of the DSM-III category Psychogenic Pain Disorder. *Journal of Nervous and Mental Disease, 170,* 415–419.

Williamson, P.S. & Yates, W.R. (1989). The initial presentation of depression in family practice and psychiatric outpatients. *General Hospital Psychiatry, 11,* 188–193.

Wilson, P.M.J., Kusumakar, V., McCartney, R.A., & Bell, E.J. (1989). Features of Coxsackie B virus (CBV) infection in children with prolonged physical and psychological morbidity. *Journal of Psychosomatic Research, 33,* 29–36.

Wulsin, L.R., Hillard, J.R., Geier, P., Hissa, D., & Rouan, G.W. (1988). Screening emergency room patients with atypical chest pain for depression and panic disorder. *International Journal of Psychiatry in Medicine, 18,* 315–323.

Yousef, G.E., Bell, E.J., Mann, G.F., Marugesan, V., Smith, D.G., McCartney, R.A., & Mowbray, J.F. (1988). Chronic enterovirus infection in patients with postviral fatigue syndrome. *Lancet, 1,* 146–150.

Yunus, M., Masi, A.T., Calabro, J.J., Miller, K.A., & Feigenbaum, S.L. (1981). Primary fibromyalgia (fibrositis): Clinical study of 50 patients with matched normal controls. *Seminars in Arthritis and Rheumatism, 11,* 151–171.

Yunus, M.B. (1983). Fibromyalgia syndrome: A need for uniform classification [editorial]. *Journal of Rheumatology, 10,* 841–844.

4

Course and Complications

The course of major depression may be influenced by a number of factors. These include specific vulnerabilities of the patient, precipitating events, the severity of the syndrome, the social and familial environment, and the provision of and response to treatment (Scott, Barker, & Eccleston, 1988). Symptoms may fluctuate in severity during the course of major depression, and without treatment, the full syndrome may last for up to one year or longer. Certain symptoms (e.g., social apprehension, lack of confidence) may persist following resolution of acute symptoms. In 12 percent to 15 percent of patients, major depression may not fully resolve, but rather continue in a milder form (Robins & Guze, 1972). In some cases, there are specific factors that perpetuate the depression. At least one study has found that chronic treatment with some antihypertensive drugs is associated with chronic depression (Akiskal et al., 1981). The course and duration of a medical condition may also strongly influence the course of depression. Longitudinal studies of major depression have most commonly been undertaken in subjects from psychiatric settings. The small number of studies that have specifically examined the course of depression in patients with physical illness are discussed in this chapter.

Symptoms of depression that interfere with the quality of life include dysphoria, anhedonia, and agitation. In addition, depression itself may produce other adverse effects due to associated psychological, social, and behavioral impairment. For example, reduced interest and concentration may interfere with work or academic functioning, and, in medical patients, with their ability to comply with rehabilitation or other treatment programs. Anhedonia, irritability, and lack of sexual interest may strain patients' personal relationships and compromise the

/ 129

availability of social support at a time when it is most needed. This is most likely to occur when patients or their families are unaware that a depressive disorder is the cause of the changes in the patient. Feelings of hopelessness and self-recrimination may result in self-harm behavior. In the medical patient, this may be manifest with overt suicidal intent, passive death wishes, neglect of self-care, or with a request to discontinue a life-sustaining medical treatment.

This chapter reviews the literature regarding the onset, course, and complications of depression in medically ill patients. Some of the complications are illustrated through case examples. Not all of the potential complications of depressive disorders are reviewed here. Emphasis is placed on the negative effects that are most likely to occur when depression coexists with physical illness.

ONSET OF DEPRESSION

Depression Predating Physical Illness

Depression may precede a physical illness, or it may arise following its diagnosis. Both Carter (1968) and Moffic and Paykel (1975) found that symptoms of depression in hospitalized medical patients predated the recognition of physical illness as recalled by the patients in approximately one-quarter of cases, and followed the onset of physical illness in three-quarters of patients. In a study of the lifetime prevalence of major depression in 60 renal dialysis subjects, Hong et al. (1987) found that major depression preceded the onset of renal disease in 17 percent of patients. Craven et al. (1987) found that six (30 percent) of 20 dialysis patients with a lifetime history of major depressive episode, experienced their first episode prior to the onset of renal disease. Lloyd and Cawley (1978) found that of 18 patients diagnosed with depressive neurosis following a first myocardial infarction, six (33 percent) had been depressed prior to the event. It should be noted, however, that each of these studies were retrospective in design. There may be imperfect recall with regard to the time of onset and sequence of depression and physical illness. Further, depression in some patients may occur following onset of subclinical medical illness, but prior to diagnosis and awareness of illness. However, there is some consistency to the results that suggest that in approximately 20 to 30 percent of depressed medical patients, a history of depression preceded the clinical manifestations of physical illness. From the studies cited, it appears that, in some cases, depressive symptoms were present both prior to and following the onset of illness. In other cases, there was a history of major depression and a subsequent episode was precipitated by physical illness.

Depression preceding physical illness may arise due to a number of mechanisms (see Table 4.1). The relationship may be coincidental when physical illness arises in a person with major depression, dysthymic disorder, or another mood disorder. Alternatively, physical illness may arise as a direct complication of depressive symptoms (e.g., apathy and suicidal thoughts leading to self-neglect, noncompliance with medical treatment, overt self-harm, or lack of self-care), or as a result of treatment for depression (e.g., hepatic complications with tricyclic an-

TABLE 4.1. *Postulated Mechanisms for Depression Associated with Physical Illness*

When depression precedes physical illness

immunologic or physiologic changes due to depression

depression as an early symptom of the illness

self-neglect or self-harm leading to physical illness

coincidental co-occurrence

When physical illness precedes depression

biological mechanisms

depressogenic drugs used in treating the illness

effects upon neurochemical pathways mediating mood

immunological or endocrine effects

psychological mechanisms

damaged self-esteem, self-efficacy, self-worth

alterations in body image, sense of identity

social mechanisms

loss of social roles, activities

isolation, stigma, alienation

financial and/or loss

coincidental co-occurrence

tidepressant medications). Depressed patients who delay seeking help when physical symptoms arise may have a greater likelihood of more severe complications. A number of authors have either documented or speculated upon associations between depression and specific medical illnesses. For example, with coronary artery disease depression has been found to be a risk factor of similar magnitude to cigarette smoking (Friedman & Booth-Kewley, 1987). A history of major depressive episode has also been associated with a greater likelihood of myocardial infarction in patients with preexisting coronary artery disease (Stern, Pascale, & Ackerman, 1977; Carney et al., 1988). The physiological mechanisms by which this relationship is mediated are discussed in greater detail later in this chapter.

An association between depression and subsequent malignancy has been less well substantiated. In a study by Shekelle et al. (1981), increased risk of malignancy was reported in patients who were depressed. This finding was interpreted as evidence that depression contributes to the development of a cancer. However, two other studies that found an increased mortality rate among depressed cancer patients reported that death was not due to carcinoma (Evans, Baldwin, & Gath, 1974; Innes & Millar, 1970). Indirect evidence that depression does not contribute to cancer incidence or mortality also arises from two longitudinal studies. First, veterans disabled by "psychoneurosis" in 1944 did not show an increased risk of developing cancer 24 years later (Keehn, Goldberg, & Beebe, 1984). Second, cancer-associated deaths were not significantly increased in 4,905 widows in England during a five-year period following their bereavement (Jones, Goldblatt, & Leon, 1984). Finally, Fox (1989), in an extensive review of the literature on the connection between depression and cancer risk, concluded that the evidence for such a relationship is very weak.

Alteration of immune status has been proposed as a mechanism by which depression may contribute to the development of physical illness. Most controlled studies have now documented impairment of immune function in drug-free patients with major depression (Kronfol et al., 1983; Schleifer et al., 1984; Calabrese et al., 1986), showing a reduction of mitogen-induced lymphocyte stimulation. Cappel et al. (1978) followed patients with depression and found a significantly increased mitogen response after recovery from depression. In addition, Schleifer et al. (1985) reported both a generalized reduction in the number of peripheral blood lymphocytes and a reduction in the numbers of both of the major lymphocyte subclasses (T and B cells). In this study, there was no difference in the proportion of these cell groups in depressed patients compared with controls matched for age and sex. Changes in lymphocyte function have also been demonstrated in bereaved persons with a symptom profile similar to that of patients with depressive disorders (Bartrop et al., 1977; Schleifer et al., 1983).

There are several pathways by which depression might be associated with changes in immune parameters. Hypercortisolemia, which may occur in depression, has long been recognized as an immunosuppressant. Depression has also been associated with changes in growth hormone, luteinizing hormone secretion, and in the hypothalamic-pituitary-thyroid axis, all of which may themselves be related to alteration of immune parameters (Schleifer et al., 1984). The specific immunologic changes associated with depression continue to be an active area of investigation.

Although laboratory tests have documented that immune changes are associated with depression, it has been much more difficult to demonstrate that these changes are causally related to the occurrence of physical illness or dysfunction. There have been some reports that depression tends to be associated with infection (Rimon et al., 1971; Lycke, Norby, & Roos, 1974) and allergic disorders (Nasr, Altman, & Meltzer, 1981), but, even with these conditions, results are conflicting. With the possible exception of relatively minor infections or allergies, there is little direct data to confirm the hypothesis that depression is associated with the onset of physical illnesses due to impaired immune function. In fact, Hall (1987) has argued that the effect of psychological factors on the immune response is always marginal and inconsequential. He suggested that the only reliable indicator of immune deficit is an increased incidence of serious infection. However, all studies of the effect of depression on immunity have relied upon laboratory indicators of immune activity. The association of depression with impaired immune status and physical illness deserves further investigation. Conclusions about the clinical relevance of these findings are premature at this time.

With some medical conditions, depressive symptoms or a depressive disorder preceding a physical illness may be an early manifestation of the illness, rather than a risk factor for its development. A study by Santamaria, Tolosa, and Valles (1986) suggested that depression may be an early presenting feature of at least one subgroup of patients with Parkinson's disease. Of 34 Parkinson patients, they found one with major depression and 10 with minor depression. Interestingly, 10 of the 11 depressed patients became depressed prior to the onset of motor symptoms, suggesting that depression was not a secondary result of disability. Based on a review of the literature, Brown and Paraskevas (1982) suggested that depression may also be an initial manifestation of malignancy. In particular, depressive symptoms or a major depressive episode may be an early presenting feature of cancer of the pancreas (Joffe et al., 1986) and lung (Hughes, 1985). The mechanisms by which depression may occur in this context remain unclear (see Chapter 8), but may include the production of psychotropic neuroendocrine substances by the malignancy, or the psychological response of a patient to undifferentiated somatic experiences related to the undetected tumor.

Davies, Davies, and Delpo (1986) designed an interesting predictive study to determine if symptoms of depression were an early presenting feature of head and neck cancer. They administered the Leed's Scale for Anxiety and Depressive Symptoms (SAD) to 72 consecutive admissions to an assessment unit for head and neck carcinoma. Moderate depression was defined by a score of six or more on the SAD. All patients had lesions that could potentially represent malignancies, although this diagnosis was later substantiated in only 38 patients. Patients who were subsequently found to be biopsy-positive for malignancy had a greater prevalence of moderate depression (29 percent) than those who were biopsy negative (17 percent). These results suggest that depressive symptoms in these patients were related to the physical effects of the illness and were not due entirely to worry about it.

When depression occurs before the somatic presentation of a physical illness, there is a risk that the medical diagnosis will be delayed or even missed. For example, there have been reports that mood changes and other psychiatric symptoms early in the course of normal pressure hydrocephalus contribute to a delay in the recognition of potentially reversible neurological deficits (Rosen & Swigar, 1976). Others have suggested that a delay in the diagnosis of cancer of the pancreas may occur when depression is the presenting feature and becomes the initial focus of treatment (Savage & Noble, 1954). Several series of cases have been reported in which the diagnosis of a physical illness was delayed when depression dominated the clinical picture (Rossman, 1969; Wingfield, 1967; Stokes et al., 1954; Herridge, 1960). Hall (1980) has compiled an extensive list of physical illnesses that may present with symptoms of mood disturbance including epilepsy, multiple sclerosis, porphyria, neurofibromatosis, amyotrophic lateral sclerosis, carcinoma, thyrotoxicosis, myxedema, and endocarditis. Hoffman and Koran (1984) proposed some guidelines designed to optimize the detection of physical illness in patients presenting with psychiatric disorders. They suggested that the evaluation of the depressed patient should include consideration of certain organic conditions in combination with medical functional enquiry, physical examination, and laboratory testing as indicated.

A minority of medical patients who are depressed have a previous history of depressive disorder. These patients may or may not be depressed at the time of onset or diagnosis of a physical illness. Craven et al. (1987) diagnosed a current major depressive episode in 8 percent of a sample of 99 renal dialysis patients. Almost all of the depressed patients had been on dialysis less than two years, and 50 percent had a past history of MDE. This suggests that the initiation of renal dialysis sometimes precipitated depression, particularly in those with a past history of depression. Lustman, Griffith, and Clouse (1988) found that adults with diabetes who met DSM-III criteria for major depressive episode at initial assessment were far more likely to have recurrent major depression during a five-year follow-up period than were patients without depression at the time of initial assessment. Of course, nonmedically ill persons with a previous history of major depression are also at increased risk of recurrent depressive disorder (Amenson & Lewinsohn, 1981; Zeiss & Lewinsohn, 1988). Thus, the connection between medical illness and recurrent depression may be coincidental. However, the stressful circumstances facing an individual with a chronic illness may compound other factors predisposing to depression. It has also been hypothesized that an episode of depression may "scar" an individual in some manner that increases subsequent susceptibility to depression.

Preexisting personal vulnerabilities may help explain why the presence of depression or other psychiatric disorders prior to the onset of an illness-related event appears to have important implications for subsequent adjustment. Lloyd and Cawley (1983) administered a clinical psychiatric interview to assess maladjustment in 100 men who had survived one week following myocardial infarction. The group with a psychiatric disorder prior to myocardial infarction had significantly greater psychiatric morbidity following the infarction. By contrast, men whose emotional disturbances were precipitated by the infarction largely recovered during follow-up. After one year, they resembled patients who had no substantial psychiatric morbidity either before or immediately following infarction. The authors concluded that the patients with a preexisting psychiatric disturbance were most likely to demonstrate persistent emotional disturbance following myocardial infarction. For the remainder, the event tended not to be associated with severe or persistent emotional disability. Indeed, it is not surprising that individuals who are psychiatrically more vulnerable will experience increased psychiatric morbidity following any stressful life event.

The following case illustrates some of the implications of major depression that predates the onset of a physical illness.

Case Example

■ Mrs. Q. was a 42-year-old woman who was referred for depression six weeks following the diagnosis of an intrahepatic malignancy. She reported, and her family confirmed, that she had been depressed for approximately one year prior to the diagnosis of cancer. The patient also reported a lengthy previous history of recurrent but untreated major depressive episodes. Mrs. Q. was initially pessimistic about the possible benefit of chemotherapy and was reluctant to begin such treatment. However, this point of view seemed due, at least in part, to her depressed mood. With the encouragement of family and friends, she finally agreed to begin chemotherapy. Because of major depression, nortriptyline was also started in a low dosage of 10 milligrams orally at bedtime. Unfortunately, due to medical complications unrelated to antidepressant treatment, the drug dosage was not increased so that therapeutic levels were not obtained for another six weeks.

During the period of untreated depression, Mrs. Q. was plagued by feelings of hopelessness and guilt, and she reported fantasies of passive death. Psychotherapeutic interventions were ineffective in the face of her emotional detachment and her abject feelings of worthlessness and hopelessness. It was subsequently possible to increase the nortriptyline to 30 mg daily. This oral dose resulted in plasma levels within the therapeutic range for this drug. Within four weeks after this increase, her medical condition stabilized and her mood improved. At this time, she decided to return to her home in a distant city and to continue both the chemotherapy and the nortriptyline. ■

This case illustrates some implications of major depression developing prior to the diagnosis of a malignancy. In view of the relatively long period of time between the onset of depressive symptoms and the medical diagnosis, the co-occurrence of cancer with depression may have been coincidental. Alternatively, a subclinical physical disturbance may have triggered her depression on a psychological or biological basis before the malignancy had openly declared itself. In view of her previous episodes of major depression, Mrs. Q. may have been predisposed to develop depression with the onset of a malignancy. In any case, the presence of depression at the time of onset of the tumor complicated the initial management of the medical condition. Without the support of family members, she may well have declined life-saving chemotherapy as a result of her depressed mood. This patient appeared to have had a positive therapeutic response to relatively low doses of nortriptyline, although it is also possible that her depressive symptoms remitted because of the improvement in her medical condition.

Physical Illness Predating Depression

The mechanisms by which depression may follow the onset of physical illness are the primary focus of several chapters in this text. Biological, psychological, and social pathways may be involved in this process (see Table 4.1.). Additional illness-related situations that may be associated with the occurrence or exacerbation of depression in physically ill patients are listed in Table 4.2.

The onset, diagnosis, or exacerbation of a life-threatening physical illness such as coronary artery disease or carcinoma may directly contribute to depression in some patients. Roth and Kay (1956) found that the onset or exacerbation of physical illness was a prominent factor associated with the development of depression in the elderly. Similarly, substantial changes in prognosis (e.g., discovery of bony metastases in a woman with a history of breast cancer), or the occurrence of significant complications of an ongoing illness (e.g., retinopathy in patients with insulin dependent diabetes mellitus), are highly disturbing events that may precipitate depression. In other cases, a substantial change in medical treatment may be associated with depression. For example, prescription medications such as reserpine, propranolol, and methyldopa have been implicated in the pathogenesis of organic depressive syndromes (see Chapter 8). The prevalence of depression in patients with endstage renal disease is highest during the first two years after initiation of renal dialysis, a treatment associated with dramatic physical and psychosocial changes (Craven et al., 1987). For patients with chronic obstructive lung disease, the initiation of continuous ambulatory oxygen therapy may be associated with deterioration in social activity and

TABLE **4.2.** *Illness-Related Situations That May Trigger Depression*

Onset or diagnosis of a physical illness

Change in treatment modality

Change in prognosis

Intensive treatment regimen

Other negative life events secondary to illness

Significant medical complications

overall quality of life (Marchionno et al., 1985). These changes in physical health may contribute to depression.

A major series of studies have examined the onset and course of depression following stroke (Robinson & Price, 1982; Robinson et al., 1983). During a preliminary investigation using the General Health Questionnaire, Robinson and Price (1982) found that 30 percent of patients demonstrated moderately severe depressive symptoms following stroke. These symptoms were most common six to twenty-four months following the stroke, and, in two-thirds of the patients, were still present at follow-up examination seven to eight months later. In a replication study, this same group used the Present State Examination (PSE), Hamilton Rating Scale for Depression (HAM-D), and the Zung Self-Rating Depression Scale (SDS) to make DSM-III diagnoses of depressive disorders and to determine the time of onset of the disorders (Robinson et al., 1983). They found that 27 percent of 103 subjects demonstrated a major depressive episode (MDE) and 20 percent had dysthymic disorder (DD). The depressive syndrome most commonly began within two weeks of the stroke. At six-month follow-up, three-quarters of the patients with MDE still met criteria for this disorder, and over 40 percent of those with DD had developed MDE.

Interestingly, major depression may follow an intensive treatment regardless of the medical outcome of the treatment. This "paradoxical depression" has been described by Blacher (1987) following a successful surgical procedure in which psychological mechanisms such as survivor guilt may be involved. Medical staff may be slow to identify such "paradoxical" depression, or to recognize biological mechanisms which may be contributory. This delayed onset of depression may occur because denial and other defensive operations during the immediate stress of acute illness may have postponed the opportunity to reflect upon the implications of the illness. In such cases, a full awareness of the meaning of the illness may occur only after the acute phase has passed. More serious symptoms of depression may then be triggered.

Case Example

■ Mrs. L., a 47-year-old woman with acute myelogenous leukemia of five months duration, obtained a remission of her illness with intermittent chemotherapy. Prior to the remission, Mrs. L. had periodically voiced concerns about dying and about being unable to look after her five-year-old grandson for whom she was the official guardian. However, she did not demonstrate other signs or symptoms of clinical depression and persistently declined any psychotherapeutic interventions that were offered. She feared that discussing her worries would lead to depression and that it would then be "all over for me."

Several days after being told that she was in remission, Mrs. L. became profoundly depressed. She lost all interest in her medical care and she was plagued by guilty ruminations and the fear of dying at any moment. She lost her appetite, was reluctant to accept visitors into her room, and felt unable to enjoy any of her previous activities or social relationships. Mrs. L. felt that her mood would improve if she were discharged home and medical staff agreed to this plan. However, at oncology follow-up clinic one month later, it was evident that her depressive symptoms had not resolved and that she felt increasingly frustrated at "not feeling myself." Nortriptyline 50 mg qhs was started at this time and, within two weeks at this dose, she reported an improved mood. She now felt able to face her greatest worry about the future of her grandson, and was able to proceed with practical arrangements to ensure that he would be well looked after if she were to die. Following one month of nortriptyline treatment, Mrs. L. stated that she was feeling herself again. She continued this treatment for three subsequent months and then discontinued the antidepressant on her own and without recurrence. ■

This case illustrates the paradoxical occurrence of depression after a successful treatment for a serious medical condition. It may be that the immediate concerns of treatment permitted this patient to avoid temporarily the more global implications of her illness. It may also be that the cumulative effect of illness-related stress finally led to the onset of a depressed state. Supportive psychotherapeutic interventions in such cases during the period of acute medical illness can have a prophylactic effect with regard to the occurrence of clinical depression. However, the patient described was too fearful that she would be overwhelmed by feelings that would emerge, to consider any form of psychotherapy. Her blunted affect may have been a manifestation, not only of her depression, but of the emotional constriction in the medically ill referred to as "secondary alexithymia" (see Chapter 3). Major depression in this woman was understandable in terms of her severe medical illness, and limited capacity to tolerate distressing affects. However, pharmacologic treatment was eminently successful and facilitated the patient's capacity to face her fears.

COURSE OF DEPRESSION

In the physically ill, evaluating the course of depression is especially important in determining its clinical significance. Because mild or even severe symptoms of depression may fluctuate depending upon the medical state, Ford (1988) has raised a valid concern that cross-sectional surveys of depression in medical patients may be identifying those who are only transiently depressed. This is most likely to occur in studies that employ, for case definition or screening purposes, self-report measures of depressive symptoms at a single point in time (see Chapter 1). When standardized diagnostic criteria incorporating a threshold for duration of symptoms (i.e., DSM-III-R) are used, patients with more persistent syndromes can be identified. However, the degree to which the course of depressive disorders in medical patients parallels that in psychiatric samples remains unclear. Observations about the course of major depression in nonmedical samples cannot necessarily be generalized to the medically ill.

A few longitudinal studies have examined specifically the course of depressive symptoms and depressive disorders in medical patients. Moffic and Paykel (1975) followed general medical inpatients until the time of hospital discharge. They found that the symptoms of depression had not resolved completely by the time of discharge in 72 percent of cases with at least moderate symptoms of depression. Of the 28 percent who did demonstrate full recovery by the time of discharge, most had experienced a dramatic improvement in depressive symptoms concomitant with recovery from an acute life-threatening illness. Hankin and Locke (1982) found that 50 percent of general practice patients who were depressed based on Center for Epidemiologic Studies Depression Scale (CES-D) scores of greater than 15 continued to have elevated scores 12 months after the initial assessment. They found that persistent depressive symptoms were associated with current physical illness, initial reporting of cognitive-affective symptoms of depression, and more severe initial depressive symptoms. Sociodemographic characteristics did not predict which of the depressed patients would continue to have elevated scores at follow-up.

Stern, Pascale, and Ackerman (1977) followed 68 patients for one year following myocardial infarction. They found that 22 percent of patients had at least mild depressive symptoms (SDS >40) during their hospital admission, and that 70 percent of these patients continued to demonstrate substantial depressive symptoms throughout a one-year follow-up period. During a controlled treatment study of mianserin for depression in postmastectomy patients, Maguire et al. (1980) found no evidence in untreated subjects that mood disorders remitted spontaneously. Lalinec-Michaud, Engelsmann, and Marino (1988) administered the SDS and HAM-D to 152 presurgical hysterectomy patients, 72 patients awaiting other pelvic surgeries, and 36 patients awaiting cholecystectomy. A follow-up with these same measures carried out 12 months after surgery found that the mean SDS scores for all patient groups decreased over the year following surgery. However, over 60 percent of patients who initially scored greater than 63 on the SDS continued to have high ratings at one or more follow-up assessments.

An additional three studies have included follow-up assessment of cases who were assigned categorical diagnoses of depressive disorders. Parker, Holmes, and Manicavasagar (1986) screened 564 general practice outpatients with the Beck Depression Inventory and the Zung Self-Rating Depression Scale. Of the 35 high-risk patients who were subsequently interviewed, 61 percent had an adjustment disorder, 11 percent had major depression, 14 percent had dysthymic disorder, 11 percent had uncomplicated bereavement, and 3 percent had atypical depression. As would be expected, given the large proportion of patients diagnosed with the less severe syndromes of adjustment disorder, only 26 percent of the participants remained depressed at six week follow-up. Alternatively, Robinson, Starr, and Price (1984) followed up poststroke patients diagnosed with major depression based on Research Diagnostic Criteria (RDC) during their initial hospital stay. At six-month follow-up, 95 percent of these patients continued to be depressed. These and other studies of poststroke patients show that both major and minor depression occurring during the few months following stroke may persist for up to 24 months (Parikh et al., 1988).

Lustman, Griffith, and Clouse (1988) obtained five-year follow-up data on 37 subjects with diabetes who had been included in a previous study (Lustman et al., 1986). In their initial study, they administered the Diagnostic Interview Schedule (DIS) to 114 patients with diabetes. They found that 33 percent had a lifetime history of major depression. The follow-up assessment, which included readministration of the DIS, was striking in that of 28 patients who reported a previous history of major depression at the initial evaluation, 64 percent reported a major depressive episode during the one year prior to follow-up assessment, 43 percent reported a current major depressive episode, and 14 percent met DSM-III criteria for current dysthymic disorder. By contrast, only 10 percent of those without a previous affective disorder at index evaluation developed depression during the follow-up period. No association was found between the likelihood of depression and the occurrence of diabetic complications. These authors suggested that major depression may have a particularly malevolent course when associated with diabetes.

The need for longitudinal or follow-up studies of depression in the physically ill is highlighted by a series of studies by Rimon (1969). Based on interviews with 100 female patients with rheumatoid arthritis, he found that 29 percent were suffering from a "depressive reaction." Follow-up interviews 15 years later showed that 45 percent of the remaining sample became depressed during the follow-up period (Rimon & Laakso, 1984). These findings suggest that cross-sectional studies of depressive disorders in persons with persistent illness may actually underestimate the proportion of persons who become depressed at some time during the course of their illness.

A substantial number of depressed medical patients continue to demonstrate a disturbance in mood at follow-up assessment. The proportions of patients with persistent depression vary from a low of 26 percent in general practice patients (Parker, Holmes, & Manicavasagar, 1986), to a high of 95 percent in poststroke patients (Robinson, Starr, & Price, 1984). In addition, at least one series of studies has shown that diabetes patients with MDE may be at high risk for recurrent depression. It is not known whether this finding can be replicated in longitudinal studies of patients with other chronic or recurring physical illnesses. However, current research suggests that the course of depressive disorders in the medically ill is not necessarily either transient or benign. To some extent, these findings validate the construct of major depression in these patients and underscore its clinical relevance.

The severity, prognosis, and persistence of medical illness all serve to influence the course of depression. Physical illness may delay recovery from depression and psychological disorders (Mann, Jenkins, & Belsey, 1981). In addition, depression has been observed to persist or recur in patients with continuing illness and to recede with remission of the medical illness (Moffic & Paykel, 1975). The persistence of major depression in medical outpatients was predicted by the number of physical diagnoses at initial assessment (Schulberg, McClelland, & Gooding, 1987), and by level of physical disability in stroke patients (Starkstein, Robinson, & Price, 1988). In a longitudinal study of elderly general medical clinic patients, Kukull et al. (1986) found that the number of new physical diagnoses during the 33-month follow-up period was the best predictor of depression at the final retest. It is likely that for certain conditions, the relationship between persistent depression and persistent disability is bidirectional. Chronic disability may lead to persistent depression in some patients, but the reverse may also be true (Robinson et al., 1984; Parikh et al., 1987).

It is probable that other factors also contribute to the persistence of depression in some patients with physical illness. Although difficult to substantiate without a large prospective study, previous psychiatric disability and certain personality features may impair adjustment to illness and thereby be associated not only with a greater likelihood of depression, but also with a more protracted course. For some patients, physical illness may trigger a series of social, financial, or psychological events that are not necessarily resolved when the overt manifestations of the physical illness remit. These changes may indirectly contribute to the persistence of depression.

In summary, although many patients who become depressed during the course of a physical illness will recover spontaneously with remission of the illness, a substantial proportion will suffer from persistent or recurrent depression. All medical patients who demonstrate symptoms of depression should be closely monitored, and it should not be assumed that depression associated with a medical illness will necessarily resolve without specific antidepressant treatment. In fact, as the following case may illustrate, unexplained persistent somatic symptoms may be an important indication of the presence of a depressive disorder in need of specific treatment.

Case Example

■ Mrs. S. was a 54-year-old woman with a four-year history of idiopathic thrombocytopenic purpura (ITP). She tended to report fatigue, moodiness, and poor concentration during exacerbations of her illness when her platelet count would fall below 40,000 platelets/milliliter. The patient herself regarded these symptoms as indications of her illness activity and was reassured by her previous experience that these symptoms improved with resolution of thrombocytopenia. However, during the year prior to the most recent assessment, she noticed that these symptoms persisted between exacerbations of her ITP. In addition, she experienced decreased ability to work, loss of appetite, loss of sexual interest, marked irritability, persistent loss of energy, passive thoughts of death, and she was preoccupied with worry regarding her prognosis. At the time of psychiatric assessment, when a major depression was diagnosed, ITP had been inactive for over six months. ■

In this case, the persistence of mild depressive symptoms even after the remission of the medical illness, and the progression of depressive symptoms without progression of the disease, led to the suspicion that a major depressive episode had complicated the course of her illness. This patient was successfully treated with a tricyclic antidepressant, and at two-month follow-up stated that she was feeling within 90 percent of herself again.

COMPLICATIONS OF DEPRESSION IN THE MEDICALLY ILL

Increased Morbidity and Mortality

Whether depression presents prior to the onset of physical illness, or as a complication of it, the combined effect can be devastating. Dysphoria, anhedonia, and social withdrawal due to depression may reduce even further the poor quality of life produced by the illness itself. Several studies have demonstrated that both psychiatric and social factors are related to outcome in patients with physical illness (Querido, 1959; Huxley et al., 1979; Hawton, 1981; Mann, Jenkins, & Belsey, 1981). It should be noted, at the outset, that the few studies that have carefully examined the association of increased morbidity and depression in medical samples have found that depression is a likely result, rather than a cause, of poorer medical outcome. However, the work discussed in this chapter on the relationship between depression and poorer medical outcome suggests that it is likely bidirectional. Specific mechanisms have still been shown to account for increased medical morbidity in certain clinical situations involving depression and some physical illnesses. These are discussed in turn, but it will be apparent to the reader that further research is required in this area.

We describe here several studies that have examined, in some depth, the implications of coexisting depression and physical illness. The first of these studies examined the association between depression and increased morbidity and/or mortality in medical inpatients with a variety of physical illnesses. Moffic and Paykel (1975) followed 150 medical inpatients until the time of hospital discharge. Twenty-four percent of these patients were found to have at least mild depressive symptoms as defined by a Beck Depression Inventory score of greater than 13. Ninety-three percent of the patients who were not depressed were discharged home, whereas only 67 percent of the depressed patients were discharged home. Twelve percent of the depressed patients had died and 21 percent were transferred to other hospitals. Although the authors did not include a formal measure of illness severity, they concluded from their findings that depression was most likely to occur in patients with a poorer prognosis.

Maguire et al. (1974) surveyed a group of general medical inpatients for depression using the GHQ. Patients with a GHQ score of greater than 11 were administered the Standardized Psychiatric Interview (SPI). Cases of psychiatric disorder were identified with SPI scores of 2 to 4. Of 45 cases identified in total, 25 (56 percent) had depressive disorders. Hawton (1981) obtained follow-up information 18 months after completion of the initial study on a subgroup of these patients. He found that, in many cases, the psychiatric disorder persisted throughout the follow-up period, and that there was a higher subsequent mortality rate in patients initially demonstrating a psychiatric disorder. The presence of a psychiatric disorder was associated with increased mortality, not only during the hospital admission when the initial study was undertaken, but for several months following discharge from hospital. However, the causal direction of the association could not be determined in this study.

In a later study, Mayou, Hawton, and Feldman (1988) specifically examined the relationship of depression to outcome in a large sample of hospital admissions. These investigators randomly selected subjects from daily lists of emergency and elective hospital admissions. They excluded patients who were too ill to take part in the assessment, patients who were admitted following a suicide attempt, and patients who had stayed in hospital for less than 24 hours. All other patients were administered the GHQ-30 as a screening instrument, and those scoring above a threshold for mild symptoms were interviewed with the Present State Examination (PSE). Those individuals with an affective disorder, and an age and sex-matched group of nondepressed controls were reassessed four and 12 months later with the GHQ-30, the PSE, and a review of clinical status. The investigator responsible for follow-up assessments was blind to the initial findings. The 54 patients who were diagnosed with a mood disorder at initial assessment were found to have a significantly worse outcome at four-month follow-up assessment compared with the control group. Specifically, depressed patients were less likely to have shown recovery or improvement in their physical disorder, and were more likely to have been readmitted. In addition, one-half of the depressed group continued to demonstrate a mood disorder at the time of follow-up. At one-year follow-up, the depressed patients continued to have a poorer physical and psychiatric outcome, and their mortality rate was twice that of the control group. Persistence of the mood disorder was predicted only by the severity of the initial psychiatric disorder, but not by other medical, social, or demographic criteria. However, the authors noted that the patients with a psychiatric disorder had more severe and more chronic physical illnesses at the time of admission to the protocol. They concluded that this initial difference between the groups may have accounted for the poorer medical outcome in the group of patients with mood disorders. They did not find direct evidence that psychiatric or social variables were a direct cause of higher mortality in this group, although they noted that it was not possible with their research design to exclude this possibility.

Indirect evidence that depression may negatively influence the course of physical illness is provided by treatment studies that show a reduction in the indices of medical disease severity following resolution of depression. For example, in a study of 37 women with rheumatoid arthritis, Rimon (1974) found that successful treatment of a depressed mood with antidepressants and/or psychotherapy not only resulted in improved general well-being, but also in decreased activity of rheumatoid disease. Disease activity was measured in this study by clinical examination of affected joints, body weight, hemoglobin levels, and erythrocyte sedimentation rate. Similar findings in depressed patients with rheumatoid arthritis have been reported by Lieb (1983) following treatment with monoamine oxidase inhibitors. However, Lieb (1983) postulated a biological mechanism to account for this effect.

A relationship between depression and mortality has been found in oncology patients. Davies et al. (1973) found that oncology patients with high scores on an "apathetic-given up" scale derived by factor analysis, were more likely to have reduced survival time. Achute and Vauhkonen (1970) found that cancer patients who survived less than one year reported depressive symptoms more frequently than those who survived for more than two years. Plumb and Holland (1981) however, did not find any link between depressive symptoms and increasing nearness to death in their survey of oncology inpatients.

Depression has been associated with poorer outcome following different types of surgical procedures. Tufo and Ostfeld (1968) and Kimball (1969) both found an increased postoperative mortality rate in patients who were depressed prior to open heart surgery. Powers et al. (1988) administered a clinical psychiatric interview and the BDI to 29 patients undergoing psychosocial assessment prior to bariatric surgery for morbid obesity. These investigators found that a preoperative DSM-III-R Axis I diagnosis of a mood disorder or an anxiety disorder prior to surgery was associated with an increased rate of postsurgical medical complications, dietary noncompliance, subclinical bulimia, poor sexual adjustment, and social adjustment difficulties. A BDI score of greater than 10 before surgery was associated with an increased rate of postoperative complications including infection and staple-line dehiscence. Other studies have shown that a history of depression and/or other psychiatric difficulties prior to a clinical event (e.g., myocardial infarction) or surgery (e.g., mastectomy) are associated with increased risk of psychiatric morbidity following the event (Dean, 1987).

Several studies have shown that patients with coronary artery disease (CAD) who are depressed demonstrate poorer psychosocial rehabilitation (Stern, Pascale, & Ackerman, 1977; Mayou, Foster, & Williamson,

1978) and increased mortality (Lebovits et al., 1967; Bruhn, Chandler, & Wolf, 1969; Garrity & Klein, 1975; Stern, Pascale, & Ackerman, 1977) compared with nondepressed patients with CAD. In addition, Greene, Goldstein, and Moss (1972) found that over one-third of patients who die following a first myocardial infarction were significantly depressed for some time prior to the infarction. However, these studies did not systematically control for severity of illness and therefore cannot be used to determine the influence of this factor upon outcome. Carney et al. (1988) reported a 12-month follow-up of 52 patients with CAD who were administered the DIS and measures of clinical status at the time of coronary angiography. They found that the nine patients with major depressive disorder demonstrated a two-fold increase in the incidence of significant cardiac events (e.g., myocardial infarction) during follow-up. Depression was the single best predictor of these events, independent of other risk factors or overall illness severity.

Wai et al. (1981) analyzed a large number of factors that might influence the survival of 285 home-dialysis patients followed for a minimum of 18 months. They compared 204 survivors with 37 dialysis patients who died during the course of the study and found that increased age and higher BDI scores were the two factors most highly associated with increased mortality. Berrios and Samuel (1987) compared the outcome of 43 subjects with both major depression and neurological disease to that of patients with either neurological disease or major depression, but not both. Telephone interviews were conducted between 14 and 65 months following initial assessment. They found that, on both neurologic and mood parameters, patients with both conditions had a poorer course than did those with either condition alone.

Although depression may negatively influence the course of medical illness and increase the risk of death from some illnesses, the causal connection among these factors is unclear. The most likely explanation for the association between depression and poorer medical outcome is that more severe depressive symptoms occur in response to more severe physical illness. Most studies do not control adequately for severity of physical illness. One study that did so (Mayou, Hawton, & Feldman, 1988) indicated that illness severity was most likely responsible for the association of depression with poorer medical outcome and increased mortality. However, in patients with coronary artery disease, at least one study that documented physical state adequately demonstrated that depression contributed to increased morbidity and mortality independent of illness severity (Carney et al., 1988). Several authors have examined psychophysiological mechanisms that may underlie this association. These studies are discussed later in this chapter.

Other investigators have assessed specifically the influence of depression on the functional and/or psychosocial outcome of illness. These studies have most commonly been undertaken in patients with well defined illness events (e.g., myocardial infarction, stroke) that require participation in a recovery/rehabilitation program to optimize functional outcome. As early as 1967, Wynn studied the emotional effects of ischemic heart disease in 400 patients and concluded that depression was a contributing factor to disability in 40 percent. Stern, Pascale, and McLoone (1976) followed 68 patients with diagnosed myocardial infarction for one year after infarction to determine factors which predicted psychosocial adjustment. Of the 15 patients with depression (SDS >40), 70 percent continued to report substantial depressive symptomatology throughout the one-year follow-up. After one year, this group was less likely to have returned to work, and to be sexually active, and was more likely to have been readmitted to a hospital. Mossey et al. (1989) reported that following hip fractures in women, elevated depression scores were associated with poorer functional recovery at 12-month follow-up.

Sinyor et al. (1986) examined the effect of poststroke depression on functional outcome in 64 patients who presented to a rehabilitation facility within weeks of a first stroke. Twenty-two percent of patients demonstrated at least moderate symptoms of depression as indicated by a score of greater than 59 on the Zung Self-Rating Depression Scale. Patients who were depressed demonstrated lower functional ability, as assessed by physiotherapy and occupational therapy staff at admission, at the time of discharge from the program, and at three-month follow-up. The rate of improvement in depressed and nondepressed patients was similar during involvement with the program. However, at follow-up assessment, euthymic patients demonstrated slight improvement or no change in functional status, whereas patients with depression demonstrated marked reductions in functional status. The authors suggested that intensive involvement in the treatment program compensated for the symptoms of depression during the initial phase of rehabilitation, but that after discontinuation of this program, depressive symptoms may have contributed to a decrease in functional level.

Channer et al. (1988) examined the influence of psychological symptoms, including depression and anxiety, on the degree of symptomatic recovery from coronary artery bypass surgery. Forty-one preoperative patients were administered the GHQ-28 and the Clinical Interview Schedule, among other measures of psychosocial status. Patients were defined as "cases" if they scored greater than 9 on the GHQ-28 and reported depressive symptoms when interviewed. These authors found that postoperative exercise tolerance was equal in both groups, but that patients with psychological distress were more likely to report persistent physical symptoms following surgery. In a survey of 11,242 medical clinic attendees, Wells et al. (1989) found strong evidence for an association of depressive symptoms with poor functional outcome in a variety of chronic conditions. Compared with euthymic patients, those with depression tended to have poorer physical and social functioning, poorer perceived current health, and greater bodily pain. Strikingly, the degree of impaired functioning independently associated with depressive symptoms was at least as great as that associated with the chronic medical condition itself.

It is likely that the association of depression with increased morbidity, increased mortality, and impaired psychosocial outcome is due, in some cases, to the presence of more severe physical disorders. In other cases, this association may result from the negative influence of depression on medical course. The latter may be more common for those with persistent or recurrent major depressive disorder. There are several specific mechanisms by which a major mood disorder could result in increased morbidity or mortality in a physically ill patient. These are briefly discussed in the final section of this chapter.

Reduced Compliance with Medical Recommendations

It has been suggested that "emotional factors," including depressed mood or impaired self-worth, may interfere with patients' self-care behavior (DeWys & Herbst, 1977; Schmale, 1979). The majority of studies in this area have examined the relationship of depressive symptoms and impaired compliance. For example, Blumenthal et al. (1982) documented a lower rate of adherence to a structured rehabilitative regimen in depressed patients recovering from myocardial infarction. Studies which investigate specifically the influence of major depression on the ability of patients to adhere to medical recommendations have not been reported. However, in a clinical context, a decreased ability to comply with medical recommendations is a common reason for patients to be referred for psychiatric assessment, and many of these referrals result in a diagnosis of major depression. Loss of interest, hopelessness, and loss of energy may interfere with physical, functional, or vocational rehabilitation. A decreased sense of self-worth and excessive feelings of guilt may inhibit a patient from asking for or accepting assistance. Other symptoms may interfere more directly with specific treatment regimens. For example, loss of appetite may make it difficult to follow dietary recommendations, and the diminished ability of depressed patients to concentrate and to think clearly may impair their ability to self-medicate or to take part in educative programs.

Channer and Rees (1987) have shown that depressed patients with coronary artery disease were able to walk on a standard treadmill for a significantly shorter time and had lower exercise tolerance than similar nondepressed patients. Findings from this study emphasize that mood disturbances in cardiac patients may affect the objective assessment of physical status. This must be considered in cardiac patients, whose ability to exercise is impaired as a result of depression, to prevent them from being inappropriately referred for coronary artery surgery. Depression may similarly adversely affect the exercise tolerance and functional capabilities of patients with COPD (Agle et al., 1973; Dudley et al., 1980). Specifically, Agle et al. (1973) demonstrated, in patients with COPD, that mild symptoms of depression were alleviated by pulmonary rehabilitation, but that more severe symptoms of depression interfered with rehabilitation and were associated with prolonged psychological and functional impairment. Light et al. (1986) demonstrated, over a six-week period, that the distance walked by COPD patients in 12 minutes was more closely related to changes in depression and anxiety scores than to changes in pulmonary status.

Others have studied the mechanisms responsible for the association of depression and impaired performance (Rutter, 1970; Morgan et al., 1983). Depressed mood, pessimism, and low energy are symptoms that appear to be most associated with discrepancies between functional capacity based on exercise testing results and objective measures of pulmonary function. Similarly, depression in poststroke patients has been found to contribute both to cognitive impairment and to the need for long-term rehabilitation to recover from a stroke. Robinson et al. (1986) found, in 38 patients with left hemispheric lesions, that, independent of lesion size, depression was associated with cognitive impairment and decreased performance during rehabilitation. Performance improved in these patients only with amelioration of depression scores. Cognitive impairment may have been one of several mechanisms by which depression and poorer performance were related. Parikh et al. (1988) found that functional activity following stroke was inversely related to depression. This group proposed that depression may lead to diminished motivation to participate in rehabilitative therapies during a critical period of recovery and that this may contribute to impaired functional outcome in the long term. Sinyor et al. (1986) found that depressive symptoms in poststroke patients were associated with coping responses that impaired the level of participation in a rehabilitative program. Treatment directed toward changing these responses included increasing behavioral activity and rational cognition, and reducing feelings of hopelessness.

Case Example

■ Ms. D. was a 21-year-old student with a 15-year history of insulin dependent diabetes mellitus. During her first year away from home attending university, she was admitted to hospital in diabetic ketoacidosis. Following treatment of her hyperglycemia, she was discharged home and returned to live with her parents. She was also referred for psychiatric consultation because of depressed mood.

When seen in psychiatric assessment, the patient reported a two-month history of progressively worsening depressed mood, loss of interest, and feelings of decreased self-worth. She began to seclude herself in her university dormitory, and although she continued to administer her insulin on a regular basis, she did not test her urine or adhere to her diabetic diet. She binged periodically on high caloric food, a behavior which she had not engaged in prior to the onset of the depressive episode. She was started on a tricyclic antidepressant and was followed frequently to monitor and to encourage appropriate medical self-care. Parental assistance in monitoring insulin requirements was necessary for approximately one month. However, after recovery from the depressive episode, she successfully assumed responsibility for her diabetic management.

In spite of a favorable response to treatment, Ms. D. was not convinced that she required psychiatric follow-up or antidepressant treatment, and she discontinued both. Over the next several months, she began to neglect her diabetes, and she was referred back for psychiatric assessment, again profoundly depressed and in very poor metabolic control. She was restarted and successfully treated with a tricyclic antidepressant and this time she was more convinced of the need for ongoing help. She remained on the antidepressant for several months following remission of her depression and she subsequently agreed to be referred to a group intervention for young adults with diabetes mellitus. ■

Noncompliance with the diabetic protocol was intimately associated with depression in this patient. It appeared that the onset of major depression repeatedly resulted in neglect of self-care and subsequent metabolic dyscontrol. As Lustman et al. (1986) concluded in their study of the influence of psychiatric disorders on metabolic control in diabetes, depression may either cause, or result from, poor glucose regulation.

Self-harm Activity

Suicidal ideation has frequently been reported to be less common in depressed medical patients than in depressed psychiatric patients. Nevertheless, acquired medical disability does appear to be a clinical risk factor for a completed suicide. Suicidal ideation in physically ill patients may represent the consideration of a rational alternative to current suffering and/or may arise from frustration, demoralization, or the lack of social support. Major depression may also be associated with suicidal ideation that is active (i.e., the wish to take action to end one's life) or passive (i.e., the wish that life would end without taking an active role in hastening this outcome). However, with a medical illness that requires regular attention to ensure survival, passive suicidal ideation may lead to a fatal outcome if associated with self-neglect. Also, the mood of patients may affect treatment decisions that are made. Rodin et al. (1981) discussed the role of depressed mood in the decision of some patients with endstage renal disease to discontinue dialysis. The death of such a patient would not necessarily be classified as a suicide, although in some cases, the motivation may be similar. Active and passive suicidal actions likely represent part of a continuum of suicidal ideation. Passive self-destructive behavior may occur when other self-harm behavior is unacceptable to the individual or is difficult to act upon.

Surveys of particular physical illnesses have documented a rate of suicide that is higher than in the general population. Abrams, Moore, and Westervelt (1971) reported a high suicide rate in patients with endstage renal disease being treated with maintenance renal dialysis. Other surveys have shown increased suicide rates in oncology patients (Louhivuori & Hakama, 1979; Fox et al., 1982; Marshall, Burnett, & Brasure, 1983). Each of these latter studies has utilized tumor registries with follow-up of death certificates. The risk of suicide for women with cancer ranged from 0.9 to 1.9 times that in the general population, and the risk of suicide for men ranged from 1.3 to 2.3 times the risk in the general population. Fox et al. (1982) derived the suicide rates for all 144,530 cancer patients in the Connecticut Tumor Registry between 1940 and 1973. They found that the suicide rate in males was increased compared with the general population and that the likelihood of death by suicide was greatest soon after the diagnosis. No significant findings were found for women with cancer. However, suicide in men with cancer cannot necessarily be assumed to be associated with clinical depression. AIDS has recently been shown to be associated with a high risk of suicide. Marzuk et al. (1988) found that the relative risk of suicide in men aged 20–59 with AIDS was 36 times that of men this age without this diagnosis, and 66 times that of the general population.

Miller (1987) has discussed etiological factors that may be involved in death from acute episodes of asthma. Psychosocial factors may be implicated in lethal outcomes from acute episodes of asthma as a result of denial that produces delayed treatment, noncompliance with medical treatment, or poor self-care. Some authors have also suggested that the improper use of asthma medications in some patients may represent a suicidal equivalent (Strunk et al., 1985; Wood & Lecks, 1976). Although the proportion of these patients who suffered from depressive symptoms or a depressive disorder prior to death is not known, Miller (1987) argues convincingly that at least some of the maladaptive behavior reported could be secondary to depression. He also suggested that increased cholinergic tone associated with depression could contribute to worsening of the clinical state and even death in the asthmatic patient. This hypothesis is discussed further in the next section.

Case Example

■ Ms. W., a 67-year-old widow, was admitted to the coronary care unit with unstable angina over the preceding 48 hours. She had been diagnosed with angina and severe coronary artery disease several years ago, but her symptoms were previously well controlled with medical treatment. Now that she had apparently become unresponsive to her drug regimen, she was considered a potential candidate for coronary artery bypass grafting.

Following admission to the coronary care unit, her symptoms were easily controlled. However, shortly after transfer to a general medical ward, Ms. W.'s symptoms of pain returned. The treatment team believed that she had surreptitiously been hoarding the prescribed medication. Psychiatric consultation was requested to assess the patient.

Ms. W. was only minimally cooperative during the psychiatric interview. She stated that she had no emotional problems and that there was "no use" wasting time with her as she was going to die soon anyway. From the few questions that she was willing to answer, it became apparent that Ms. W. felt lonely and detached from life since her husband's death three years earlier. Since then, she had withdrawn from activities, had lost interest in food, and had lost 10 pounds. She was cognitively intact and clearly understood the importance of taking her drugs properly. Ms. W. adamantly denied any suicidal ideation and clearly stated that at no time had she ever wished to die. She said that discussion of such things contradicted her religious beliefs, and she asked that the interview be discontinued after these issues were raised. Ms. W. described a lifelong and intense involvement with a fundamentalist religious group.

Later that evening, Ms. W. died following the onset of a cardiac arrythmia. After her death, nursing staff found a quantity of pills at her bedside that were determined to be medications prescribed and brought to her over the previous few days on the hospital ward. She had apparently ingested a large quantity of these pills. A family interview that had been planned prior to Ms. W.'s death was undertaken. Several family members stated that they had suspected that Ms. W. was not taking her drugs but that she had always denied this when approached. She had been living alone and the family could provide little other information regarding her symptoms. They believed that she had "given up" on life three years earlier after her husband had died. ■

This case illustrates unacknowledged suicidal actions in a woman who had some features of a depressive disorder. It seemed likely that her self-harm behavior was related to depression and unresolved grief related to her husband's death. However, her strict religious beliefs prevented her from fully acknowledging or reporting her noncompliance or its lethal motivation.

Physiologic or Immunologic Alterations with Major Depression

Major depression has been associated with alterations in the autonomic nervous system (e.g., increased peripheral sympathetic and parasympathetic activity), in hormonal systems (e.g., growth hormone, luteinizing hormone, and alteration of the hypothalamic-pituitary-thyroid axis with hypercortisolemia), and in the immune system (e.g., diminished mitogen response, lowered levels of circulating T and B lymphocytes). Although these biological alterations may be particularly relevant in the medically ill, their clinical significance is variable. For example, the negative influence of autonomic nervous system changes upon the medical course of coronary artery disease is well established, but the evidence is much less convincing that the immunologic alterations found with depression affect clinical outcome. This literature is more fully discussed in the remainder of this section.

Studies demonstrating an increased morbidity and mortality in depressed patients with coronary artery disease (CAD) are referred to earlier in this chapter. Further evidence of an association between CAD and depression was found in a follow-up study of 62 elderly patients. In this study, patients with major depression based on DSM-III criteria suffered nearly twice the expected mortality due to cardiovascular diseases (Rabins, Harvis, & Koven, 1985). Dreyfuss, Dasberg, and Assael (1969) found that 23 of the 29 inpatients at a psychiatric facility who had experienced a myocardial infarction in hospital had previously suffered from a depressive disorder. In each of the 23 cases, depression had preceded the infarction, usually by several years. In a study of depression during the first 48 hours following myocardial infarction, Silverstone (1987a) found depression was associated with an increased risk of early death, reinfarction, or myocardial arrest. They concluded that depression following infarction was an indication for more prolonged monitoring than is the standard practice. Although it could not be entirely ruled out, Silverstone (1987b) concluded that this association was not simply a result of more extensive infarction or a poorer clinical course.

The strength of the relationship between depression and coronary artery disease has led a number of investigators to postulate specific mechanisms by which depression may contribute to the development of, or worsening of, coronary artery disease. Medically well patients with major depressive disorder have been shown to have increased sympathetic nervous system activity (Esler et al., 1982), elevated catecholamines (Roy et al., 1985), and higher resting heart rates than nondepressed controls (Lahmeyer & Bellier, 1987). Carney et al. (1987) administered the DIS to 77 consecutive patients undergoing elective cardiac catheterization for evaluation of suspected coronary artery disease. They found that heart rate was significantly higher in depressed patients with coronary artery disease than in nondepressed patients. Interestingly, increased mortality in patients with myocardial infarction has been associated with both increased heart rate (Kannel et al., 1987) and with decreased heart rate variability (Kleiger et al., 1987).

Miller (1987) has described some of the preliminary evidence that major depression may be associated with increased parasympathetic activity, or increased "cholinergic tone." Although these changes may be inconsequential for most depressed patients, individuals with asthma may be at particular risk due to changes in their airways that may occur with increased cholinergic sensitivity. Miller has suggested that depression or any other condition that contributes to a preponderance of cholinergic tone in the airways increases the likelihood in asthmatic patients of a compromised clinical state or a neurologically mediated sudden death. However, this hypothesis has not been confirmed by comparisons of cholinergic tone and pulmonary function in depressed asthmatic patients and similar nondepressed patients. As an aside, Miller (1987) noted that tricyclic antidepressants may have a beneficial effect on the airways of asthmatic patients due to the anticholinergic or antihistaminic effects of these drugs.

The neurohormonal changes associated with depression may affect adversely metabolic control in patients with insulin dependent diabetes mellitus (Sachar et al., 1980). Major depression has been associated with both cortisol hypersecretion and elevated plasma catecholamines, both of which may antagonize the actions of insulin. There have been at least two reports of insulin resistance in depressed patients (Mueller, Heninger, & McDonald, 1969; Sachar et al., 1980). Insulin resistance in depressed patients with IDDM could contribute to increased insulin requirements. This would be most dramatic during the afternoon and evening hours when cortisol secretion with depression is greatest. However, to our knowledge, this effect has not been systematically demonstrated in a sample of patients with insulin dependent diabetes mellitus.

As noted earlier in this chapter, immune impairment is one mechanism postulated to account for an increased prevalence of physical illness in patients with depression. For instance, it has been suggested that psychiatric patients with mood disorders may have more frequent active infections with herpes virus accompanied by immune dysfunction (Rimon et al., 1971; Lycke, Norby, & Roos, 1974). One could speculate that immune dysfunction contributes to complications, such as postoperative infections, in patients who were depressed prior to surgery (Powers et al., 1988). However, although depression accompanied by immune impairment is thought by some to have a negative influence on infections, allergies, and malignancies, we are aware of no systematic reports to confirm this speculation.

Many immune changes are not specific to depression but have also been found with stress (Schleifer et al., 1985) and with other psychiatric disorders (Delisi & Crow, 1986). Nevertheless, a depressive response to a stressful event may be the one most strongly associated with immune impairment. In one study, men who were most depressed after either bereavement or serious family illness, had the lowest mitogen response (Linn, Linn, & Jensen, 1984). Another study of immune function in women who had experienced stressful life events found that the severity of depressive symptoms was positively associated with impairment of natural killer cell activity (Irwin et al., 1987). Thus, the individual response to stress, particularly when associated with depression, may be the most important determinant of the degree of immune impairment. Patients with physical illness and depression may be at greatest risk of impaired immune function and its negative consequences. Although still speculative, psychological treatments to optimize coping and to minimize depression have been used as adjunctive therapy based on the rationale that depression suppresses the immune response in life-threatening disease (Ader & Cohen, 1982) and in less serious disorders (Surman et al., 1973). In addition, psychological interventions have been examined in the hope that the immune system might be enhanced in patients particularly vulnerable to immune dysfunction (Kiecolt-Glaser et al., 1985).

It has not yet been convincingly demonstrated that the immune impairment that occurs with depression has significant clinical consequences, particularly for patients with only mild to moderate depressive symptoms. There is, at present, no convincing evidence that enhancing immune functioning should take precedence over facilitating the process of adjustment to a physical illness.

Depression in Specific Medical Situations

The negative influence of depression on the course of physical illness may be due in part to the clinical setting in which it occurs. For example, a profound depressive syndrome occurring during the postoperative course of major surgery may negatively influence rehabilitative care, weight gain, educative efforts, and reintegration into active life (Blacher, 1987). Also, inactivity in the postsurgical patient may increase the risk for postoperative complications such as deep vein thrombosis and pulmonary embolus. Poststroke depression may interfere with physical and occupational therapeutic rehabilitation, which are necessary activities both for optimal medical and functional outcome. Other medical situations in which major depression may particularly influence outcome include depression in the intensive care unit, in burn units, and in patients recovering from disabling medical events (e.g., myocardial infarction, stroke) who require extensive rehabilitative programs.

CONCLUSIONS

Further research is clearly needed with regard to the course and complications of depression in the physically ill. In particular, the routine quantification of both depression and the severity of medical illness over time would contribute to our understanding of the causal relationship between poorer medical outcome and depression. Nevertheless, some preliminary conclusions may be drawn.

Although many patients may experience depressive symptoms that are transient or that may be resolved with alleviation of physical distress, other patients with depressive disorders are at risk of persistent or recurrent depression. The course of depression in these patients may be influenced by factors related to the illness, the person, and the depressive syndrome itself. Clearly, increased severity of medical illness contributes in some patients both to depressed mood and poorer medical outcome. However, a select number of studies have also demonstrated that major depression has a negative influence on medical and functional outcome of a variety of illnesses. More research is needed to substantiate the mediating mechanisms including impaired performance in rehabilitation programs, diminished compliance, active or passive self-harm intent, and alteration of influential physiological or immune parameters.

REFERENCES

Abrams, H.S., Moore, G.L., & Westervelt, F.B. (1971). Suicidal behaviour in chronic dialysis patients. *American Journal of Psychiatry, 127,* 1199–1204.

Achute, K. & Vauhkonen, M.L. (1970). *Cancer and Psyche.* Helsinki: Kunnallispaino.

Ader, R. & Cohen, N. (1982). Behaviourally conditioned immunosuppression and murine systemic lupus erythematosus. *Science, 215,* 1534–1536.

Agle, D.P., Baum, L.G., Chester, E.G., & Wendt, M. (1973). Multidiscipline treatment of chronic pulmonary insufficiency: 1. Psychological aspects of rehabilitation. *Psychosomatic Medicine, 35,* 41–49.

Akiskal, H.S., King, D., Rosenthal, T.L., Robinson, D., & Scott-Strauss, A. (1981). Chronic depressions: Part 1. Clinical and familial characteristics in 137 probands. *Journal of Affective Disorders, 3,* 297–315.

Amenson, C.S. & Lewinsohn, P.M. (1981). An investigation into the observed sex differences in prevalence of unipolar depression. *Journal of Abnormal Psychology, 90,* 1–13.

Bartrop, R.W., Lazarus, L., Luckhurst, E., Kiloh, L.G., & Penny, R. (1977). Depressed lymphocyte function after bereavement. *Lancet, 1,* 834–836.

Berrios, G.E. & Samuel, C. (1987). Affective disorder in the neurological patient. *Journal of Nervous and Mental Disease, 175,* 173–176.

Blacher, R.S. (1987). General surgery and anesthesia: The emotional experience. In R.S. Blacher (Ed.), *The Psychological Experience of Surgery.* (pp. 1–25). New York: John Wiley & Sons.

Blumenthal, J.A., Williams, R.S., Wallace, A.G., Williams, R.B., & Needles, T.L. (1982). Physiological and psychological variables predict compliance to prescribed therapy in patients recovering from myocardial infarction. *Psychosomatic Medicine, 44,* 519–527.

Brown, J.H. & Paraskevas, F. (1982). Cancer and depression: Cancer presenting with depressive illness: An autoimmune disease? *British Journal of Psychiatry, 141,* 227–232.

Bruhn, J.G., Chandler, B., & Wolf, S. (1969). A psychological study of survivors and nonsurvivors of myocardial infarction. *Psychosomatic Medicine, 31,* 8–19.

Calabrese, J.R., Skwerer, R.G., Barna, B., Gulledge, A.D., Valenzuela, R., Butkus, A., Subichin, S., & Krupp, N.E. (1986). Depression, immunocompetence, and prostaglandins of the E series. *Psychiatry Research, 17,* 41–47.

Cappel, R., Gregiore, F., Thirley, L., & Sprecher, S. (1978). Antibody and cell-mediated immunity to herpes simplex virus in psychotropic depression. *Journal of Clinical Psychiatry, 29,* 266–268.

Carney, R.M., Rich, M.W., Freedland, K.E., Saini, J., teVelde, A., Simeone, C., & Clark, K. (1988). Major depressive disorder predicts cardiac events in patients with coronary artery disease. *Psychosomatic Medicine, 50,* 627–633.

Carney, R.M., Rich, M.W., teVelde, A., Saini, J., Clark, K., & Freedland, K.E. (1987). Prevalence of major depressive disorder in patients receiving beta-blocker therapy versus other medications. *American Journal of Medicine, 83,* 223–226.

Carter, F.S. (1968). Treatment of depression associated with chronic gastrointestinal and cardiovascular disorders. *Psychosomatics, 9,* 314–318.

Channer, K.S., O'Connor, S., Britton, S., Walbridge, D., & Rees, J.R. (1988). Psychological factors influence the success of coronary artery surgery. *Journal of the Royal Society of Medicine, 81,* 629–632.

Channer, K.S. & Rees, J.R. (1987). Affect and angina. *Stress Medicine, 3,* 141–146.

Craven, J.L., Rodin, G.M., Johnson, L., & Kennedy, S.H. (1987). The diagnosis of major depression in renal dialysis patients. *Psychosomatic Medicine, 49,* 482–492.

Davies, A.D.M., Davies, C., & Delpo, M.C. (1986). Depression and anxiety in patients undergoing diagnostic investigations for head and neck cancers. *British Journal of Psychiatry, 149,* 491–493.

Davies, R.K., Quinlan, D.M., McKegney, F.P., & Kimball, C.P. (1973). Organic factors and psychological adjustment in advanced cancer patients. *Psychosomatic Medicine, 35,* 464–471.

Dean, C. (1987). Psychiatric morbidity following mastectomy: Preoperative predictors and types of illness. *Journal of Psychosomatic Research, 31,* 385–392.

Delisi, L.E. & Crow, T.J. (1986). Is schizophrenia a viral or immunological disorder? *Psychiatric Clinics of North America, 9,* 115–132.

DeWys, W.K. & Herbst, S.H. (1977). Oral feeding in the nutritional management of the cancer patient. *Cancer Research, 37,* 2429–2431.

Dreyfuss, F., Dasberg, H., & Assael, M.I. (1969). The relationship of myocardial infarction to depressive illness. *Psychotherapy and Psychosomatics, 17,* 73–81.

Dudley, D.L., Glaser, E.M., Jorgenson, B.N., & Logan, D.L. (1980). Psychosocial concomitants to rehabilitation in chronic obstructive pulmonary disease: Part 2. Psychosocial treatment. *Chest, 77,* 544–551.

Esler, M., Turbott, J., Schwarz, R., Leonard, P., Bobik, A., Skews, H., & Jackman, G. (1982). The peripheral kinetics of norepinephrine in depressive illness. *Archives of General Psychiatry, 39,* 285–300.

Evans, N.J.R., Baldwin, J.A., & Gath, D. (1974). The incidence of cancer among in-patients with affective disorders. *British Journal of Psychiatry, 124,* 518–525.

Ford, D.E. (1988). Principles of screening applied to psychiatric disorders. *General Hospital Psychiatry, 10,* 177–188.

Fox, B.H. (1989). Depressive symptoms and risk of cancer. *Journal of the American Medical Association, 262,* 1231.

Fox, B.H., Stanek III, E.J., Boyd, S.C., & Flannery, J.T. (1982). Suicide rates among cancer patients in Connecticut. *Journal of Chronic Diseases, 35,* 89–100.

Friedman, H.S. & Booth-Kewley, S. (1987). The "disease-prone personality": A meta-analytic view of the construct. *American Psychologist, 42,* 539–555.

Garrity, T.F. & Klein, R.F. (1975). Emotional response and clinical severity as early determinants of six-month mortality after myocardial infarction. *Heart and Lung, 4,* 730–737.

Greene, W.A., Goldstein, S., & Moss, A.J. (1972). Psychosocial aspects of sudden death: A preliminary report. *Archives of Internal Medicine, 129,* 725–731.

Hall, J.G. (1987). Depression, stress, and immunity. *Lancet, 2,* 221.

Hall, R.C.W. (1980). Depression. In R.C. Hall (Ed.), *Psychiatric Presentations of Medical Illness: Somato Psychic Disorders.* (pp. 37–63). New York: Spectrum Publications, Inc.

Hankin, J.R. & Locke, B.Z. (1982). The persistence of depressive symptomatology among prepaid group practice enrollees: An exploratory study. *American Journal of Public Health, 72,* 1000–1007.

Hawton, K. (1981). The long-term outcome of psychiatric morbidity detected in general medical patients. *Journal of Psychosomatic Research, 25,* 237–243.

Herridge, C.F. (1960). Physical disorders in psychiatric illness: A study of 209 consecutive admissions. *Lancet, 2,* 949–951.

Hoffman, R.S. & Koran, L.M. (1984). Detecting physical illness in patients with mental disorders. *Psychosomatics, 25,* 654–660.

Hong, B.A., Smith, M.D., Robson, A.M., & Wetzel, R.D. (1987). Depressive symptomatology and treatment in patients with end-stage renal disease. *Psychological Medicine, 17,* 185–190.

Hughes, J.E. (1985). Depressive illness and lung cancer. *European Journal of Surgical Oncology, 11,* 15–20.

Huxley, P.J., Goldberg, D.P., Maguire, P., & Kincey, V. (1979). The prediction of the course of minor psychiatric disorder. *British Journal of Psychiatry, 135,* 535–543.

Innes, G. & Millar, W.M. (1970). Mortality amongst psychiatric patients. *Scottish Medical Journal, 15,* 143–148.

Irwin, M., Daniels, M., Bloom, E.T., Smith, T.L., & Weiner, H. (1987). Life events, depressive symptoms, and immune function. *American Journal of Psychiatry, 144,* 437–441.

Joffe, R.T., Rubinow, D.R., Denicoff, K.D., Maher, M., & Sindelar, W.F. (1986). Depression and carcinoma of the pancreas. *General Hospital Psychiatry, 8,* 241–245.

Jones, D.R., Goldblatt, P.O., & Leon, D.A. (1984). Bereavement and cancer: Some data on deaths of spouses from the longitudinal study of Office of Population Censuses and Surveys. *British Medical Journal, 289,* 461–464.

Kannel, W.B., Kannel, C., Paffenbarger, R.S., Cupples, P.H., & Cupples, L.A. (1987). Heart rate and cardiovascular mortality: The Framington Study. *American Heart Journal, 113,* 1489–1494.

Keehn, R.J., Goldberg, I.D., & Beebe, G.W. (1984). Twenty-four year follow-up of army veterans with disability separations for psychoneurosis in 1944. *Psychosomatic Medicine, 36,* 27–46.

Kiecolt-Glaser, J.K., Glaser, R., Williger, D., Stout, J., Messick, G., Sheppard, S., Ricker, D., Romisher, S.C., Briner, W., Bonnell, G., & Donnerberg, R. (1985). Psychosocial enhancement of immunocompetence in a geriatric population. *Health Psychology, 4,* 25–41.

Kimball, C.P. (1969). Psychological responses to the experience of open heart surgery: I. *American Journal of Psychiatry, 126,* 348–359.

Kleiger, R.E., Miller, J.P., Bigger, J.T., & Moss, A.J. (1987). Decreased heart rate variability and its association with mortality after myocardial infarction. *American Journal of Cardiology, 59,* 256–262.

Kronfol, Z., Silva Jr., J., Greden, J., Dembinski, S., Gardner, R., & Carroll, B. (1983). Impaired lymphocyte function in depressive illness. *Life Sciences, 33,* 241–247.

Kukull, W.A., Koepsell, T.D., Inui, T.S., Borson, S., Okimoto, J., Raskind, M.A., & Gale, J.L. (1986). Depression and physical illness among elderly general medical clinic patients. *Journal of Affective Disorders, 10,* 153–162.

Lahmeyer, H.W. & Bellier, S.N. (1987). Cardiac regulation and depression. *Journal of Psychiatric Research, 21,* 1–6.

Lalinec-Michaud, M., Engelsmann, F., & Marino, J. (1988). Depression after hysterectomy: A comparative study. *Psychosomatics, 29,* 307–314.

Lebovits, B.Z., Shekelle, R.B., Ostfeld, A.M., & Paul, O. (1967). Prospective and retrospective psychological studies of coronary heart disease. *Psychosomatic Medicine, 29,* 265–272.

Lieb, J. (1983). Remission of rheumatoid arthritis and other disorders of immunity in patients taking monoamine oxidase inhibitors. *International Journal of Immunopharmacology, 5,* 353–357.

Light, R.W., Merrill, E.J., Despars, J., Gordon, G.H., & Mutalipassi, L.R. (1986). Doxepin treatment of depressed patients with chronic obstructive pulmonary disease. *Archives of Internal Medicine, 146,* 1377-1380.

Linn, M.W., Linn, B.S., & Jensen, J. (1984). Stressful events, dysphoric mood, and immune responsiveness. *Psychological Reports, 54,* 219-222.

Lloyd, G.G. & Cawley, R.H. (1978). Psychiatric morbidity in men one week after first acute myocardial infarction. *British Medical Journal, 2,* 1453-1454.

Lloyd, G.G. & Cawley, R.H. (1983). Distress or illness? A study of psychological symptoms after myocardial infarction. *British Journal of Psychiatry, 142,* 120-125.

Louhivuori, K.A. & Hakama, M. (1979). Risk of suicide among cancer patients. *American Journal of Epidemiology, 109,* 59-65.

Lustman, P.J., Griffith, L.S., & Clouse, R.E. (1988). Depression in adults with diabetes: Results of 5-year follow-up study. *Diabetes Care, 11,* 605-612.

Lustman, P.J., Griffith, L.S., Clouse, R.E., & Cryer, P.E. (1986). Psychiatric illness in diabetes mellitus: Relationship to symptoms and glucose control. *Journal of Nervous and Mental Disease, 174,* 736-742.

Lycke, E., Norby, E., & Roos, B.E. (1974). A serological study of mentally ill patients with particular reference to the prevalence of herpes virus infections. *British Journal of Psychiatry, 124,* 273-279.

Maguire, G.P., Julier, D.L., Hawton, K.E., & Bancroft, J.H.J. (1974). Psychiatric morbidity and referral on two general medical wards. *British Medical Journal, 1,* 268-270.

Maguire, G.P., Tait, A., Brooke, M., Thomas, C., Howat, J.M.T., Sellwood, R.A., & Bush, H. (1980). Psychiatric morbidity and physical toxicity associated with adjuvant chemotherapy after mastectomy. *British Medical Journal, 281,* 1179-1180.

Mann, A.H., Jenkins, R., & Belsey, E. (1981). The twelve-month outcome of patients with neurotic illness in general practice. *Psychological Medicine, 11,* 535-550.

Marchionno, P.M., Kirilloff, L.H., Openbrier, D.R., & Dauber, J.H. (1985). Effects of continuous oxygen therapy on body image and lifestyle in patients with COPD. *American Review of Respiratory Disease, 131,* A163.

Marshall, J.R., Burnett, W., & Brasure, J. (1983). On precipitating factors: Cancer as a cause of suicide. *Suicide and Life-Threatening Behavior, 13,* 15-27.

Marzuk, P.M., Tierney, H., Tardiff, K., Gross, E.M., Morgan, E.B., Hsu, M.A., & Mann, J.J. (1988). Increased risk of suicide in persons with AIDS. *Journal of the American Medical Association, 259,* 1333-1337.

Mayou, R., Foster, A., & Williamson, B. (1978). The psychological and social effects of myocardial infarction on wives. *British Medical Journal, 1,* 699-701.

Mayou, R., Hawton, K., & Feldman, E. (1988). What happens to medical patients with psychiatric disorder? *Journal of Psychosomatic Research, 32,* 541-549.

Miller, B.D. (1987). Depression and asthma: A potentially lethal mixture. *Journal of Allergy and Clinical Immunology, 80,* 481–486.

Moffic, H.S. & Paykel, E.S. (1975). Depression in medical inpatients. *British Journal of Psychiatry, 126,* 346–353.

Morgan, A.D., Peck, D.F., Buchanan, D.R., & McHardy, G.J.R. (1983). Effect of attitudes and beliefs on exercise tolerance in chronic bronchitis. *British Medical Journal, 286,* 171–173.

Mossey, J.M., Mutran, E., Knott, K., & Craik, R. (1989). Determinants of recovery 12 months after hip fracture: The importance of psychosocial factors. *American Journal of Public Health, 79,* 279–286.

Mueller, P.S., Heninger, G.R., & McDonald, R.K. (1969). Insulin tolerance test in depression. *Archives of General Psychiatry, 21,* 587–594.

Nasr, S., Altman, E.G., & Meltzer, H.Y. (1981). Concordance of atopic and affective disorders. *Journal of Affective Disorders, 3,* 291–296.

Parikh, R.M., Lipsey, J.R., Robinson, R.G., & Price, T.R. (1987). Two-year longitudinal study of post-stroke mood disorders: Dynamic changes in correlates of depression at one and two years. *Stroke, 18,* 579–584.

Parikh, R.M., Lipsey, J.R., Robinson, R.G., & Price, T.R. (1988). A two year longitudinal study of poststroke mood disorders: Prognostic factors related to one and two year outcome. *International Journal of Psychiatry in Medicine, 18,* 45–56.

Parker, G., Holmes, S., & Manicavasagar, V. (1986). Depression in general practice attenders: "Caseness", natural history and predictors of outcome. *Journal of Affective Disorders, 10,* 27–35.

Plumb, M. & Holland, J. (1981). Comparative studies of psychological function in patients with advanced cancer: II. Interviewer-rated current and past psychological symptoms. *Psychosomatic Medicine, 43,* 243–254.

Powers, P.S., Rosemurgy, A.S., Coovert, D.L., & Boyd, F.R. (1988). Psychosocial sequelae of bariatric surgery: A pilot study. *Psychosomatics, 29,* 283–288.

Querido, A. (1959). Forecast and follow-up: An investigation into the clinical, social, and mental factors determining the results of hospital treatment. *British Journal of Preventive and Social Medicine, 13,* 33–49.

Rabins, P.V., Harvis, K., & Koven, S. (1985). High fatality rates of late-life depression associated with cardiovascular disease. *Journal of Affective Disorders, 9,* 165–167.

Rimon, R. (1969). A psychosomatic approach to rheumatoid arthritis. *Acta Rheumatologica Scandinavica [Suppl], 13,* 1.

Rimon, R. (1974). Depression in rheumatoid arthritis. *Annals of Clinical Research, 6,* 171–175.

Rimon, R., Halonen, P., Anttinen, E., & Evola, K. (1971). Complement fixing antibody to herpes simplex virus in patients with psychotic depression. *Diseases of the Nervous System, 32,* 822–824.

Rimon, R. & Laakso, R.L. (1984). Overt psychopathology in rheumatoid arthritis: A fifteen-year follow-up study. *Scandinavian Journal of Rheumatology, 13,* 324–328.

Robins, E. & Guze, S.B. (1972). Classification of affective disorders: The primary-secondary, the endogenous-reactive, and the neurotic-psychotic concepts. In T.A. Williams, M.M. Katz, & J.A. Shield Jr. (Eds.), *Recent Advances in the Psychobiology of the Depressive Illnesses.* (pp. 283–293). Washington, D.C.: US Government Printing Office.

Robinson, R.G., Bolla-Wilson, K., Kaplan, E., Lipsey, J., & Price, T.R. (1986). Depression influences intellectual impairment in stroke patients. *British Journal of Psychiatry, 148,* 541–547.

Robinson, R.G. & Price, T.R. (1982). Post-stroke depressive disorders: A follow-up study of 103 outpatients. *Stroke, 13,* 635–641.

Robinson, R.G., Starr, L.B., Kubos, K.L., & Price, T.R. (1983). A two-year longitudinal study of post-stroke mood disorders: Findings during the initial evaluation. *Stroke, 14,* 736–741.

Robinson, R.G., Starr, L.B., Lipsey, J.R., Rao, K., & Price, T.R. (1984). A two-year longitudinal study of post-stroke mood disorders: Dynamic changes over the first six months of follow-up. *Stroke, 15,* 510–517.

Robinson, R.G., Starr, L.B., & Price, T.R. (1984). A two-year longitudinal study of mood disorders following stroke: Prevalence and duration at six months follow-up. *British Journal of Psychiatry, 144,* 256–262.

Rodin, G.M., Chmara, J., Ennis, J., Fenton, S., Locking, H., & Steinhouse, K. (1981). Stopping life-sustaining medical treatment: Psychiatric considerations in the termination of renal dialysis. *Canadian Journal of Psychiatry, 26,* 540–544.

Rosen, H. & Swigar, M.E. (1976). Depression and normal pressure hydrocephalus: A dilemma in neuropsychiatric differential diagnosis. *Journal of Nervous and Mental Disease, 163,* 35–40.

Rossman, P.L. (1969). Organic disease resembling functional disorders. *Hospital Medicine, 5,* 72–76.

Roth, M. & Kay, D.W.K. (1956). Affective disorder arising in the senium: II. Physical disability as an etiological factor. *Journal of Mental Science, 102,* 141–150.

Roy, A., Pickar, D., Linnoila, M., & Potter, W.Z. (1985). Plasma norepinephrine level in affective disorders: Relationship to melancholia. *Archives of General Psychiatry, 42,* 1181–1185.

Rutter, B.M. (1970). The prognostic significance of psychological factors in the management of chronic bronchitis. *Psychological Medicine, 9,* 63–70.

Sachar, E.J., Asnis, G., Halbreich, W., Nathan, R.S., & Halpern, F. (1980). Recent studies in the neuroendocrinology of major depressive disorders. *Psychiatric Clinics of North America, 3,* 313–326.

Santamaria, J., Tolosa, E., & Valles, A. (1986). Parkinson's disease with depression: A possible subgroup of idiopathic parkinsonism. *Neurology, 36,* 1130–1133.

Savage, C. & Noble, D. (1954). Cancer of the pancreas: Two cases simulating psychogenic illness. *Journal of Nervous and Mental Disease, 120,* 62–65.

Schleifer, S.J., Keller, S.E., Camerino, M., Thornton, J.C., & Stein, M. (1983).

Suppression of lymphocyte stimulation following bereavement. *Journal of the American Medical Association, 250,* 374–377.

Schleifer, S.J., Keller, S.E., Meyerson, A.T., Raskin, M.J., Davis, K.L., & Stein, M. (1984). Lymphocyte function in major depressive disorder. *Archives of General Psychiatry, 41,* 484–486.

Schleifer, S.J., Keller, S.E., Siris, S.G., Davis, K.L., & Stein, M. (1985). Depression and immunity: Lymphocyte function in ambulatory depressed patients, hospitalized schizophrenic patients, and patients hospitalized for herniorrhaphy. *Archives of General Psychiatry, 42,* 129–133.

Schmale, A.H. (1979). Psychological aspects of anorexia: Areas of study. *Cancer, 43,* 2087–2092.

Schulberg, H.C., McClelland, M., & Gooding, W. (1987). Six month outcome for medical patients with major depressive disorders. *Journal of General Internal Medicine, 2,* 312–317.

Scott, J., Barker, W.A., & Eccleston, D. (1988). The Newcastle Chronic Depression Study: Patient characteristics and factors associated with chronicity. *British Journal of Psychiatry, 152,* 28–33.

Shekelle, R.B., Raynor, W.J., Ostfeld, A.M., Garron, D.C., Biliauskas, L.A., Liu, S.C., Maliza, C., & Paul, O. (1981). Psychological depression and 17-year risk of death from cancer. *Psychosomatic Medicine, 43,* 117–125.

Silverstone, P.H. (1987a). Depression and outcome in acute myocardial infarction. *British Medical Journal, 294,* 219–220.

Silverstone, P.H. (1987b). Depression and outcome in acute myocardial infarction. *British Medical Journal, 294,* 645.

Sinyor, D., Amato, P., Kaloupek, D.G., Becker, R., Goldenberg, M., & Coopersmith, H. (1986). Post-stroke depression: Relationships to functional impairment, coping strategies, and rehabilitation outcome. *Stroke, 17,* 1102–1107.

Starkstein, S.E., Robinson, R.G., & Price, T.R. (1988). Comparison of patients with and without poststroke major depression matched for size and location of lesion. *Archives of General Psychiatry, 45,* 247–252.

Stern, M.J., Pascale, L., & Ackerman, A. (1977). Life adjustment postmyocardial infarction: Determining predictive variables. *Archives of Internal Medicine, 137,* 1680–1685.

Stern, M.J., Pascale, L., & McLoone, J.B. (1976). Psychosocial adaptation following an acute myocardial infarction. *Journal of Chronic Diseases, 29,* 513–526.

Stokes, J.F., Nabarro, J.D., Rosenheim, M.L., & Dunkley, E.W. (1954). Physical disease in a mental observation unit. *Lancet, 2,* 862–863.

Strunk, R.C., Mrazek, D.A., Wolfson, G.S., & LaBrecque, J.F. (1985). Physiologic and psychological characteristics associated with deaths due to asthma in childhood: A case-controlled study. *Journal of the American Medical Association, 254,* 1193–1198.

Surman, O.S., Gottlieb, S.K., Hackett, T.P., & Silverberg, E.L. (1973). Hypnosis in the treatment of warts. *Archives of General Psychiatry, 28,* 439–441.

Tufo, H.M. & Ostfeld, A.M. (1968). A prospective study of open-heart surgery. *Psychosomatic Medicine, 130,* 552–553.

Wai, L., Richmond, J., Burton, H., & Lindsay, R.M. (1981). Influence of psychosocial factors on survival of home-dialysis patients. *Lancet, 2,* 1155–1156.

Wells, K.B., Stewart, A., Hays, R.D., Burnam, M.A., Rogers, W., Daniels, M., Berry, S., Greenfield, S., & Ware, J. (1989). The functioning and well-being of depressed patients: Results from the Medical Outcomes Study. *Journal of the American Medical Association, 262,* 914–919.

Wingfield, R.T. (1967). Psychiatric symptoms that signal organic disease. *Virginia Medical Monthly, 94,* 153–157.

Wood, D. & Lecks, H. (1976). Deaths due to childhood asthma. *Clinical Pediatrics, 15,* 677–687.

Wynn, A. (1967). Unwarranted emotional distress in men with ischaemic heart disease (IHD). *Medical Journal of Australia, 2,* 847–851.

Zeiss, A.M. & Lewinsohn, P.M. (1988). Enduring deficits after remissions of depression: A test of the scar hypothesis. *Behaviour Research and Therapy, 26,* 151–158.

PART II

ETIOLOGY AND PATHOGENESIS

5

The Nature of Affect

It is our goal in this text to address both the clinical and conceptual issues related to depression in the medically ill. We emphasize especially the underlying principles regarding the etiology, diagnosis, and management of this perplexing condition. However, what is fundamental to our subject, namely an understanding of depressive affect, still remains clouded.

Why are depression and other affective experiences so poorly understood? Is the uncertainty due, as Green (1977) suggested, to the inherently diffuse and subjective nature of affective experience? Perhaps. However, a comprehensive theory of affects also requires the integration of concepts that lie at the interface of biology and psychology. As Reiser (1984) noted, approaches based on the psychological construct of the mind and those based on the brain-body are separated by semantic, conceptual, and methodological discontinuities. The development of an integrated theory requires bridging the gaps, divisions, and barriers to communication that exist among theoreticians, clinicians, psychodynamicists, basic scientists, and empirical investigators.

Most conceptualizations of affect describe an interactive process among the neurobiological aspects of affects, the expressive motor components, and the subjective experience of emotion. From this point of view, emotions may be seen to arise from an adaptive biological base that is modified by social learning. As expressed by Knapp (1983), emotional experience may be conceived of as a neuropsychological core with an automatic connection to bodily processes, surrounded by a matrix of imagery and ideation.

It is beyond our capacity at this time to resolve the ambiguity which persists in the literature regarding the nature of affect. However, as background to our discussion of the etiology of depression, we briefly review here some of the current concepts of affect. Recent contributions to the understanding of affect have been made from diverse areas including neurobiology, social and cognitive psychology, and psychoanalysis. Theories of the nature of affect, and formulations involving various factors that may produce depressive affect are briefly summarized in the following section. This may add a helpful perspective to the understanding of the origin of depressive disorders in the medically ill and in other populations.

PSYCHOANALYTIC CONCEPTS OF AFFECT

From the time of Freud, there has been speculation in the psychoanalytic literature regarding the fundamental nature of affect. The evolution of psychoanalytic concepts of affect has been previously reviewed by a number of authors (Rapaport, 1953; Green, 1977; Arlow, 1977; Whybrow, Akiskal, & McKinney, 1984) and is outlined here only briefly. However, an attempt is made in the section on psychodynamics in Chapter 6 to integrate traditional psychoanalytic formulations with some recent observations about depressive affect.

Rapaport (1953) documented what he regarded as three phases in Freud's elaboration of affect theory. In the first phase, affect was viewed as a quantity of psychic energy requiring discharge. According to this model, symptoms such as conversion disorders arose when affects were blocked from discharge; the goal of treatment was to discharge "dammed up" affect. In the second phase of theory development, affect was seen in more psychological terms and was related to such concepts as drive representations and intrapsychic conflict. In the third phase, affects were viewed as danger signals that warned of potential psychic trauma and that called defensive operations into play. This view is evident in current concepts of affect within both psychoanalysis and other theoretical perspectives.

Although Freud emphasized the signal function of anxiety, others subsequently postulated that depressive affect also serves as a signal function to bring coping strategies and defense mechanisms into operation to maintain self-esteem (Bibring, 1953; Brenner, 1975; Emde, 1988a, 1988b) and to avoid more severe depressive states (Emde, 1988b). Brenner (1982) postulates that whereas anxiety is a signal to warn of impending danger or calamity, depression is the response to a calamity that has already occurred. This view of depression as a response to an existing rather than potential calamity may have explanatory value with regard to the psychological significance of depression associated with serious medical illness.

Much of the psychiatric literature on depression is concerned with discrete depressive disorders which can be diagnosed at a particular moment in time. This cross-sectional perspective may be associated with the tendency among clinicians to regard depression and other affect states in relatively static terms. However, developmental theorists have recently reminded us that affects are continuous rather than intermittently disruptive states related to the ongoing adaptation of the individual to the internal and external environment (Emde, 1983; Demos & Kaplan, 1986). From this perspective, affects are vital ingredients in such diverse functions as establishing social relations, responding to the internal and external environment, and providing signals for new plans, thoughts, and actions. Emde (1988b) summarized this view of affects as composite states rooted in biology that function consciously as well as unconsciously to organize mental functioning and behavior. Whereas early psychoanalytic affect theory relied heavily upon the postulated existence of drives, more recent formulations have regarded affects as closely related to subjective experience. Stolorow, Brandchaft, and Atwood (1987) suggest that disorders of affect arise when the subjective experience associated with affective arousal cannot be tolerated. This point of view is elaborated upon further in the section on psychodynamics in Chapter 6.

COGNITION AND EMOTION

Several theories have emphasized the cognitive components of affective experience (Arnold, 1960; Averill, 1980; Lang, 1983, 1984; Lazarus, 1966, 1968; Leventhal, 1982, 1984; Schachter & Singer, 1962; Weiner, 1986). This perspective assumes that a cognitive process of evaluation underlies the perception of emotion. Two influential theoretical approaches that integrate the cognitive with the physiological components of emotion are cognitive physiological-arousal theory (Schachter & Singer, 1962) and the cognitive appraisal-coping theory (Arnold, 1960; Lazarus, 1966, 1968). These approaches are discussed briefly below. In addition, a third approach, psychoevolutionary theory (Plutchik, 1980a, 1980b), is addressed. Cognitive evaluative processes are also considered as a part of this discussion. Finally, the evolutionary expressive models (Izard, 1977; Plutchik, 1980a; Zajonc, 1985) are mentioned.

Cognitive Physiological-Arousal Theory

This approach, which built upon the early physiological theories of emotion such as the James-Lange theory, postulated that emotional experience derives from the cognitive interpretation of physiological states. From this point of view, the individual's subjective experience of emotion is determined by his or her interpretation of situational cues. Signals of physiological arousal, such as rapid heartbeat, flushing, or trembling, were thought to be interpreted in different ways, depending upon the situation at hand. In support of this view, Schachter and Singer (1962) reported, in a study using undergraduates, that the perceived affective response to epinephrine was influenced not only by information provided to subjects, but also by the social context in which it was delivered. Although initially quite influential, this theory has not been substantiated over time. The experimental manipulation on which it was based has been criticized as being too artificial and too difficult to reproduce (Reisenzein, 1983). Furthermore, later findings contradicted the position that emotional experience is determined solely by external cues. For example, both Marshall and Zimbardo (1979) and Maslach (1979) reported that unexplained physiological arousal is more likely to be interpreted as negative emotion, independent of the situation. Shaver and Klinnert (1982) challenged the assumption that physiological arousal necessarily precedes emotional experience and Brewin (1988) observed that the experience of emotion can occur swiftly, well before peripheral physiological changes take place. Finally, and most importantly, subsequent research has shown that rather than being a generalized response, physiological arousal is specific to the emotion experienced (Ekman, Levenson, & Friesen, 1983). For these and other reasons, the cognitive physiological-arousal model is no longer a dominant theory of emotion. Nevertheless, the situational context is likely one important determinant of emotional experience for patients with chronic disease. Awareness of their illness could cause patients to interpret physiological experiences, such as fatigue or anorexia, as manifestations of a negative affective state such as depression.

Cognitive Appraisal-Coping Theory

The appraisal theorists proposed that the specific meaning attached to emotion arises from cognitive appraisal of the situation, and that a physiological response is secondary to this appraisal process. An early proponent of this model was Arnold (1960) who viewed emotion as a sequential process beginning with an automatic and unconscious perceptive awareness, or "intuitive appraisal." This appraisal was thought to encompass both current subjective and physiological components as well as past experiences, or "affective memories," thought to be a revival of the affect associated with earlier appraisals. Intuitive appraisal was seen to produce a tendency to act to deal with the immediate situation, as well as to interact with higher level cognition, referred to as the "reappraisal process." This process consisted of attributions about the original appraisal and evaluations regarding a course of action. The interaction between the two levels of appraisal was thought to affect ongoing behavior.

Strongly influenced by Arnold (1960), Lazarus and his colleagues (Lazarus, Averill, & Opton, 1970; Lazarus, Kanner, & Folkman, 1980) defined emotions as complex, organized, psychophysiological reactions consisting of: (1) cognitive appraisals, (2) action impulses, and (3) patterned somatic reactions. These three components were seen to operate as a unit rather than as separate responses, with the quality and intensity of the emotion determining the patterning of the components (Folkman & Lazarus, 1988). From this perspective, cognitive appraisal (e.g., the evaluation of events in terms of their potential impact on the individual) is a cornerstone of the emotional process. According to this formulation, "primary appraisal" is the immediate evaluation of the threat value of the situation. This is determined by factors related to the person (e.g., personality, previous experiences, health, resources) and by factors related to the environment (e.g., type and imminence of danger). The situation is evaluated with regard to its potential for present or future harm or for mastery or gain. "Secondary appraisal" refers to the evaluation of the individual's options and resources to cope with the threat. This evaluation leads to the choice of particular coping strategies to deal with the situation.

Problem-focused coping strategies (i.e., interpersonal and strategic problem-solving actions) tend to be undertaken when the situation is evaluated as amenable to change. Emotion-focused strategies (i.e., distancing, escape-avoidance, acceptance of responsibility or blame, self-control, seeking out others for support, and positive reappraisal) are useful at any time but they are especially helpful when the situation is seen as unchangeable. Both primary and secondary appraisal are thought to be constantly modified by reappraisal of the success of the coping effort and of the continuing impact of the situation on the person. Lazarus and his colleagues regard cognitive appraisal and reappraisal as an integral part of the emotion state (Folkman & Lazarus, 1988). This process leads to "action impulses" that in turn contribute to characteristic physiological response patterns that correspond to particular emotions. This theory has generated a great deal of research interest, and its relevance to the development of depression in medical patients is discussed in Chapter 6.

Psychoevolutionary Theory

Plutchik (1980a, 1980b) advocated a psychoevolutionary perspective on affects. He proposed that emotions evolved in response to particular problems of adaptation that were confronted by early Homo sapiens, and that cognitions evolved "in the service of emotions" (Plutchik, 1980b, p. 12). Plutchik suggested that a primary function of cognition is to predict the future. His view of the cognitive-emotional process is quite similar to that proposed by the appraisal theorists. Like them, he proposed that input is initially processed at a sensory level, compared with information stored in memory, evaluated, and followed by the emotional response. Continuous feedback among the various elements was thought to occur during this process, much of which may be unconscious. Action was the final common pathway of this inferred process and the appropriateness of the action was thought to determine survival. This view is compatible with the idea that depression that occurs in association with medical illness may have some adaptive value.

Facial Expression and Emotion

Since Darwin, the role of facial expressions in emotional experience has generated a great deal of research interest. Differential emotions theory (Izard, 1977) proposed that events trigger innately determined facial expressions by stimulating change in the level or pattern of neural activity. From this point of view, the subjective experience of emotion is secondary to sensory feedback from the face. Izard and Buechler (1980) suggested that cognitive factors may contribute to this process but that the "entire experience of an emotion, from its neural activation through its behavioral expression, can occur without cognitive mediation" (p. 180). Zajonc (1985), in an updated version of a vascular theory of emotion developed by Waynbaum (1907), also proposed that the subjective experience of emotion results from, rather than leads to, facial expression and that cognitive factors are a nonessential part of the process.

Plutchik (1980a) placed facial expressions within the context of a larger innate display system that, along with postural changes, vocalizations, and movements, communicates information to others. Cross-cultural research suggests that the facial expressions that correspond to the basic emotions (i.e., happiness, surprise, sadness, fear, disgust, and anger) are innate (Ekman et al., 1987). Also, research with children who are blind and deaf from birth has demonstrated that they display the same emotional reactions as those who are not similarly impaired (Eibl-Eibesfeldt, 1973). Within Plutchik's (1980a, 1980b) model, cognitive appraisal mediates these behavioral displays.

In summary, debate continues about whether affect or cognition is primary in the experience of emotion (cf., Brewin, 1988; Greenberg & Safran, 1987). Zajonc (1980) contended that higher order cognitive processes are not necessary for affective experience to occur. Lazarus (1982) argued that some degree of preconscious cognitive processing must be involved in the experience of affect, and that affect and cognition are inseparable. However, Lazarus (1984) and others (e.g., Leventhal, 1984; Watts, 1983) include unconscious processing in their view of cognition, whereas Zajonc (1984) limits his definition to material that is in conscious awareness. Overall, the prevailing assumption in experimental psychology is that cognition is not necessarily primary, but that cognitions and affects are interrelated (Greenberg & Safran, 1987).

NEUROBIOLOGIC FACTORS

Some of the greatest recent advances in our understanding of depressive affect and depressive disorders have come from an improved understanding of the biological basis of depression. Studies of central nervous system neurotransmitters, neuroendocrine and sleep changes, and inheritance patterns associated with depression have each provided remarkable findings relevant to the biology of depression. Selected findings are briefly summarized here, but the interested reader is referred to more comprehensive reviews of this subject (Baldessarini, 1983; Rothschild, 1988).

The most prominent biological hypotheses of depression emphasize the altered function of one or more monoamine neurotransmitter systems in the central nervous system. Support for these hypotheses arose from studies of the effects on behavior and mood of drugs that act via these neurotransmitters. Some of the earliest evidence of this kind led to the "catecholamine hypothesis" of depression, as described in two influential papers, one by Schildkraut (1965) and the other by Bunney and Davis (1965). The initial hypothesis, simply stated, proposed that depression results from underactivity of norepinephrine in the central

176 / DEPRESSION IN THE MEDICALLY ILL

nervous system. Subsequent parallel hypotheses implicated other mono-amines (e.g., indoleamines) and monoamine receptors in depression. Studies suggesting that antidepressant agents cause down-regulation of beta-receptors led to an influential proposal that depression is a state of noradrenergic hyperactivity. This hypothesis directly contradicted the original catecholamine hypothesis.

To resolve some of the contradictory evidence regarding the role of catecholamines in the production of depression, Siever and Davis (1985) proposed their "dysregulation hypothesis." As summarized by Roths-child (1988), this hypothesis states that the dysregulated neurotrans-mitter system is characterized by: impairment in one or more hom-eostatic mechanisms, erratic basal output, disruption in the normal periodicities of output, less selective responses to environmental stimuli, a slower return to basal activity following a perturbation, and a return to efficient regulation when clinically efficacious antidepressant agents are prescribed. This hypothesis proposes that depression arises from a failure in the regulation of these systems, rather than from too little or too much central catecholaminergic activity.

Depression has also been associated with numerous endocrine changes including those in the hypothalamic-pituitary-adrenal axis, the hypo-thalamic-pituitary-thyroid axis, and in growth hormone and prolactin. The hyper-responsivity of the hypothalamic-pituitary-adrenal axis in depression is the basis for the dexamethasone suppression test. The utility of this test in the medically ill is further discussed in Chapter 2. However, the neuroendocrine and sleep changes observed in de-pressed patients appear to be characteristics of depression rather than etiologic factors.

Strong support for the biological basis of depression has been provided by genetic studies of mood disorders. Research indicates that individual risk rates for depression exceed 25 percent when a sibling and one parent are affected, and 40 percent when a sibling and both parents have a primary mood disorder (Tsuang, 1975). Twin studies, which show a higher concordance rate for depression between identical or monozygotic twins than between fraternal or dizygotic twins, also suggest a possible genetic component to depressive illness (Baldessarini, 1983). Adoption studies, used to differentiate environmental from ge-netic factors, also confirm that inherited factors are important. These studies show that subjects develop depression in accordance with their biological inheritance, rather than their adoptive experience (Cadoret, 1978; Mendlewicz & Rainer, 1977). However, preliminary attempts to determine genetic linkage for depression have led to conflicting and poorly reproducible results (Rothschild, 1988). Future investigation in this area will benefit from the remarkable developments that have occurred in the area of molecular biology research.

Research into the biology of depression has benefitted greatly from the utilization of standardized methodology to diagnose depressive disorders. However, this research on major depression has contributed little thus far, to an understanding of the full range of depressive affect. Specific biological alterations may yet be defined in association with subsyndromal levels of depressive symptomatology. However, more likely, the biological alterations that characterize major depressive syndromes may help to distinguish these disorders from more transient and/or subclinical depressive states. The presence of genetic or other biological vulnerabilities in combination with situational and other factors, may also help to predict individual vulnerability to major depressive syndromes.

CONCLUSIONS

The etiological factors that may contribute to depression in the medically ill are discussed in greater detail later in this section. Nevertheless, it is evident that depressive affect derives its essence from each of the biological, psychological, and social spheres. Medical illness may produce profound changes in a variety of biological and psychosocial systems, and thus may create multiple risk factors for depression. This fits with Akiskal and McKinney's (1975) formulation of depression as a final common pathway. However, much more needs to be understood about the interrelationship between factors in one category (e.g., neurobiological) with those in another (e.g., cognitive), in order to develop a more comprehensive and integrative understanding of depressive affect.

REFERENCES

Akiskal, H.S. & McKinney Jr., W.T. (1975). Overview of recent research in depression: Integration of ten conceptual models into a comprehensive clinical frame. *Archives of General Psychiatry, 32,* 285–305.

Arlow, J.A. (1977). Affects and the psychoanalytic situation. *International Journal of Psychoanalysis, 58,* 157–170.

Arnold, M.B. (1960). *Emotion and Personality (Volumes 1 & 2).* New York: Columbia University Press.

178 /   DEPRESSION IN THE MEDICALLY ILL

Averill, J.R. (1980). A constructivist view of emotion. In R. Plutchik & H. Kellerman (Eds.), *Emotion: Theory, Research, and Experience Volume 1: Theories of Emotion.* (pp. 305–339). New York: Academic Press, Inc.

Baldessarini, R.J. (1983). *Biomedical Aspects of Depression.* Washington, DC: American Psychiatric Press.

Bibring, E. (1953). The mechanism of depression. In P. Greenacre (Ed.), *Affective Disorders: Psychoanalytic Contributions to their Study.* (pp. 13–48). New York: International Universities Press, Inc.

Brenner, C. (1975). Affects and psychic conflict. *Psychoanalytic Quarterly, 44,* 5–28.

Brenner, C. (1982). *The Mind in Conflict.* New York: International Universities Press, Inc.

Brewin, C.R. (1988). *Cognitive Foundations of Clinical Psychology.* Hove, U.K.: Lawrence Erlbaum Associates, Inc.

Bunney, W.E. & Davis, J.M. (1965). Norepinephrine in depressive reactions. *Archives of General Psychiatry, 13,* 483–494.

Cadoret, R.J. (1978). Evidence for genetic inheritance of primary affective disorder in adoptees. *American Journal of Psychiatry, 135,* 463–466.

Demos, V. & Kaplan, S. (1986). Motivation and affect reconsidered: Affect biographies of two infants. *Psychoanalysis and Contemporary Thought, 9,* 147–221.

Eibl-Eibesfeldt, I. (1973). The expressive behaviour of the deaf-and-blind-born. In M. von Cranach & I. Vine (Eds.), *Social Communication and Movement.* (pp. 163–194). New York: Academic Press, Inc.

Ekman, P., Friesen, W.V., O'Sullivan, M., Chan, A., Diacoyanni-Tarlatzis, I., Heider, K., Krause, R., LeCompte, W.A., Pitcairn, T., Ricci-Bitti, P.E., Scherer, K., Tomita, M., & Tzavaras, A. (1987). Universals and cultural differences in the judgments of facial expressions of emotion. *Journal of Personality and Social Psychology, 53,* 712–717.

Ekman, P., Levenson, R.W., & Friesen, W.V. (1983). Autonomic nervous system activity distinguishes among emotions. *Science, 221,* 1208–1210.

Emde, R.N. (1983). The prerepresentational self and its affective core. *Psychoanalytic Study of the Child, 38,* 165–192.

Emde, R.N. (1988a). Development terminable and interminable I. Innate and motivational factors from infancy. *International Journal of Psychoanalysis, 69,* 23–42.

Emde, R.N. (1988b). Development terminable and interminable II. Recent psychoanalytic theory and therapeutic considerations. *International Journal of Psychoanalysis, 69,* 283–296.

Folkman, S. & Lazarus, R.S. (1988). The relationship between coping and emotion: Implications for theory and research. *Social Science and Medicine, 26,* 309–317.

Green, A. (1977). Conceptions of affect. *International Journal of Psychoanalysis, 58,* 129–156.

Greenberg, L.S. & Safran, J.D. (1987). *Emotion in Psychotherapy.* New York: Guilford Press.

Izard, C.E. (1977). *Human Emotions.* New York: Plenum Press.
Izard, C.E. & Buechler, S. (1980). Aspects of consciousness and personality in terms of differential emotions theory. In R. Plutchik & H. Kellerman (Eds.), *Emotion: Theory, Research, and Experience Volume 1: Theories of Emotion.* (pp. 165–187). New York: Academic Press, Inc.
Knapp, P.H. (1983). Emotions and bodily changes: A reassessment. In L. Temoshok, C. Van Dyke, & L.S. Zegans (Eds.), *Emotions in Health and Illness: Theoretical and Research Foundations.* (pp. 15–27). New York: Grune & Stratton.
Lang, P.J. (1983). Cognition in emotion: Concept and action. In C.E. Izard, J. Kagan, & R.B. Zajonc (Eds.), *Emotions, Cognition, and Behavior.* (pp. 192–226). Cambridge: Cambridge University Press.
Lang, P.J. (1984). The cognitive psychophysiology of emotion: Fear and anxiety. In A.H. Tuma & J.D. Maser (Eds.), *Anxiety and the Anxiety Disorders.* (pp. 131–170). Hillsdale, N.J.: Lawrence Erlbaum Associates, Inc.
Lazarus, R.S. (1966). *Psychological Stress and the Coping Process.* New York: McGraw-Hill.
Lazarus, R.S. (1968). Emotions and adaptation: Conceptual and empirical relations. In W.J. Arnold (Ed.), *Nebraska Symposium on Motivation, XVI [papers].* (pp. 175–270). Lincoln: University of Nebraska Press.
Lazarus, R.S. (1982). Thoughts on the relations between emotion and cognition. *American Psychologist, 37,* 1019–1024.
Lazarus, R.S. (1984). On the primacy of cognition. *American Psychologist, 39,* 124–129.
Lazarus, R.S., Averill, J.R., & Opton Jr., E.M. (1970). Towards a cognitive theory of emotion. In M.B. Arnold (Ed.), *Feelings and Emotions.* (pp. 207–232). New York: Academic Press, Inc.
Lazarus, R.S., Kanner, A.D., & Folkman, S. (1980). Emotions: A cognitive-phenomenological analysis. In R. Plutchik & H. Kellerman (Eds.), *Emotion: Theory, Research, and Experience Volume 1: Theories of Emotion.* (pp. 189–217). New York: Academic Press, Inc.
Leventhal, H. (1982). The integration of emotion and cognition: A view from the perceptual-motor theory of emotion. In M.S. Clark & S.T. Fiske (Eds.), *Affect and Cognition: The Seventeenth Annual Carnegie Symposium on Cognition.* (pp. 121–156). Hillsdale, N.J.: Lawrence Erlbaum Associates, Inc.
Leventhal, H. (1984). A perceptual-motor theory of emotion. In L. Berkowitz (Ed.), *Advances in Experimental Social Psychology (Vol. 17).* (pp. 117–182). Orlando: Academic Press, Inc.
Marshall, G.D. & Zimbardo, P.G. (1979). Affective consequences of inadequately explained physiological arousal. *Journal of Personality and Social Psychology, 37,* 970–988.
Maslach, C. (1979). Negative emotional biasing of unexplained arousal. *Journal of Personality and Social Psychology, 37,* 953–969.
Mendlewicz, J. & Rainer, J.D. (1977). Adoption study supporting genetic transmission of manic-depressive illness. *Nature, 268,* 327–329.

Plutchik, R. (1980a). *Emotion: A Psychoevolutionary Synthesis.* New York: Harper & Row.

Plutchik, R. (1980b). A general psychoevolutionary theory of emotion. In R. Plutchik & H. Kellerman (Eds.), *Emotion: Theory, Research, and Experience Volume 1: Theories of Emotion.* (pp. 3–33). New York: Academic Press, Inc.

Rapaport, D. (1953). On the psycho-analytic theory of affects. *International Journal of Psychoanalysis, 34,* 177–198.

Reisenzein, R. (1983). The Schachter theory of emotion: Two decades later. *Psychological Bulletin, 94,* 239–264.

Reiser, M.F. (1984). *Mind, Brain, Body: Toward a Convergence of Psychoanalysis and Neurobiology.* New York: Basic Books, Inc.

Rothschild, A.J. (1988). Biology of depression. *Medical Clinics of North America, 72,* 765–790.

Schachter, S. & Singer, J.E. (1962). Cognitive, social, and physiological determinants of emotional state. *Psychology Review, 69,* 379–399.

Schildkraut, J.J. (1965). The catecholamine hypothesis of affective disorders: A review of supporting evidence. *American Journal of Psychiatry, 122,* 509–522.

Shaver, P. & Klinnert, M. (1982). Schachter's theories of affiliation and emotion: Implications of developmental research. In L. Wheeler (Ed.), *Review of Personality and Social Psychology (Volume 3).* (pp. 37–72). Newbury Park, CA: Sage Publications, Inc.

Siever, L.J. & Davis, K.L. (1985). Overview: Toward a dysregulation hypothesis of depression. *American Journal of Psychiatry, 142,* 1017–1031.

Stolorow, R.D., Brandchaft, B., & Atwood, G. (1987). *Psychoanalytic Treatment: An Intersubjective Approach.* Hillsdale, N.J.: The Analytic Press.

Tsuang, M.T. (1975). Genetics of affective disorder. In J. Mendels (Ed.), *The Psychobiology of Depression.* (pp. 85–100). New York: Spectrum.

Watts, F. (1983). Affective cognition: A sequel to Zajonc and Rachman. *Behaviour Research and Therapy, 21,* 89–90.

Waynbaum, I. (1907). *La Physionomie Humaine: Son Mechanisme et son Role Social.* Paris: Alcan.

Weiner, B. (1986). *An Attributional Theory of Motivation and Emotion.* New York: Springer-Verlag.

Whybrow, P.C., Akiskal, H.S., & McKinney, W.T. (1984). *Mood Disorders: Toward a New Psychobiology.* New York: Plenum Press.

Zajonc, R.B. (1980). Feeling and thinking: Preferences need no inferences. *American Psychologist, 35,* 151–175.

Zajonc, R.B. (1984). On the primacy of affect. *American Psychologist, 39,* 117–123.

Zajonc, R.B. (1985). Emotion and facial efference: A theory reclaimed. *Science, 228,* 15–21.

6

Psychological
Factors

"That this search for meaning is a human universal, that there is a compulsion to attribute meanings, is only doubted by those who do not want to and cannot see" (GRODDECK, 1925, p. 202).

The psychological response to a particular illness is variable and highly dependent on the personality, life stage, emotional conflicts and vulnerabilities, and social milieu of the person affected. This chapter focuses on the relationship between the psychological response to illness and the development of clinically significant depression. We emphasize here the personal meaning of the illness for the individual, and the associated psychodynamic and cognitive alterations that may lead to depression. Psychological factors that determine whether depression results following the onset of a serious medical illness include the capacity of the individual to tolerate the thoughts and feelings that accompany the illness, the ability to integrate the illness into the self-concept and life-plan without an undue fall in self-esteem, and the capacity to elicit and to use constructively the support of others to assist with this process. Other chapters in this section focus on the biological predisposition to depression, the neurobiological effects of the illness, and the supportive and buffering effects of the social environment. Any or all of these factors may predispose to, or protect from, depression.

To understand depression in the medically ill, we have extrapolated from the broader range of human experiences. For example, we draw on current thinking about adjustment to stressful life events other than a medical illness, and include observations not only from patients with major mood disorders but also from those with nonpathological dysphoria or distress. Psychological responses such as grief, sadness, guilt, shame, self-blame, and lowered self-esteem may all occur with medical illness, in the absence of a diagnosable psychiatric disorder. Obviously, when such symptoms are severe and persistent, a depressive disorder must be considered. However, at times, subclinical emotional states may also warrant intervention, even when they are not manifestations of an overt depressive disorder. We concur with Breslau and Davis (1986), that psychiatric nomenclature does not capture exhaustively the phenomenon of psychological suffering.

In the discussion that follows, we have drawn freely on theory and data from psychoanalytic, cognitive, personality, and coping perspectives. Although the use of multiple models adds complexity, we believe that it also enhances the understanding of depression in the medically ill. Finally, we have drawn some general conclusions about the psychology of illness and of depression in medical patients. However, we have no doubt that the response to a major life stress such as a medical illness is a unique and individual process.

THE PERSONAL MEANING OF ILLNESS

A central factor in the psychological response to illness may be the personal meaning of the illness for that individual (Figure 6.1). As Kleinman (1988) recently observed, the personal meaning of illness derives from the inner world of the patient and is affected by, but is not necessarily synonymous with, its biomedical or social meaning. Therefore, for both explanatory and psychotherapeutic purposes, illness must be understood in terms of the patient's own "narrative" (Kleinman, 1988).

In this chapter, as illustrated in Figure 6.1, we emphasize how the personal meaning of the illness is influenced by the psychodynamic equilibrium, self-structure, personality, and cognitive disposition of the individual affected. Personal meaning contributes not only to the subsequent affective response but also to the adaptive mechanisms and coping strategies that are brought into play. With milder medical illnesses, the psychological response may be heavily determined by such individual factors. However, with illnesses that are more disabling and/ or disfiguring, there may be greater commonality in the personal experience.

Our text is mainly concerned with the psychological response to chronic medical illness. Others, such as Horowitz et al. (1984), have outlined more precisely the response to a more sudden life event. Their

The Psychological Response to Illness

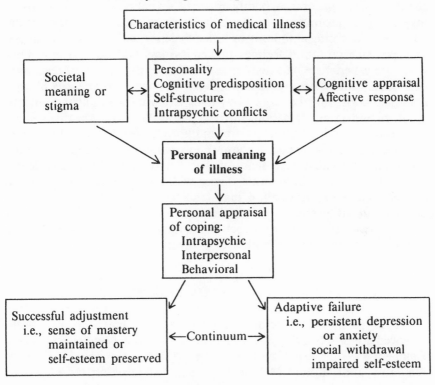

FIGURE 6.1.

observations may be relevant to the acute phase of illness onset. They observed that the typical immediate response to a serious life event is an outcry and the shattering of the illusion of invulnerability. Adaptive defenses including denial are soon brought into operation. The clinical state that follows may alternate between denial of the event and intrusive images of it. Optimally, there is a gradual adjustment to the personal meaning of the event. Dangers or problems in this process of adjustment are thought to include maladaptive avoidances such as the use of drugs or alcohol, persistent flooding of affects, or emotional constriction with somatization (Horowitz et al., 1984). The inability to adjust to the meaning of a medical illness and to tolerate the associated affect may lead to more persistent states of dysphoria and depression.

The distress associated with a chronic illness also depends upon other factors. The life stage of the individual may be a major determinant.

For example, when a major illness occurs during adolescence, anxieties about physical appearance, bodily integrity, sexuality, and stigmatization may be most prominent. In the elderly, or in those with preexisting anxieties concerning autonomy or self-sufficiency, serious medical illness may provoke profound feelings of helplessness and dependency. Previous life experiences also help to determine the psychological response. Individuals who have previously suffered traumatic experiences of separation and loss may be more likely to experience fears of abandonment following the onset of a serious medical illness. Similarly, the preexisting self-structure and psychodynamic equilibrium of the individual are important determinants of response. Those whose self-concept and body image are permeated by a sense of defect may be likely to experience a medical illness in these terms. Those who tend to experience feelings of guilt and self-recrimination may tend to perceive their illness as a punishment for perceived misdeeds. Some of these specific meanings will be discussed in the next section in relation to three of the most common psychodynamic models of depression.

PSYCHODYNAMIC MODELS OF DEPRESSION

The psychodynamic factors associated with depression have been reviewed admirably by a variety of authors including Mendelson (1974), Goldberg (1975), Arieti and Bemporad (1978), Gaylin (1983), and Whybrow, Akiskal, and McKinney (1984). We focus on three mechanisms that have formed the cornerstone of psychoanalytic theories about depression (Goldberg, 1975). These mechanisms are: (1) aggression directed against the self; (2) loss and mourning; and (3) narcissism and lowered self-esteem. These mechanisms and their applicability to the understanding of depression in the medically ill are briefly described here.

Aggression Directed Against the Self

The model of depression based upon aggression directed toward the self was put forth by Freud (1917) and Abraham (1924), who observed differences between normal grief and the pathological condition of melancholia. They suggested that grief regularly follows loss or bereavement, but that the morbid state of melancholia occurs following the experience of loss only in individuals with a pathological predisposition and a tendency to form ambivalent attachments. It was hypothesized that such individuals identify with the introjected lost object to minimize the sense of loss. Anger that cannot be directly acknowledged or expressed following the loss is instead directed inward toward the introjected lost object. This self-directed anger contributes to a lowering of self-esteem that, at times, reaches the point of self-hatred. Self-hatred also derives, according to this formulation, from guilt about the aggressive feelings with a subsequent need for self-punishment.

The need for self-punishment based upon guilt has been regarded in the psychoanalytic literature as a central mechanism leading to depression and lowered self-esteem (Beres, 1966). However, the hypothesis that self-directed anger and guilt leads to depression in medical patients has not been substantiated by current research. In fact, a number of studies (Moffic & Paykel, 1975; Lansky et al., 1985; Emmons, Fetting, & Zonderman, 1987) suggest that medical patients who are depressed actually tend to report fewer feelings of guilt than depressed psychiatric patients. On the other hand, depressed medical patients have been observed to report more feelings of helplessness, more somatic symptoms, and more anxiety than depressed psychiatric patients (Lansky et al., 1985; Emmons, Fetting, & Zonderman, 1987). Thus, while the hypothesis that guilt related to illness leads to depression is theoretically appealing, support for it has not been found in most observations of the medically ill. However, there may be subgroups of depressed medically ill individuals in whom this mechanism is predominant.

Lowered Self-Esteem

Bodily experience is the precursor of the psychological sense of self and likely contributes to self-experience throughout life. It may be because of the life-long association between one's body and one's sense of self that medical illness is so commonly associated with lowered self-esteem. Individuals whose sense of self is particularly fragile, or is closely tied to their physical integrity or bodily appearance, may be most vulnerable to loss of self-esteem in response to a medical illness. In this regard, Muslin (1984) suggested that the extent of damage to the sense of self and the degree of depression associated with the diagnosis of cancer depends significantly upon the preexisting integrity of the self-structure. The nature of the illness may also affect its impact on the sense of self. Medical illnesses associated with marked disability, disfigurement, or physical distress may be particularly likely to have a negative impact on self-concept. Also, unstable or refractory medical conditions may undermine the patient's sense of mastery over the condition.

Lowering of self-esteem has been regarded from the time of Freud

(1917) as a core aspect of depression. Bibring (1953) postulated that the basic mechanism of depression is a partial or complete collapse of self-esteem related to the feeling that one has not lived up to one's expectations. Others (Rado, 1928; Jacobson, 1946) have emphasized that disappointment with one's self and with parental figures in early childhood results in lowered self-esteem and a predisposition to subsequent depression in adult life. More recently, Kohut (1984) and his followers in the school of self-psychology have suggested that not only depressive states, but most other psychological disturbances as well, arise from defects in the structure of the self. A defective sense of self, from this point of view, is considered to arise from faulty parental responsiveness early in life and to be associated with subsequent impairment in the capacity to regulate self-esteem, and in a propensity to depression. Even when the sense of self has been firmly consolidated, a serious medical illness may result in what Kohut (1977) termed a secondary disorder of the self, with similar consequences in terms of mood.

Physical illness may be emotionally catastrophic for individuals in whom a sense of defectiveness or inadequacy is a prominent aspect of the self, and/or when bodily integrity or physical strength are necessary to maintain self-esteem. In such cases, the physical illness may reinforce and concretize preexisting feelings of defectiveness. In effect, the physical defect is experienced as if it were a flaw in the personhood of the individual. This symbolic aspect of the illness is not necessarily related to the severity of the medical condition. Indeed, some have postulated that defects, illnesses, or disabilities that are not visible to others, may be particularly likely to be incorporated into the private symbolic world of the individual (Castelnuovo-Tedesco, 1981). When vigorous efforts to maintain physical health and attractiveness have been necessary to compensate for or defend against underlying feelings of defectiveness and low self-esteem, a physical illness, defect, or disability that is objectively relatively minor, may be psychologically devastating. Depression may follow in this context due to a lowering of self-esteem, a pervasive sense of defect, and/or from the perception that relationships with others who are needed to maintain the sense of self are no longer available.

Although the onset of a physical illness may be damaging to the sense of self, successful experiences of coping with it may eventually bolster self-esteem (Adams & Weaver, 1986). In such cases, feelings of weakness, defectiveness, or ineffectiveness may be compensated for, or even overcome, when the individual is able to achieve a sense of mastery over the condition, particularly when success is perceived to arise from the individual's own efforts. For example, arthritis patients who have greater confidence in their ability to control their illness have been found to be less depressed and less anxious, and to exhibit less impairment in daily living (Nicassio et al., 1985). Similarly, patients with spinal cord injury who believed that their medical prognosis was more likely to be determined by their own efforts than by powerful others or by chance factors also tended to be less depressed (Frank et al., 1987). In addition, breast cancer patients and their husbands who were given a choice regarding type of surgery reported less depressive symptoms both before and after surgery than those not given a choice (Morris & Royle, 1987). On the other hand, the failure to manage a medical condition adequately, even when due to circumstances beyond the individual's realistic control, may intensify feelings of ineffectiveness and contribute to overt depression. For instance, among nearly 1,000 noninstitutionalized persons with a variety of physical disabilities and chronic illnesses, the single best predictor of depressive symptoms was a tendency to be fatalistic rather than to regard life events as under personal control (Turner & Wood, 1985).

The process through which unsuccessful coping might lead to depression may be illustrated by a disease such as insulin-dependent diabetes mellitus. In this condition, caregivers usually place great emphasis on the importance of diet, self-monitoring of blood sugars, and administering insulin reliably. However, control of blood sugars involves many other factors beyond the patient's voluntary control. When metabolic control is impaired, lower self-esteem and depression may result from the perceived failure to master the condition. This may lead, in a self-reinforcing circular fashion, to feelings of futility, noncompliance, poor metabolic control, increased worry about the illness and the future, and ultimately, even lower self-esteem. This sequence of events likely contributes to the association of depression with poor metabolic control in some patients with diabetes mellitus (Mazze, Lucido, & Shamoon, 1984).

A sense of mastery and control over a progressive illness may help to maintain self-esteem and to protect from depression. Previous experiences of mastery in response to challenging situations are clearly important in determining the response to the challenge of a medical illness. Some have suggested that it may be adaptive to be able to relinquish control to powerful others in the face of an uncontrollable stressor (e.g., Burish et al., 1984; Miller, 1980; Rothbaum, Weisz, & Snyder, 1982). However, whether patients derive comfort from this more dependent state depends both on its meaning for them, and on their perception of their relationship with significant others. Those whose self-esteem is more fragile, or who are more sensitive to being disappointed by others, may lack the trust and flexibility necessary to depend upon other people in an adaptive fashion.

Loss and Mourning

Interest in the association between depression and loss has a long history in psychiatry. Psychoanalytic theorists including Abraham (1924), Klein (1940), Benedek (1946), and Mahler (1961), emphasized that early experiences of loss and deprivation may lead to depression in adult life. However, the relevance of these formulations to clinical depression is not clear, and these theorists did not always distinguish universal and nonpathological depressive feelings associated with the inevitable losses of childhood, from the effects of unexpected major separations or losses, or from the manifestations of overt depressive disorders. Nonetheless, the concept that experiences of loss lead to depression both in childhood and in adult life has been the focus of much investigation and speculation in the more recent psychiatric literature.

Bowlby (1980) is credited with drawing most attention in recent years to the impact on children of early parental loss. He challenged the assumption that guilt is intrinsic to mourning and suggested that the despair and detachment observed in children exposed to prolonged separations from their mothers is similar to the depression in adults following experiences of loss. Spitz and Wolf (1946) similarly observed that infants cared for in institutional settings without consistent maternal figures failed to thrive. They considered such failure to thrive to be a manifestation of so-called anaclitic depression. However, there have been some criticisms of the assumption that certain childhood states can be equated with depression. For example, it has been suggested that the withdrawn or "frozen" states (Fraiberg, 1982) observed following separations and losses in infancy and childhood may not be analogues of depression in adults, but may reflect the lack of sensory and affective stimulation that characterized institutional settings at the time these observations were made (Scarr, Phillips, & McCartney, 1989). Also, the conclusions of Bowlby (1961) and Brown and Harris (1978) that the loss of parents in childhood is necessarily associated with depression in adult life has been challenged on methodological grounds (Akiskal & McKinney, 1975). At the very least, it appears that other factors must be present for subsequent depression to occur following a loss. For example, the quality of home life subsequent to a loss has been found to be critical (Breier et al., 1988). Recent reviewers have concluded that, on balance, the weight of evidence supports the notion that both early loss and undesirable losses in adult life are associated with or precipitate of clinical depression in adults (Lloyd, 1980a, 1980b; Rutter, 1985). These associations are very likely mediated by the personal strengths and vulnerabilities of the individual, together with the circumstances surrounding the loss and its aftermath.

Early loss, particularly when followed by inadequate care, may create dependency needs that are unlikely to be satisfied. Similarly, medical illness may increase the need for support from others, but simultaneously interfere with the capacity to maintain supportive interpersonal relationships. A sense of helplessness and depression may result. Medical illness and other symbolic and actual losses in adult life may also activate underlying unresolved feelings of abandonment. However, it should be noted that the pathogenic effects of loss are not necessarily specific for depression, and that early losses are also associated with other psychiatric disorders (Rutter, 1985).

Although most of the literature on depression and loss refers to experiences of actual bereavement, there may be significant parallels between the reaction of an individual to the loss of a significant other, and the reaction to the symbolic and practical losses associated with a chronic physical illness. The latter are certainly no less real and no less distressing than the loss of a significant other. As Pollock (1978) noted, all change involving the "loss" of something entails a mourning process. Medically ill patients may lose their sense of physical well-being, and/or their ability to work, to perform sexually, or to maintain family and social relationships. Even before there is any objective disability associated with a medical illness, the symbolic sense of loss related to the sudden dissolution of one's idealized view of one's self and one's future possibilities may be profound.

The likelihood that depressive symptoms will persist following the onset of a serious medical illness may depend upon the extent to which the individual is able to tolerate and work through feelings of loss associated with the disease. This process of working through feelings may be analagous to that observed in bereavement. The phases and tasks of mourning following bereavement, as outlined by Worden (1982), can be modified to apply to the mourning process associated with a significant physical illness. These modified phases might include: (1) accepting the reality of the loss; (2) experiencing the pain of grief; (3) adjusting to an environment in which one's objective and/or symbolic position is drastically altered; and (4) withdrawing emotional energy from the former perception of the self and investing it in an altered self-concept and level of adaptation. Prominent symptoms of depression may normally be present at certain phases of this mourning process.

Grief and mourning may be part of the normal process of adaptation to a serious medical illness and do not necessarily imply the presence of psychopathology or the need for therapeutic intervention. The mourning process may begin when an illness is first diagnosed or may be delayed until later in the course of the disease, especially when its manifestations are less visible or symptomatic and/or denial of its implications more likely. It may not be until the onset of a serious complication, such as a retinal hemorrhage or renal impairment in patients with diabetes, or the appearance of the first indications of AIDS in an individual who has tested HIV positive, that the sense of loss associated with the illness begins to be experienced. Optimally, resolution of the mourning leads to a constructive reorganization, described by Pollock (1978) as a renewed capacity to be involved with others, to experience feelings, and to engage in creative work and play. However, the medical course of the illness is a major determinant of the likelihood of this favorable outcome.

Although denial may be beneficial in certain circumstances associated with acute medical illness (Lazarus, 1982; Levenson et al., 1989), adaptation to chronic medical illness is usually more effective when the sense of loss can be acknowledged and tolerated (Krantz & Deckel, 1983). In this regard, Keltikangas-Jarvinen (1986) found that patients who tended to experience their illness as a loss, and who felt rational sorrow over lost health, demonstrated a higher degree of psychological health. Similarly, McFarlane, Kalucy, and Brooks (1987) found that patients with rheumatoid arthritis who reported symptoms of depression and anxiety, and who tended to acknowledge the emotional problems associated with having an illness at the time of initial assessment, had a better outcome three years later in terms of their medical disease. In the same vein, Leigh et al. (1987) found that symptoms of depression and anxiety were actually associated with better survival in cancer patients who had dealt realistically with their disease. However, they noted that milder depressive symptoms in this context should be distinguished from more severe depressive symptoms which reflect massive defensive failure. The latter, they suggest, may prove to be associated with diminished survival.

In conclusion, depressive symptoms may occur with medical illness when it is experienced as an actual or symbolic loss. A mourning process, typically involving transient depressive symptoms, normally follows this experience of loss. Resolution of this process may lead to a decrease in dysphoria and even to constructive reorganization and to personal growth in the individual. However, more severe or more persistent depression may occur when there have been previous traumatic experiences of loss and/or when other factors arrest the process of mourning. When the process of mourning does not proceed, or when the sense of loss is profound, depressive symptoms of clinical significance may occur.

The Dynamics of Depression

The following two cases illustrate how the psychology of chronic illness interacts with the sense of self, and how early developmental experiences may contribute both to the meaning of illness and to the affective response in adult life. In these cases, the specific effect of the medical illness on either the psychological development of the individual or on the precipitation of depressive symptoms cannot be determined with certainty. However, there is little doubt that the course of events would have been different in both cases if medical illness had not been present.

Case A

■ Ms. A., a 24-year-old single woman with insulin dependent diabetes mellitus (IDDM) since age 11, was referred for assessment of symptoms of depression. These symptoms had been present in low-grade intensity for two to three years, but had become more severe and more continuous during the three months prior to assessment. This recent worsening of her depression coincided with the break-up of a romantic relationship and with the onset of persistent pain in her right forearm. Although the medical assessment of this pain was inconclusive, she believed that it was due to neuropathy, a complication of her diabetes.

Ms. A. described herself as an individual who tended to put aside her own needs and instead felt drawn to help others. She observed that this pattern became exaggerated in her recent relationship with her boyfriend. Although she found him to be inconsiderate of her, she felt some satisfaction in being needed by him and she feared being alone. It was after she finally broke up with him, that her symptoms of depression worsened and coincidentally, that her arm pain began. Whereas she had previously tended to avoid thinking about her diabetes, she now became preoccupied with the possibility of diabetes-related medical complications.

In her background, Ms. A. suffered two major separations from parental figures and a subsequent adoption during the first year of her life. She was "in and out of hospitals" throughout her childhood because of frequent respiratory infections, and she felt that her adoptive mother experienced her and her problems as burdensome. She was thought to be a slow learner in school and recalls that her adoptive mother regarded her as "dumb and lazy," although psychological testing subsequently revealed that she was bright.

Ms. A. found that the dietary and other demands of her diabetes intensified her sense of being a burden to her mother. When her mother coincidentally developed the same illness two years later, Ms. A. blamed herself, believing that the stress of her illness actually caused her mother's diabetes. Ms. A. aspired to study photography but had postponed applying to a training program because she doubted her abilities. She was temporarily working as a security guard which provided her with some sense of strength but which also contributed to her sense of underachievement and inadequacy.

Ms. A.'s need to care for and to protect others was evident in all of her personal relationships. During the preceding couple of years, she felt increasingly responsible for and worried about her mother's health. Her mother suffered frequent hypoglycemic reactions, some of which were associated with loss of consciousness or convulsions. Ms. A. was fearful that her mother would die daring one of these spells and that she would feel devastated by this loss. As a result, she took on considerable personal responsibility for her mother's well-being. Whereas she had previously tried to exclude from awareness her fears of her illness, the pain in her arm, with its foreboding personal implications, now made it less possible for her to avoid these fears.

When interviewed, Ms. A. was a somewhat tomboyish woman who appeared mildly depressed and who reported longstanding feelings of depression that had become worse during the past three months. She also reported some sleep and appetite disturbance, although these symptoms were not prominent. She was tearful when speaking of her mother's illness and of the recent loss of her boyfriend. She denied suicidal ideation or vegetative symptoms of depression. She was psychologically minded and themes of loss were prominent in her recounting of events. ■

The psychiatric diagnosis in Ms. A. was that of an adjustment disorder with depressed mood. It was evident that her diabetes had played a role both in the predisposition to, and in the precipitation of, her depressive symptoms. The separations from parental figures during her first year, and the sense of being a burden to her adoptive parents left her with low self-esteem and fears of abandonment. The medical illness in this patient heightened and concretized her feelings of helplessness and inadequacy, which "explained" her perception that others found her burdensome. She regarded her own needs as unacceptable to others and increasingly felt called upon to be a caregiver to others, particularly her mother. This role enhanced her self-esteem in some respects, but it interfered with her ability to obtain meaningful support for herself. Although she obtained some vicarious satisfaction by caring for others with whom she apparently identified, she found it difficult to acknowledge her own needs or to rely on others more directly for support. She seemed to believe that relationships could be maintained only if her own needs were set aside. This means of adjustment preserved her psychological equilibrium until the past few years when she became increasingly aware of her own needs and of the absence in her life of meaningful support. Her tendency to surrender altruistically to the needs of others was now maladaptive in the presence of a chronic illness with potentially life-threatening complications. The loss of a relationship, the threat to her mother's life, and the onset of an apparent diabetes-related complication brought into awareness fears that now seemed overwhelming. Her inability to calm these fears or to disavow their significance amplified her feelings of helplessness. Depressive symptoms soon followed and persisted to the time of assessment.

Ms. A. was referred for expressive psychotherapy both because of her current symptoms and because of her more longstanding difficulties related to self-esteem, personal relationships, and a coping style that seemed unlikely to protect her from further depression in response to the vicissitudes of her diabetes or other life events.

Case B

■ Ms. B., a 22-year-old single woman with sickle cell disease diagnosed in infancy, was referred for assessment because of symptoms of depression that followed an unplanned pregnancy and therapeutic abortion one year before the time of assessment. During that year, she reported symptoms of depression that had become worse over the preceding four months. She now complained of anorexia, weight loss of 5 lbs., loss of energy, social withdrawal, and difficulty falling asleep. She also reported crying frequently and, finally, she felt unable to return to work. She denied a past history of depression or psychiatric illness in herself or in any family members. Her last hospitalization due to her sickle cell disease occurred four months earlier, and she had previously required hospitalization up to six times per year.

Prior to the onset of her depressive symptoms, Miss B. described having been in a relationship with a man whom she regarded as handsome and popular, but unfaithful to her. She felt angry that he seemed uncaring and unreliable, although she tried so hard to please him. She described a more positive relationship with her current boyfriend whom she felt was attentive and kind. However, she still felt reluctant to trust any man with her personal feelings, and she had recently retreated into an even more dependent relationship with her family. She felt shame about her recent pregnancy and therapeutic abortion and was distressed that her family seemed so disappointed with her when they learned of it.

Ms. B.'s childhood was punctuated by multiple crises of abdominal pain and hospitalization. She felt stigmatized by her illness, which was known to everyone at her school because recurrent attacks of pain often required her to be taken by ambulance to hospital. Although others regarded her as attractive, she felt insecure about her appearance, particularly since her teenage years.

When interviewed, Ms. B. was an attractive woman who was sophisticated in her appearance but child-like in her manner. She appeared moderately depressed and reported frequent crying at home, wondering "Why am I here on earth? I feel different from everybody else. I don't fit in with anybody." She wanted treatment to relieve her feelings of depression and to overcome her fears of becoming involved with a man. ■

Ms. B. was diagnosed with major depression on axis I and with a dependent personality disorder on axis II of the DSM-III-R. She was started on antidepressant medication and referred for supportive-expressive psychotherapy. The life-long hematologic disease from which she suffered was not an immediate precipitant either of her depression or of the referral for psychiatric assessment. However, it was evident that her feelings of stigmatization and her low self-esteem were due, at least in part, to the psychological impact of her chronic medical disease and the associated episodes of pain. Her recent unwanted pregnancy activated the feelings of shame and embarrassment that she had earlier experienced in relation to her medical condition. It also seemed likely that her sickle cell disease contributed to her sense of helplessness, and to her tendency to retreat into a more dependent state following a stressful life event.

COGNITIVE THEORIES

Cognitive disposition is an aspect of personality that directly affects the meaning that is attached to illness. Cognitions may be defined as "representation(s) of knowledge" or the processes whereby "information is categorized, stored, and integrated with knowledge that is already present" (Brewin, 1988, p. 14). According to cognitive theorists, cognitive activity (i.e., evaluative perceptions, thoughts, and inferences) guides "every adaptational interchange with the environment" (Lazarus, 1982, p. 164). For individuals who are susceptible to depression, the cognitive set may be such that a medical illness is more likely to be regarded in more negative or damaging terms.

The major cognitive theorists (i.e., Beck, 1967; Abramson, Seligman, & Teasdale, 1978; Peterson & Seligman, 1984) suggest that depression may arise secondary to cognitive distortions, negative beliefs and attributions, and dysfunctional attitudes. According to Beck (1967, 1976), three cognitive constructs are implicated in the etiology of depression: (1) the negative cognitive triad (i.e., a negative view of self, the world, and the future); (2) depressogenic schemata (i.e., rigid and inappropriate beliefs and attitudes about the self and the world); and (3) cognitive distortions or errors (i.e., catastrophizing, overgeneralizing, personalizing, and selectively attending to negative aspects of experience). Some of these concepts have been incorporated in the reformulated learned helplessness theory of depression (Abramson, Seligman, & Teasdale, 1978; Peterson & Seligman, 1984). This theory postulates that vulnerability to depression is due to a negative attributional style that includes the belief that desirable outcomes are highly improbable, that aversive outcomes are very probable, and that one is helpless to change the probability of these outcomes (Alloy & Ahrens, 1987).

These theories postulate that negative cognitions develop as a result of earlier life experiences and become activated in the face of stress. Most of the cognitive theories of depression encompass both automatic cognitive processing that operates outside of awareness, and that which is conscious and voluntary. For example, the "core assumptions" described by Beck et al. (1979) refer to unarticulated rules by which the individual evaluates and integrates new information and generates "automatic thoughts" about self, others, and the world. Cognitive therapy is directed toward bringing these thoughts and assumptions into conscious awareness in order to rectify the faulty processing of information. This may be particularly relevant with illness-related information. For example, medical patients often misremember and distort information given to them by their physicians, perhaps due to a block in the processing of information that is perceived as threatening (Smith et al., 1988). The cognitions associated with a medical illness influence not only the meaning ascribed to it, but likely the patient's subsequent vulnerability to depression as well. Some of these cognitive factors are discussed in the next section.

Attributional Style

Attributional or explanatory style refers to the explanations that individuals habitually assign to uncontrollable negative events that befall them (Peterson, Seligman, & Vaillant, 1988). This concept, which emerged from the reformulated learned helplessness theory (Abramson, Seligman, & Teasdale, 1978), postulates that people who attribute unpleasant events to causes which are stable (e.g., "it will always be like this"), global (e.g., "it will ruin everything"), or internal (e.g., "it's me"), will experience more helplessness than persons who explain such events with causes which are unstable (e.g., "it was a fluke"), specific (e.g., "it won't affect my life"), or external (e.g., "it was the weather"). Depression is the primary deficit that is thought to follow from the former explanatory styles. Other factors that have been found to correlate with such explanatory styles include poor physical health in males (Peterson, Seligman, & Vaillant, 1988), poor academic performance in university students (Peterson & Barrett, 1987), and low productivity and quitting in the workplace (Seligman & Schulman, 1986).

A recent meta-analysis of over 100 studies found a reliable relationship between current depressive symptoms and the attribution of negative events to global, stable, and internal causes such as lack of personal ability (Sweeney, Anderson, & Bailey, 1986). Although the concept of attributional style is theoretically distinct from locus of control, greater internality for negative events also tends to be associated with depression (Benassi, Sweeney, & Dufour, 1988). For medical patients, an internal locus of control may help to preserve a sense of mastery, but, at least theoretically, may also increase self-blame when adverse events occur. Sweeney, Anderson, and Bailey (1986) suggested that the evidence that attributions play a causal role in depression is "promising." Attributional style may influence patients' assessment of their illness and contribute to depressed mood. However, Barnett and Gotlib (1988) concluded that it should be considered a symptom rather than a cause of depression since depressive attributional style has not been found to precede depression or to be more common in patients in remission. This caution regarding causation is warranted because a depressive style may be activated in response to adverse life events, but not be evident prior to or following the episode. The following case example illustrates how cognitive factors may influence the psychological response to medical illness and reoccurrence of clinical depression.

Case Example

■ Ms. E. is an obese 47-year-old single mother working at a midlevel position at a large printing company. She had been diagnosed some years previously with irritable bowel syndrome and degenerative disc disease. She complained of chronic pain associated with both of these conditions. However, she sought psychotherapy not because of these medical conditions, but because she was experiencing difficulty managing the demands of her job. She had been transferred recently to a new position as a middle manager, and she found this position to be challenging. At the same time, her supervisor left, and she also had insufficient support staff.

When she began therapy, Ms. E. was struggling not only with her job, but also with a correspondence course to complete her college degree. She described herself as a "workaholic," and it seemed evident that she needed to be regarded by others as competent and efficient to maintain her self-esteem. She experienced considerable distress when she perceived that others at work were not satisfied with her performance. She felt unable either to continue juggling all of the demands on her, or to give up any of her activities.

She described an episode of depression 15 years previously that had lasted about two weeks. This, too, was related to difficulty managing the multiple demands of work, of school, and of her then two-year-old daughter. Her mood at that time improved after calling a telephone help-line for depression. She had sought psychotherapy on four other occasions in her life but had not completed these treatments for various reasons.

When interviewed, Ms. E. presented as a well-dressed, articulate woman of above-average intelligence. She appeared to be mildly depressed and she was somewhat guarded in her approach to the interviewer. She presented herself as an "informed consumer" who wished to be an active participant in determining the course that therapy took. There was no evidence of a major psychiatric disorder at this time, although she did demonstrate longstanding problems with self-esteem and a tendency to become periodically depressed.

Ms. E. agreed to begin time-limited psychotherapy with a cognitive focus. Shortly after this treatment began, she developed Type II diabetes mellitus, a condition to which she was predisposed because of her obesity and her family history. She was advised to lose weight, but she found it difficult either to do this or to achieve adequate control of her blood sugars. She felt victimized by life in general and by the health care system in particular. She became increasingly preoccupied with somatic complaints and felt unready to terminate therapy.

Ms. E. experienced a loss of personal freedom and choice because of her diabetes. She also felt as though a vital part of her had been damaged by this diagnosis, that the "free spirit" in her had been broken. Although she felt responsible for her illness because of her longstanding obesity, she felt angry toward the medical team for what she perceived to be their blaming attitude. For example, she interpreted her referral to a diabetes education program as a "punishment" by her physician. She felt hopeless about her health and said: "It doesn't matter what I do, something else will break down. It's like my body is haunted—as though my body is dead but my mind won't quit." Ms. E. also reported vegetative symptoms of depression at this time including sleep disturbance. A diagnosis of major depression was made and she was started on antidepressant medication and continued in psychotherapy. ■

Ms. E. demonstrated Beck's negative cognitive triad with her negative view of herself, the world, and her future. These negative cognitions affected her response to the subsequent onset of diabetes. She believed that the negative aspects of her physical illness would continue unabated into the future, she blamed herself for its onset, and she generalized the negative aspects of the illness to all areas of her life. These features became prominent when she became clinically depressed. She saw herself as permanently damaged by this condition, powerless to improve her situation, and she questioned the value of life if she was no longer "free." Finally, she saw herself as less competent in all areas of her life because of her illness, and she felt that everyone else was blaming her for her condition.

Dysfunctional Attitudes

Dysfunctional attitudes include "unrealistic, often perfectionistic, standards by which the self is judged" (Barnett & Gotlib, 1988, p. 106). These attitudes have been found to be more common among both depressed college students (Dobson & Breiter, 1983; Gotlib, 1984) and psychiatric patients (Zimmerman et al., 1986) than among nondepressed controls. Similarly, medical patients who have rigid expectations about their own abilities and performance that cannot be modified in spite of the restrictions of the illness, may be more vulnerable to depression. For example, individuals who develop renal failure and must begin dialysis will necessarily find that their appearance and lifestyle are altered considerably. If the same standards of attractiveness and performance are expected, disappointment, frustration, depression, and lowered self-esteem may be the consequences.

Cognitive Distortions

Cognitive distortions are errors in the processing of information (Beck, 1976). Such errors include catastrophizing, overgeneralization, personalization, and selective attention. They are thought to lead to dysphoric affect and maladaptive behaviors in the face of negative life events such as medical disease (Smith et al., 1988). Medical patients who tend to catastrophize might experience their disease in far more devastating terms than is warranted by their physical condition. Those who overgeneralize may assume that a specific outcome, such as a poor response to a particular medication, indicates that other treatments will also be ineffective. With personalization, negative events such as the recurrence of cancer, may be interpreted to mean that the patient is in some way responsible, or is being punished for imagined transgressions. Selective attention (e.g., noticing only negative aspects of the illness to the exclusion of positive signs) may lead to focusing on the misfortune of having a disease and ignoring signs of a rapid or favorable response to treatment.

Two recent studies provide evidence that such cognitive distortions have relevance for depression in medical patients. Using the Cognitive Error Questionnaire, Smith et al. (1988) showed in 92 patients with rheumatoid arthritis that cognitive distortions added to the prediction of depression, independent of the effects of severity of disease and disability. Similarly, Keefe et al. (1987) found among 51 patients with osteoarthritis of the knees that the tendency to catastrophize and to rate as low one's ability to control and decrease pain, as measured by the Coping Strategy Questionnaire, was associated with more psychological distress on the SCL-90. Causality cannot be inferred from these correlational studies, but they do provide information about the cognitions that may be targetted in cognitive intervention programs for medical patients.

Lack of Positive Illusions

Positive illusions refer to the tendency to evaluate oneself and one's degree of control or mastery in an overly positive way, and to be unrealistically optimistic in the face of adversity. Positive illusions have been linked to psychological well-being (Taylor & Brown, 1988) and may protect persons from depression. Individuals who are more realistic in their assessment of themselves and their future circumstances tend to have lower self-esteem and to report more depressive symptoms than persons who are more positively biased (Taylor & Brown, 1988).

The inability to maintain positive illusions in the presence of a medical illness may predispose to depression. Alternatively, the maintenance of positive illusions or unrealistic hope may protect against depression, even in the face of potentially overwhelming adversity.

Case Example

■ Mr. B., a 25-year-old single man with cystic fibrosis was awaiting lung transplantation. Over the one year prior to admission to the transplant program, this patient's clinical condition had worsened dramatically to the point where he required assistance with personal care activities. It was readily apparent both to Mr. B. and to the treatment team, not only that he required a lung transplant, but that he would be unlikely to survive a prolonged wait for an available donor.

Most remarkable about this patient was his persistent good humor and his frequently stated belief that things would work out well for him. This attitude was based on a number of factors including a firm belief that he would regain his health with a transplant, that he was not meant to die yet, and that whatever did happen to him would be acceptable, as it would be the will of his God. He had stated at times that he could not imagine becoming depressed with so much to live for. The positive attitude demonstrated by this young man in the face of overwhelming stress was, in part, his response to being told by many physicians and others that he would not live past adolescence. Mr. B. took great delight in proving these people incorrect and he fully intended to do everything in his power to continue to do so. ■

This patient's positive state of mind could not, of course, protect him from the physical consequences of his condition. In fact, he died of pulmonary complications prior to receiving a transplant. However, his objectively unrealistic appraisal of his situation not only allowed him to tolerate his circumstances without being overwhelmed by depression or by anxiety, but also facilitated his participation in a demanding rehabilitation program. Furthermore, this positive appraisal was maintained without denying the fact that his life was threatened by illness. Although Mr. B. never received a transplant, his coping style nevertheless optimized his functional capacities.

In summary, this section focused on a variety of psychological factors that influence the likelihood that depression will arise in the medical patient. These factors include the premorbid psychodynamics, personality, and cognitive disposition (see Figure 6.1). The rich interplay among all of these factors determines the particular meaning that will be attached to an illness by any individual patient. However, meaning is not static, but is affected by ongoing psychological processes, the course of illness, and the success of strategies employed to cope with the medical condition. The next section elaborates on the coping process in more detail.

COPING WITH ILLNESS

Coping has been defined as the "cognitive and behavioral efforts to manage specific external and/or internal demands that are appraised as taxing or exceeding the resources of the person" (Folkman & Lazarus, 1988, p. 310). With life stress, such as that due to a medical illness, individuals who are more pessimistic about their ability to cope will likely appraise their current situation as more threatening. This appraisal may lead to maladaptive coping strategies that are ineffective in either reducing distress or alleviating illness, and that lead ultimately to the development of depressive symptoms.

Cognitive Appraisal

According to the current major theory of coping (Lazarus & Folkman, 1984), the appraisal of illness consists of two steps. First is primary appraisal in which the individual asks, "What do I have at stake in this situation?" (Folkman & Lazarus, 1988). The degree of perceived threat influences both the meaning of the illness and the emotional response. In the general community, people with a high level of depressive symptoms have been found to perceive more at stake (e.g., with regard to self-esteem, physical well-being, goals at work, financial strain) in stressful situations than nondepressed individuals (Folkman & Lazarus, 1986). Whereas primary appraisal refers to the assessment of the stressor, secondary appraisal refers to the question, "What are my options for coping?"

Research among medical patients has not adequately addressed how cognitive appraisal influences coping strategies or the occurrence of depression. Burish and Bradley (1983) and Lazarus (1982) have outlined a number of conceptual and methodological difficulties that exist in the literature on coping in the medically ill. These issues are noted briefly in the following list:

1. The term coping has been used sometimes to refer to a stable disposition and sometimes to a process. Following a particular

event, such as the diagnosis of cancer, coping immediately afterward will be different than that at other points in time.

2. Specific coping behaviors may change in response to environmental demands. For example, the attitude of a renal patient toward dialysis may depend on a variety of physical circumstances, including proximity to the dialysis center.

3. The concurrent validity of different measures of coping has not been established. Patients' ratings of their coping behaviors may differ considerably from ratings by their physicians, nurses, or families.

4. Judgments regarding the effectiveness of particular coping strategies may change depending upon the situation or course of illness. For example, in the acute phase of the illness, denial may protect myocardial infarction patients from the physiological consequences that might follow from a full awareness of their situation. However, continued denial of the implications of their condition could subsequently lead to maladaptive behaviors such as noncompliance with exercise, diet, and other medical advice.

5. It may not be valid to generalize about coping skills based on the response to a specific situation. For example, coping responses to the initial diagnosis of cancer may not predict a patient's subsequent response to a relapse in the condition.

Although the appraisal-coping process in medical patients has been insufficiently studied, we might speculate that there are clear advantages to a positive appraisal of one's physical illness. It has been suggested that persons who appraise their illness more positively may have higher morale and thus more inner resources to deal with the difficult aspects of their situation (Lazarus, 1982). This positive appraisal may be different than denial of the personal relevance of an illness, in which treatment may actually be neglected or refused. Optimistic appraisal and coping behaviors, which are clearly based on an acknowledgment of the illness, may protect from depression and preserve health. For example, a positive appraisal of the benefits of treatment may lead to excellent compliance with medical recommendations. Thus, coping strategies must be evaluated in terms of each of their psychological, medical, and social consequences.

Coping Strategies

Two main functions of coping are to solve problems and to regulate emotions (Lazarus & Folkman, 1984). Problem-solving coping is directed to improving a situation by altering one's behavior or by changing the situation. Emotion-focused coping regulates distress and preserves morale by managing one's emotional reactions. The emotional state of the individual may help to determine which coping behaviors are preferentially employed. Depressed individuals have been found to engage in more emotion-focused coping (e.g., hostile confrontation, emotional discharge) than nondepressed persons (Billings, Cronkite, & Moos, 1983; Billings & Moos, 1984; Folkman & Lazarus, 1986). However, it is unclear whether emotion-focused coping is a cause and/or an effect of the depressed state. Research is equivocal as to whether the depressed use fewer problem-focused strategies (Barnett & Gotlib, 1988).

In a recent extension of their theory, Folkman and Lazarus (1988) identified categories of cognitive activity that influence the emotional response to stress. These categories, which include deployment of attention and reframing the personal meaning of the situation, are discussed next.

Deployment of Attention

This term refers to activities that either divert attention away from the source of distress (i.e., avoidant strategies) or that focus attention on it (i.e., vigilant strategies). Avoidance includes activities such as sports, relaxation, vacations, and hobbies, when used specifically to "get away" from stressors. These strategies are thought to be adaptive when they neutralize negative emotions, provide a respite from the intensity of the emotions, or actively counter the negative effects of stress through physical activity. Chronic medical patients, depending on the nature of their disability, may also benefit from activities that enhance their sense of mastery and involvement in the outside world, such as limited physical programs, relaxation to enhance sleep, pain management, and activities related to music or crafts. All of these activities may promote well-being, and thereby help individuals to avoid depression and other less adaptive coping strategies such as excessive eating, alcohol consumption, or smoking. However, the benefits of avoidant strategies may be shortlived, and demoralization and depression may follow. For example, using the Medical Coping Modes Questionnaire, Feifel, Strack, and Nagy (1987) assessed three types of coping responses among 223 men with a variety of life-threatening and chronic illnesses. They found that cognitive avoidance (e.g., trying to forget about the illness, changing the subject) and acceptance-resignation (e.g., believing there is nothing to be done, not caring about what happens) were linked to less effective coping strategies. Such strategies may be ineffective because they accomplish neither of the primary functions of coping: they neither change the situation in any way, nor aid in the regulation of emotions.

Vigilant coping strategies focus attention on the problem at hand in order to prevent or control it. These consist of behaviors that are aimed at information gathering and problem-solving. The positive effects of this strategy are mediated both by an increased subjective sense of mastery, and by obtaining effective and timely medical treatment. These consequences might lead to improved physical and psychological well-being and to less depression. For example, vigilant coping in a woman with a family history of breast cancer might include regular breast self-examination and visits to her physician at the first sign of any breast change. This approach might not only diminish feelings of helplessness and victimization, but might lead to earlier and more effective medical treatment. In this regard, Morris and Royle (1987) showed that breast cancer patients and their husbands who were not offered a choice regarding type of surgery were significantly more anxious and depressed preoperatively and up to two months postoperatively than those who were given a choice.

Vigilance is not always the most effective coping strategy, however. It may increase distress when the information obtained is adverse, and when options to change the situation are limited or nonexistent. For example, Cohen and Lazarus (1973) found that surgical patients classified as vigilant had significantly poorer medical outcomes than those who were either avoidant or mixed. They concluded that avoidant patterns are more adaptive than vigilant ones in hospital wards where the options for active coping and mastery are limited.

In a similar vein, Miller and her colleagues (e.g., Miller, 1980, 1987; Miller, Brody, & Summerton, 1988; Miller, Leinbach, & Brody, 1989; Miller & Mangan, 1983) described a construct that they have labelled "monitoring-blunting." Monitoring refers to constant seeking out and scanning of the environment for threatening information. Blunting refers to blocking threatening information from awareness. In a study of patients visiting a primary care facility for treatment, Miller, Brody, and Summerton (1988) found that, on average, high monitors visited their physicians for less severe medical problems than low monitors, but symptoms of discomfort, dysfunction, and distress were equivalent in both groups. In addition, in the week following their visit, high monitors expressed less improvement in both physical and psychological symptoms. Overall, there was a significant and positive correlation in these patients between monitoring and depressive symptoms. However, what may be most crucial with respect to outcome is the individual's flexibility in using either of these styles. Depressed persons have been found to continue to monitor for information, rather than switch to another coping strategy, even when further information provides no benefit (Folkman & Lazarus, 1986).

Changing the Significance or Meaning of the Situation

To reframe the meaning of a situation, patients may utilize such strategies as selective attention, emotional distancing, and denial. Selective attention to the comforting or positive aspects of a situation can reduce negative emotions and generate positive ones. With this intent, Langer, Janis, and Wolfer (1975) taught surgical patients to direct their attention to more favorable aspects of their situation through cognitive reappraisal and positive self-talk, and to rehearse the positive aspects of their hospitalization. Compared with patients who were simply given information about either the surgical procedure or hospital routines, these patients were judged by their nurses to be less anxious and better able to cope with discomfort. In addition, they required fewer pain medications and sedatives postoperatively.

The beneficial effects of attending to positive aspects of a medical situation were demonstrated dramatically by Affleck et al. (1987). In this study, heart attack victims who felt that they had derived positive lessons about lifestyle, health behaviors, and life priorities within the first seven weeks following their attack, were less likely to have a subsequent heart attack over the next eight years and more likely to have better overall health with fewer symptoms of pain and discomfort. The tendency to blame others for the attack at seven weeks was related to a higher incidence of reinfarction. This study provides support for the benefits associated with positive attitudes, although it was based on a reanalysis of data originally collected for another purpose and did not include a specific measure of depression.

Distancing refers to efforts to detach oneself from the emotional significance of a situation. Humor in the face of illness or distress may be employed for this purpose. Norman Cousins (1976), who attributed his recovery from a severe collagen disease to the benefits of laughter and positive affect, is the most famous proponent of the use of humor to counteract the negative effects of illness. Research on emotional expressiveness does indicate that a change in facial expressions produces a corresponding change in physiological response (Ekman, Levenson, & Friesen, 1983). However, there is little scientific evidence to support Cousins' suggestion that laughter is actively beneficial in retarding the disease process. Further, it seems unlikely that laughter can be beneficial unless it is congruent with the individual's underlying mood and attitude.

Emotional distancing may facilitate cognitive processing and/or behavioral activity to minimize the uncertainty or the threat associated with medical illness. This may allow for the opportunity to take care of other obligations and responsibilities related to family and work. Denial may be thought of as a more extreme and sometimes unconscious form of distancing. It may help to reduce anxiety in the face of severe threat and thus, may facilitate recovery in the short term (Cassem & Hackett, 1971; Krantz & Deckel, 1983; Lazarus, 1983). In such cases, it may be adaptive to minimize the implications of the threat (Ditto, Jemmott, & Darley, 1988) to preserve morale and to maintain self-esteem. However, distancing may also have a deleterious impact on coping with illness, on the processing of feelings, and on the maintenance of interpersonal relationships. For example, when denial results in delaying or avoiding necessary treatment, worsening of the medical condition and lowering of mood may result. In this regard, Krantz and Deckel (1983) concluded that there is no evidence to suggest that the long-term use of denial is an effective protection from the depression associated with medical illness.

Changing the Situation

Efforts to cope with adversity through problem solving or confrontation can alter the perceived stressfulness of a situation and thereby minimize the emotional response. This may occur when patients act quickly to obtain effective medical treatment, or when they positively evaluate their efforts to change the situation regardless of the "objective" outcome or of the implications for the future (Folkman & Lazarus, 1988). However, when confrontive coping is associated with an aggressive style of interpersonal behavior which alienates others, a poorer outcome has been reported (Coyne, 1976). For example, patients who respond with hostility to the discovery of cancer are less likely to attract the support of others and thereby may experience more isolation and despair.

CONCLUSIONS

Grief, sadness, guilt, shame, self-blame, and lowered self-esteem may each be part of the nonpathological emotional response to a chronic physical illness. Transient depressive symptoms may be an inevitable by-product of the process of adjustment to the illness and its meaning, and should not necessarily be equated with psychopathology. Clinical or subclinical depression may occur as a complication of a breakdown in the adjustment process.

The psychological outcome in patients with a medical illness may be determined ultimately by the capacity of the individual to tolerate depressive feelings, to integrate the reality of the illness into an acceptable self-concept, and to employ alternative coping responses to deal with the changing reality associated with the medical condition. Although Felton, Revenson, and Hinrichsen (1984) concluded somewhat pessimistically that there is little that individuals can do to alter the emotional consequences of disease, our own research with chronic illness suggests that there is considerable individual variability in depressive symptoms even at the same level of disease severity (Littlefield et al., 1990). Unfortunately, the resources of some individuals will eventually be overwhelmed by the multiple and protracted stresses of severe illness. As Caplan (1964) noted, when a serious problem cannot be solved, avoided, or freshly defined, then psychological disorganization may result. Chronic illness, particularly when it is associated with prominent disability or disfigurement, may represent this kind of protracted and unavoidable stress and may lead ultimately to dysphoria and to clinical depression in some patients.

REFERENCES

Abraham, K. (1924). Theory of anal character. *International Journal of Psychoanalysis, 4,* 400–418.

Abramson, L.Y., Seligman, M.E.P., & Teasdale, J.D. (1978). Learned helplessness in people: Critique and reformulation. *Journal of Abnormal Psychology, 87,* 49–74.

Adams, J.A. & Weaver, S.J. (1986). Self-esteem and perceived stress in young adolescents with chronic disease: Unexpected findings. *Journal of Adolescent Health Care, 7,* 173–177.

Affleck, G., Tennen, H., Pfeiffer, C., & Fifield, J. (1987). Appraisals of control and predictability in adapting to a chronic disease. *Journal of Personality and Social Psychology, 53,* 273–279.

Akiskal, H.S. & McKinney Jr., W.T. (1975). Overview of recent research in depression: Integration of ten conceptual models into a comprehensive clinical frame. *Archives of General Psychiatry, 32,* 285–305.

Alloy, L.B. & Ahrens, A.H. (1987). Depression and pessimism for the future:

Biased use of statistically relevant information in predictions for self versus others. *Journal of Personality and Social Psychology, 52,* 366–378.

Arieti, S. & Bemporad, J. (1978). *Severe and Mild Depression.* New York: Basic Books, Inc.

Barnett, P.A. & Gotlib, I.H. (1988). Psychosocial functioning and depression: Distinguishing among antecedents, concomitants, and consequences. *Psychological Bulletin, 104,* 97–126.

Beck, A.T. (1967). *Depression: Clinical, Experimental and Theoretical Aspects.* New York: Harper & Row.

Beck, A.T. (1976). *Cognitive Therapy and the Emotional Disorders.* New York: International Universities Press.

Beck, A.T., Rush, A.J., Shaw, B.F., & Emery, G. (1979). *Cognitive Therapy of Depression.* New York: John Wiley & Sons.

Benassi, V.A., Sweeney, P.D., & Dufour, C.L. (1988). Is there a relation between locus of control orientation and depression? *Journal of Abnormal Psychology, 97,* 357–367.

Benedek, T. (1946). Toward the biology of the depressive constellation. *Journal of the American Psychoanalytic Association, 4,* 389–427.

Beres, D. (1966). Superego and depression. In R.M. Lowenstein, L.M. Newman, M. Schur, & A.J. Solnit (Eds.), *Psychoanalysis: A General Psychology.* (pp. 479–498). New York: International Universities Press.

Bibring, E. (1953). The mechanism of depression. In P. Greenacre (Ed.), *Affective Disorders: Psychoanalytic Contributions to their Study.* (pp. 13–48). New York: International Universities Press.

Billings, A.G., Cronkite, R.C., & Moos, R.H. (1983). Social-environmental factors in unipolar depression: Comparisons of depressed patients and nondepressed controls. *Journal of Abnormal Psychology, 92,* 119–133.

Billings, A.G. & Moos, R.H. (1984). Coping, stress, and social resources among adults with unipolar depression. *Journal of Personality and Social Psychology, 46,* 877–891.

Bowlby, J. (1961). Childhood mourning and its implications for psychiatry. *American Journal of Psychiatry, 118,* 481–498.

Bowlby, J. (1980). *Loss, Sadness and Depression.* London: The Hogarth Press.

Breier, A., Kelsoe Jr., J.R., Kirwin, P.D., Beller, S.A., Wolkowitz, O.M., & Pickar, D. (1988). Early parental loss and development of adult psychopathology. *Archives of General Psychiatry, 45,* 987–993.

Breslau, N. & Davis, G.C. (1986). Chronic stress and major depression. *Archives of General Psychiatry, 43,* 309–314.

Brewin, C.R. (1988). *Cognitive Foundations of Clinical Psychology.* Hove, U.K.: Lawrence Erlbaum Associates, Inc.

Brown, G.W. & Harris, T.O. (1978). *Social Origins of Depression: A Study of Psychiatric Disorder in Women.* London: Tavistock Publications.

Burish, T., Carey, M., Wallston, K., Stein, M., Jamison, R., & Lyles, J. (1984). Health locus of control and chronic disease: An external orientation may be advantageous. *Journal of Social and Clinical Psychology, 2,* 326–332.

Burish, T.G. & Bradley, L.A. (1983). *Coping with Chronic Disease: Research and Applications.* New York: Academic Press, Inc.

Caplan, G. (1964). *Principles of Preventive Psychiatry.* New York: Basic Books, Inc.

Cassem, N.H. & Hackett, T.P. (1971). Psychiatric consultation in a coronary care unit. *Annals of Internal Medicine, 75,* 9–14.

Castelnuovo-Tedesco, P. (1981). Psychological consequences of physical defects: A psychoanalytic perspective. *International Review of Psychoanalysis, 8,* 145–154.

Cohen, F. & Lazarus, R.S. (1973). Active coping processes, coping dispositions, and recovery from surgery. *Psychosomatic Medicine, 35,* 375–389.

Cousins, N. (1976). Anatomy of an illness (as perceived by the patient). *New England Journal of Medicine, 295,* 1458–1463.

Coyne, J.C. (1976). Depression and the response of others. *Journal of Abnormal Psychology, 85,* 186–193.

Ditto, P.H., Jemmott III, J.B., & Darley, J.M. (1988). Appraising the threat of illness: A mental representational approach. *Health Psychology, 7,* 183–201.

Dobson, K.S. & Breiter, H.J. (1983). Cognitive assessment of depression: Reliability and validity of three measures. *Journal of Abnormal Psychology, 92,* 107–109.

Ekman, P., Levenson, R.W., & Friesen, W.V. (1983). Autonomic nervous system activity distinguishes among emotions. *Science, 221,* 1208–1210.

Emmons, C.A., Fetting, J.H., & Zonderman, A.B. (1987). A comparison of the symptoms of medical and psychiatric patients matched on the Beck Depression Inventory. *General Hospital Psychiatry, 9,* 398–404.

Feifel, H., Strack, S., & Nagy, V.T. (1987). Coping strategies and associated features of medically ill patients. *Psychosomatic Medicine, 49,* 616–625.

Felton, B.J., Revenson, T.A., & Hinrichsen, G.A. (1984). Stress and coping in the explanation of psychological adjustment among chronically ill adults. *Social Science and Medicine, 18,* 889–898.

Folkman, S. & Lazarus, R.S. (1986). Stress processes and depressive symptomatology. *Journal of Abnormal Psychology, 95,* 107–113.

Folkman, S. & Lazarus, R.S. (1988). The relationship between coping and emotion: Implications for theory and research. *Social Science and Medicine, 26,* 309–317.

Fraiberg, S. (1982). Pathological defenses in infancy. *Psychoanalytic Quarterly, 51,* 612–635.

Frank, R.G., Umlauf, R.L., Wonderlich, S.A., Askanazi, G.S., Buckelew, S.P., & Elliot, T.R. (1987). Differences in coping styles among persons with spinal cord injury: A cluster-analytic approach. *Journal of Consulting and Clinical Psychology, 55,* 727–731.

Freud, S. (1917). Mourning and melancholia. *Standard Edition, 14,* 243–258.

Gaylin, W. (1983). *Psychodynamic Understanding of Depression.* New York: Jason Aronson.

Goldberg, A. (1975). The evolution of psychoanalytic concepts of depression.

In E.J. Anthony & T. Benedek (Eds.), *Depression and Human Existence.* (pp. 125-142). Boston: Little, Brown & Co., Inc.

Gotlib, I.H. (1984). Depression and general psychopathology in university students. *Journal of Abnormal Psychology, 93,* 19-30.

Groddeck, G. (1925). *The Meaning of Illness.* London: The Hogarth Press, 1977.

Horowitz, M., Marmar, C., Krupnick, J., Wilner, N., Kaltreider, N., & Wallerstein, R. (1984). *Personality Styles and Brief Psychotherapy.* New York: Basic Books, Inc.

Jacobson, E. (1946). Effect of disappointment on ego and superego formation in normal and depressive development. *Psychoanalytic Review, 33,* 129-147.

Keefe, F.J., Caldwell, D.S., Queen, K.T., Gil, K.M., Martinez, S., Crisson, J.E., Ogden, W., & Nunley, J. (1987). Pain coping strategies in osteoarthritis patients. *Journal of Consulting and Clinical Psychology, 55,* 208-212.

Keltikangas-Jarvinen, L. (1986). Psychological meaning of illness and coping with disease. *Psychotherapy and Psychosomatics, 45,* 84-90.

Klein, M. (1940). Mourning and its relation to manic-depressive states. In, *Love, Guilt and Reparation, and Other Works, 1921-1945 (Volume 1).* (pp. 344-369). London: The Hogarth Press and the Institute of Psychoanalysis, 1975.

Kleinman, A. (1988). *The Illness Narratives: Suffering, Healing and the Human Condition.* New York: Basic Books, Inc.

Kohut, H. (1977). *Restoration of the Self.* New York: International Universities Press.

Kohut, H. (1984). *How Does Analysis Cure?* Chicago: University of Chicago Press.

Krantz, D.S. & Deckel, A.W. (1983). Coping with coronary heart disease and stroke. In T.G. Burish & L.A. Bradley (Eds.), *Coping with Chronic Disease: Research and Applications.* (pp. 3-12). New York: Academic Press, Inc.

Langer, E.J., Janis, I.L., & Wolfer, J.A. (1975). Reduction of psychological stress in surgical patients. *Journal of Experimental Social Psychology, 11,* 155-165.

Lansky, S.B., List, M.A., Herrmann, C.A., Ets-Hokin, E.G., DasGupta, T.K., Wilbanks, G.D., & Hendrickson, F.R. (1985). Absence of major depressive disorder in female cancer patients. *Journal of Clinical Oncology, 3,* 1553-1560.

Lazarus, R.S. (1982). Stress and coping as factors in health and illness. In J. Cohen, J.W. Cullen, & L.R. Martin (Eds.), *Psychosocial Aspects of Cancer.* (pp. 163-190). New York: Raven.

Lazarus, R.S. (1983). The costs and benefits of denial. In S. Breznitz (Ed.), *The Denial of Stress.* (pp. 1-30). New York: International Universities Press.

Lazarus, R.S. & Folkman, S. (1984). *Stress, Appraisal and Coping.* New York: Springer Publishing Co.

Leigh, H., Percarpio, B., Opsahl, C., & Ungerer, J. (1987). Psychological predictors of survival in cancer patients undergoing radiation therapy. *Psychotherapy and Psychosomatics, 47,* 65–73.

Levenson, J.L., Mishra, A., Hamer, R.M., & Hastillo, A. (1989). Denial and medical outcome in unstable angina. *Psychosomatic Medicine, 51,* 27–35.

Littlefield, C.H., Rodin, G.M., Murray, M.A., & Craven, J.L. (1990). The influence of functional impairment and social support on depressive symptoms in persons with diabetes. *Health Psychology, 9,* 737–749.

Lloyd, C. (1980a). Life events and depressive disorder reviewed: I. Events as predisposing factors. *Archives of General Psychiatry, 37,* 529–535.

Lloyd, C. (1980b). Life events and depressive disorder reviewed: II. Events as precipitating factors. *Archives of General Psychiatry, 37,* 541–548.

Mahler, M.G. (1961). Sadness and grief in childhood. *Psychoanalytic Study of the Child, 16,* 332–351.

Mazze, R.S., Lucido, D., & Shamoon, H. (1984). Psychological and social correlates of glycemic control. *Diabetes Care, 7,* 360–366.

McFarlane, A.C., Kalucy, R.S., & Brooks, P.M. (1987). Psychological predictors of disease course in rheumatoid arthritis. *Journal of Psychosomatic Research, 31,* 757–764.

Mendelson, M. (1974). *Psychoanalytic Concepts of Depression.* New York: John Wiley & Sons.

Miller, S. (1980). Why having control reduces stress: If I can stop the roller coaster, I don't want to get off. In J. Garber & M. Seligman (Eds.), *Human Helplessness: Theory and Applications.* (pp. 71–95). New York: Academic Press, Inc.

Miller, S.M. (1987). Monitoring and blunting: Validation of a questionnaire to assess styles of information seeking under threat. *Journal of Personality and Social Psychology, 52,* 345–353.

Miller, S.M., Brody, D.S., & Summerton, J. (1988). Styles of coping with threat: Implications for health. *Journal of Personality and Social Psychology, 54,* 142–148.

Miller, S.M., Leinbach, A., & Brody, D.S. (1989). Coping style in hypertensive patients: Nature and consequences. *Journal of Consulting and Clinical Psychology, 57,* 333–337.

Miller, S.M. & Mangan, C.E. (1983). Interacting effects of information and coping style in adapting to gynecologic stress: Should the doctor tell all? *Journal of Personality and Social Psychology, 45,* 223–236.

Moffic, H.S. & Paykel, E.S. (1975). Depression in medical inpatients. *British Journal of Psychiatry, 126,* 346–353.

Morris, J. & Royle, G.T. (1987). Choice of surgery for early breast cancer: Pre- and postoperative levels of clinical anxiety and depression in patients and their husbands. *British Journal of Surgery, 74,* 1017–1019.

Muslin, H.L. (1984). Transformations of the self in cancer. *International Journal of Psychiatry in Medicine, 14,* 109–121.

Nicassio, P., Wallston, K., Callahan, L., Herbert, M., & Pincus, T. (1985). The measurement of helplessness in rheumatoid arthritis: The development of the Arthritis Helplessness Index. *Journal of Rheumatology, 12,* 462–467.

Peterson, C. & Barrett, L.C. (1987). Explanatory style and academic performance among university freshmen. *Journal of Personality and Social Psychology, 53,* 603–607.

Peterson, C. & Seligman, M.E. (1984). Causal explanations as a risk factor for depression: Theory and evidence. *Psychology Review, 91,* 347–374.

Peterson, C., Seligman, M.E.P., & Vaillant, G.E. (1988). Pessimistic explanatory style is a risk factor for physical illness: A thirty-five year longitudinal study. *Journal of Personality and Social Psychology, 55,* 23–27.

Pollock, G.H. (1978). Process and affect: Mourning and grief. *International Journal of Psychoanalysis, 59,* 255–276.

Rado, S. (1928). The problem of melancholia. *International Journal of Psychoanalysis, 9,* 420–438.

Rothbaum, F., Weisz, J., & Snyder, S. (1982). Changing the world and changing the self: A two-process model of perceived control. *Journal of Personality and Social Psychology, 42,* 5–37.

Rutter, M. (1985). Resilience in the face of adversity: Protective factors and resistance to psychiatric disorder. *British Journal of Psychiatry, 147,* 598–611.

Scarr, S., Phillips, D., & McCartney, K. (1989). Dilemmas of child care in the United States: Employed mothers and children at risk. *Canadian Psychology, 30,* 126–139.

Seligman, M.E.P. & Schulman, P. (1986). Explanatory style as a predictor of productivity and quitting among life insurance agents. *Journal of Personality and Social Psychology, 50,* 832–838.

Smith, T.W., Peck, J.R., Milano, R.A., & Ward, J.R. (1988). Cognitive distortion in rheumatoid arthritis: Relation to depression and disability. *Journal of Consulting and Clinical Psychology, 56,* 412–416.

Spitz, R.A. & Wolf, K.M. (1946). Anaclitic depression: An inquiry into the genesis of psychiatric conditions in early childhood II. *Psychoanalytic Study of the Child, 2,* 313–341.

Sweeney, P.D., Anderson, K., & Bailey, S. (1986). Attributional style in depression: A meta-analytic review. *Journal of Personality and Social Psychology, 50,* 974–991.

Taylor, S.E. & Brown, J.D. (1988). Illusion and well-being: A social psychological perspective on mental health. *Psychological Bulletin, 103,* 193–210.

Turner, R.J. & Wood, D.W. (1985). Depression and disability: The stress process in a chronically strained population. In J.R. Greenley (Ed.), *Research in Community and Mental Health, Volume 5.* (pp. 77–109). Greenwich, Ct.: Jai Press.

Whybrow, P.C., Akiskal, H.S., & McKinney, W.T. (1984). *Mood Disorders: Toward a New Psychobiology.* New York: Plenum Press.

Worden, J.W. (1982). *Grief Counselling and Grief Therapy: A Handbook for the Mental Health Practitioner.* New York: Springer Publishing Co.

Zimmerman, M., Coryell, W., Corenthal, C., & Wilson, S. (1986). Dysfunctional attitudes and attribution style in healthy controls and patients with schizophrenia, psychotic depression, and nonpsychotic depression. *Journal of Abnormal Psychology, 95,* 403–405.

7

Social Factors

This chapter addresses the relationship between social support and emotional well-being in the physically ill. To examine the protective role of social support in this context, we have drawn upon research pertaining to both clinical and subclinical depression. However, we have not included in this discussion the considerable literature on the role of social factors in the etiology of physical illness, or in mortality from it. The interested reader is directed to a number of recent articles that review the relationship between social factors and morbidity and mortality (cf., House, Landis, & Umberson, 1988). Our focus here is on the link between social support and depression among those individuals with an existing medical illness.

Research investigating the relationship between social support and life stress has blossomed over the past decade. It has become apparent from these investigations that the quality of social relationships has a profound effect on psychological functioning, especially in the face of adversity (Barnett & Gotlib, 1988; Broadhead et al., 1983; Brown & Harris, 1986; Cohen & Wills, 1985; Ganster & Victor, 1988; Kessler, Price, & Wortman, 1985). In their review of studies of social support in the medically ill, Wallston et al. (1983) concluded that naturally occurring support has a positive effect on adaptation and recovery from a number of medical illnesses, including myocardial infarction and cancer. However, less is known about the mechanisms by which social support relates more specifically to depression in the medically ill. Indeed, until recently, relatively few studies investigated social support in relation to depressive disorders in this population. Comparability across those few studies that were conducted has been problematic because there is little consistency in the self-report measures used.

However, looking to the literature on depression in nonmedical patients, it is clear that feeling cared for by others is positively associated with emotional well-being. Conversely, poor social support has been found to predict the occurrence of depressive symptoms and to distinguish remitted depressed patients from normal controls (cf. Barnett & Gotlib, 1988). Inadequate support from others is likely to be even more of a risk factor for depression in the medically ill, because of the increased needs of such individuals for various kinds of help and support. Unfortunately, little is known about how social support or its absence specifically contributes to depression in these patients. In particular, we need much more information about the effectiveness of professional support in protecting against or alleviating depression when illness strikes.

Physical illness commonly increases patients' needs for support of various kinds (Wortman & Conway, 1985). Tangible or instrumental support may be required for illness-related tasks. For example, renal patients on home dialysis may need an assistant to help them start and finish their dialysis. In fact, the availability of such a person may determine whether home dialysis is feasible, or whether treatment must be conducted in a hospital dialysis center. Some patients require practical assistance with household tasks, meals, transportation, the administration of medication, or the acquisition of information. For other patients, the availability of emotional support may be more critical than practical assistance. They may need reassurance about the illness or its treatment, empathic understanding and acceptance, and physical comfort or affection. Such support may be a powerful factor that contributes to the emotional well-being despite changes in appearance or ability to fulfill occupational or family duties.

Unfortunately, although illness heightens the need for support, it may also interfere with the individual's capacity to acquire and maintain it (Wortman & Conway, 1985). Illness may cause others to withdraw because it arouses uncomfortable fears. This withdrawal may take the form of a subtle avoidance of discussing or acknowledging the emotionally distressing aspects of the disease. Caretakers who respond in this way to a serious illness, either by maintaining a falsely optimistic posture or by distancing themselves, may thereby increase the patient's sense of isolation. Patients themselves may withdraw from contact with others because of the social stigma attached to certain illnesses or disabilities. As a result, they may avoid the very social interactions that might otherwise provide them with needed support. The perceived or feared reactions of others to illnesses such as AIDS or lung cancer may intensify feelings of self-blame or of being undeserving of help.

Finally, support may diminish if caretakers come to feel overburdened and frustrated when an illness becomes chronic or does not improve. The availability of a supportive network may be an important factor that distinguishes those medical patients who become depressed from those who do not. The increased need for social support or its decreased availability may lead some patients to feel demoralized or depressed. For others, the occurrence of illness mobilizes support from family, friends, or others in the community. We explore further in this chapter, the concept of social support and its relationship to mental health and depression in the medically ill.

THE CONCEPT OF SOCIAL SUPPORT

The need for emotional nurturance and support begins in infancy and continues throughout life. Although autonomy has come to be regarded as a particular virtue in North American society, the need for emotional connectedness is present in all individuals throughout the life cycle. But what is actually meant by the term social support as it has entered the clinical and research literature?

Definition

Contemporary researchers have tended to use a social psychological or social systems perspective to study social support, although some attention has also been paid to its intrapsychic components. According to Wallston et al. (1983), social support refers to "the comfort, assistance, and/or information one receives through formal or informal contacts with individuals or groups" (p. 369). Thoits (1986) regards social support as "functions performed for a distressed individual by significant others such as family members, friends, co-workers, relatives, and neighbors" (p. 417). Based on a survey of 60 researchers who had measured social support, O'Reilly (1988) concluded that it tended to be regarded as a process that was interactive, in which particular actions or behaviors had a positive effect on an individual's social, psychological, or physical well-being.

MEASURES OF SOCIAL SUPPORT

O'Reilly (1988) noted that there is more agreement in the literature regarding what constitutes social support than there is regarding its measurement. Indicators of support used in recent research include participation in clubs or religious organizations, satisfaction with the neighborhood, feelings about the self in relation to society, and social network dimensions such as size, frequency of contact, the reciprocalness of relationships, and the experience of significant others. These varied measures may be grouped into two categories: (1) quantitative or structural aspects, and (2) qualitative or functional components (Cohen & Wills, 1985; Ganster & Victor, 1988; Orth-Gomer & Unden, 1987; Wortman & Conway, 1985).

Structural Measures

Structural measures of social support indicate the range and interconnectedness of existing social support resources. They are generally objective, describing the presence but not the quality of relationships. Such measures include marital status, membership in organizations, and social roles. Also included are such characteristics of the social network as the frequency of interactions among persons, and the size and cohesiveness of the network (Ganster & Victor, 1988). Structural measures are used most frequently in large epidemiological surveys when more cumbersome qualitative measures are not feasible. The link between low social support and physical morbidity and mortality has most often been found in studies that employed structural measures of social support (House, Landis, & Umberson, 1988). However, these measures have generally been less reliable than functional or qualitative ones in predicting mental health and well-being (Cohen & Wills, 1985; Wethington & Kessler, 1986).

The most commonly used structural measure of social support in the medically ill is marital status. A number of studies undertaken in medical samples have reported that the married state is associated with less depression (Barnes & Prosen, 1984; Craven et al., 1987; Dean, 1987; Nielsen & Williams, 1980; Wright et al., 1980; Zung et al., 1983). On the other hand, other studies have found no difference in depression scores between those who are and those who are not married (Bukberg, Penman, & Holland, 1984; Hengeveld, Ancion, & Rooijmans, 1987; Hong et al., 1987; Littlefield et al., 1990; Moffic & Paykel, 1975; Rodin & Voshart, 1987; Rosen et al., 1987; Schwab et al., 1967; Yang et al., 1987). Because there have been no reports of more depression in married persons, on balance, it appears that marriage is associated with less depression in medical patients. Being married may in some way protect patients from becoming depressed when medical illness occurs. Alternatively, individuals who are vulnerable to depression may be less likely to marry in the first place. However, it would be a mistake to conclude that marital status tells the whole story. In fact, marital status has only a small effect on the overall likelihood of depression, indicating that many other factors are involved.

The quality of the marital relationship is likely an overriding factor when assessing the impact of marital status on depression. In a study of 122 women undergoing primary surgery for depression, Dean (1987) found that the quality of the marital relationship preoperatively was a significant predictor of depression based on RDC criteria three months postoperatively. Although depression at 12 months was predicted by marital status but not marital quality, this was likely due to the low prevalence of depression at this time, rather than because the quality of the marital relationship actually became less important. Data on marital status alone provide no information about the nature of and potential change in marital relationships over time following an illness. Such structural measures of support can, therefore, be misleading because they do not take into account interpersonal or intrapsychic processes.

Another problem with employing marital status as a measure of social support is that disturbances in support may have different implications for married patients compared with those who are unmarried. Coyne and DeLongis (1986) suggested that married and unmarried respondents should be examined separately for this reason. Low support among the unmarried may reflect isolation and difficulty in establishing interpersonal relationships, whereas among the married, it may be more likely to signal frustration or disappointment with a current nonproviding relationship. This frustration may be stressful in itself and may limit an individual's ability to obtain support elsewhere. In this regard, Brown and Harris (1986) reported that when a marital relationship is unsatisfactory, other confiding relationships do not effectively substitute. The benefits of marriage may be restricted to contented marriages; unhappily married individuals may actually be worse off than the unmarried in terms of their emotional well-being.

We found tentative support for this hypothesis in a study of patients with diabetes (Littlefield et al., 1990). In this study, there was a tendency for married individuals who reported poor social support to have more depressive symptoms than the unmarried with poor support. Marital status alone was not related to depression. Disappointed expectations may have accounted for the lower score among the unsupported married patients. In this regard, Lieberman (1986) suggested that individuals carry with them a "normative schemata" of who ought to be providing them with support, when, and under which circumstances. Violation of this expectation may be a source of distress that interferes with the acceptance of support from other sources and may itself lead to depression.

Functional Measures

Functional measures of social support tend to reflect the perceptions of the recipient. They may assess either the overall quality of social relationships and/or specific aspects of support related to self-esteem, intimacy, assistance with instrumental tasks, or the provision of information. These measures may also assess the perceived availability, quantity, and timing of social support. Functional aspects of social support have also been studied in terms of their burden to caregivers (cf., Ganster & Victor, 1988). Several recent reviews of experimental interventions have concluded that social support functions have a positive, causal impact on both mental and physical health (Ganster & Victor, 1988; Gottlieb, 1987; Kessler, Price, & Wortman, 1985; Wallston et al., 1983).

Depressive symptoms in medical patients are more clearly related to the functional than to the structural characteristics of social support. This may be illustrated by several studies of women with breast cancer. Among 151 such patients, Funch and Mettlin (1982) found that the perception of support from significant others, and satisfaction with the care provided by professional caregivers, were associated with less negative affect three to 12 months following surgery for the cancer. Similarly, Neuling and Winefield (1988) found, in 58 women recovering from breast cancer surgery, that depressive symptoms while patients were still in hospital were related to dissatisfaction with support from family members. One month after surgery, depression was associated with dissatisfaction with support from the surgeon, and three months after surgery, with dissatisfaction with support from both family members and surgeons. These findings suggest that not only is the perceived adequacy of support from others an important factor in the development of depression, but that the desired provider of support may change with the illness or treatment process.

Another approach was taken by Bloom (1982) who studied 133 women treated with surgery for breast cancer over the preceding two and a half years. Social support in this study was measured by the degree of family cohesiveness, social contact, leisure activities, and by the presence of a reported confidant. As determined by these measures, social support was inversely related to "psychological distress" based on 64 items related to depression, anxiety, anger, vigor, fatigue, and confusion.

Women who felt more supported reported fewer negative coping behaviors, and felt less psychologically distressed. Negative coping behaviors were defined here to include smoking, eating, drinking alcohol, sleeping to avoid facing difficulties, and worrying. A sense of interpersonal connectedness appears to have protected these women from depression and other manifestations of psychological distress, and from using less constructive coping strategies.

The relationship between the quality of social support and the severity of depression has been confirmed with other types of cancer (e.g., Bukberg, Penman, & Holland, 1984). Similar findings have also been reported among patients with other illnesses or disabilities. For example, in a study of 101 patients with endstage renal disease on dialysis for less than two years, Siegal, Calsyn, and Cuddihee (1987) found that psychological distress, as measured by the Brief Symptom Inventory, was negatively associated with the perceived helpfulness of significant others. Schulz and Decker (1985) assessed social support and depression in 100 middle-aged individuals with irreversible spinal-cord injuries (paraplegia and quadriplegia), with an average duration of disability of 20 years. They found that satisfaction with support from significant others was associated with fewer depressive symptoms and with greater well-being and life satisfaction, even when perceived health and income were taken into account. Other evidence suggests that the emotional tone of interpersonal interactions with others is an important determinant of depression in the medically ill. For example, in a study of 48 elderly patients who had been discharged from the hospital following a stroke during the past year, Stephens et al. (1987) found that negative interactions with family and friends were significantly related to poorer morale and to psychiatric symptoms such as depression and suicidality.

Structural vs. Functional Measures

It appears that functional measures are more informative than structural ones with respect to about how social support protects patients from depression. O'Reilly (1988) concluded that perceived social support and network structure are related but distinct constructs that should be measured independently of each other. An elaborate social network is not necessarily perceived as helpful by the patient, and support that seems minimal to others can be experienced by patients as enormously helpful. Conversely, interventions that are intended to help and support the patient may not have the desired effect. For example, Ms. E., a patient described in the previous chapter, perceived a referral by her physician to a diabetes education program to be punishing and humiliating. She described the attitude of the staff there as condescending and blaming. Other patients who have participated in the same program have found it to be informative, helpful, and supportive. It is evident that an evaluation of support must include the perception of the recipient as well as the objective characteristics of the intervention.

In their review, Barnett and Gotlib (1988) concluded from studies conducted with nonmedical samples, that poor social integration is a risk factor for depression. The same is likely true for medical patients. Although the perception of social support is usually a relatively stable characteristic of an individual (Sarason, Sarason, & Shearin, 1986), it may be altered by unusual circumstances such as those associated with a medical illness. In the medically ill, research has not yet disentangled the role of poor social support as a cause, rather than as an effect of depression. Illness may negatively affect the perception of support or may actually drive away others who could otherwise be supportive (Wortman & Conway, 1985).

A lack of precision in conceptualizing and in measuring social support, particularly with regard to its functional aspects, has hindered research in this area. In his review, O'Reilly (1988) noted that some of the items commonly used to measure functional social support were only indirectly related to it. Such related but separate constructs included social participation, social isolation, states of personal well-being, and most often, components of social networks. To clarify the relationship between social support and depression in the medically ill, standardized measures that are tailored to particular populations and health outcomes are needed.

Studies with nonmedical samples indicate that the experience of emotional support is a crucial determinant of well-being (House et al., 1985). However, what constitutes such support varies widely among individuals and circumstances. Moreover, there appears to be a critical distinction between having no social support and having at least one close confidant (Coyne & DeLongis, 1986). This threshold effect may or may not hold true with a chronic illness in which there are multiple needs related to the condition.

Finally, the impact of particular social interactions may be altered with different medical conditions. For example, with an infectious disease such as AIDS, the simple offer of a handshake may convey acceptance and a realistic understanding of the disease. Also, the relative immobility and fatigue that accompany certain illnesses may interfere with social support among those who live alone. The negative effects of being single and perhaps unsupported may appear only when this kind of disability appears.

MODELS OF SOCIAL SUPPORT

Person-Environment Fit Model

Several models have been developed to explain how social relationships affect health and well-being. Broadhead et al. (1983) proposed that support depends on the "person-environment fit." Goodness of fit in this model is thought to depend on the match between the needs of the individual and the resources available from the environment to satisfy those needs. It is the subjective perception of the goodness of fit between needs and available resources that is thought to influence mood most directly. For example, an energetic, 39-year-old man with angina will likely have very different needs for support from both family and health care providers than will a 70-year-old grandmother with the same condition. This model predicts that outcome will be optimal when individuals are able to find and to use effectively the support that fits their needs. This model emphasizes that providers of support must be sensitive to individual needs in order to provide meaningful assistance.

The goodness of fit model suggests that characteristics of the person determine not only the need for support, but also the ability to obtain it, and the perception of its adequacy. The importance of individual characteristics is supported by research that suggests that the extent to which persons feel supported tends to be stable over time (Sarason, Sarason, & Shearin, 1986). In addition, personality traits such as locus of control (Lefcourt, Martin, & Saleh, 1984; Sandler & Lakey, 1982), self-efficacy (Holahan & Holahan, 1987), and hardiness (Ganellen & Blaney, 1984) have been found to moderate the need for support from others in the face of stress. Self-reliant individuals may still need support but may be more selective in seeking and utilizing it (Lefcourt, Martin, & Saleh, 1984). Interventions designed to help patients deal with their medical conditions may be most effective when tailored to the personality or coping style of the individuals involved. For example, Martelli et al. (1987) presented 46 patients about to undergo prosthetic surgery with one of three stress management programs to help them cope with the procedure. Better adjustment during surgery, greater satisfaction with the stress management program, and less pain were all found when the intervention was matched to the patient's coping style. Those patients who typically responded to stress with a problem-solving approach did best when they were given information about the procedure and instructions on how to deal with it. Those who tended to be emotion-focused in their approach, responded best when given training in relaxation and positive imagery, but no details about the surgery. This approach to providing support assumes that there is no "correct" response to illness and no single effective intervention. Rather, it relies upon sensitivity to the individual needs of the patient. Of course, designing interventions based on an understanding of how illness and help are experienced from the perspective of the patient is more complicated than utilizing uniform approaches.

Main Effect vs. Stress-Buffering Models

Specific mechanisms by which social support protects individuals from depression have been the subject of an enormous amount of study and speculation. Two main mechanisms have been described by Cohen (1988) in some detail—the main effect and stress-buffering models. Main effect models predict that individuals with more social support will function better than those with less social support, regardless of the situation. In support of this model is the finding noted earlier that married patients tend to be less depressed, on average, than unmarried patients. Stress-buffering models, on the other hand, predict that social support will moderate the negative effects of stress, so that the benefits of social support become apparent only in the face of adversity. This effect is demonstrated by the finding that patients with good social support are less depressed than those with poor social support as illness severity increases (Littlefield et al., 1990).

In a major review of social support studies in predominantly nonmedical samples, Cohen and Wills (1985) concluded that there was evidence for both main and buffering effects. Structural measures have tended to show main effects, and functional measures, buffering effects. Cohen and Wills (1985) also concluded that there must be a "reasonable match" between the needs of the individual and the support provided in order for buffering to occur. For example, women may experience support by talking about problems and feelings, while companionship obtained through activities and task accomplishment may be more important for men. However, some researchers have been quite critical of distinctions that have been made between main effects and buffering effects, and of some of the statistical analyses used (Alloway & Bebbington, 1987). Alloway and Bebbington (1987) concluded that the evidence for the buffering model is inconsistent because the effects are not very strong. Further, they pointed out that measures of social support and depression often contain components that overlap, so that apparent "buffering" might be an artifact of measurement. Such issues become important to consider in evaluating social support studies in the medically ill.

Buffering Effects in the Medically Ill

The few published studies that have attempted to investigate whether social support acts as a buffer against depression in medical patients have produced mixed results. Each of these studies used some measure of physical health or impairment as an indicator of the degree of stress associated with the illness. Depression was measured by standardized self-report symptom inventories in each case (either the Beck Depression Inventory or the Hopkins Symptom Checklist). None of these studies examined this issue among medical patients with a clinical syndrome of depression.

In the first study, Waltz et al. (1988) followed nearly 400 male patients with myocardial infarction and their wives for five years. They found that patients with more severe health problems who reported less intimacy with their spouse, were more depressed over the entire course of the study. Those with more marital intimacy tended to be less depressed. The authors interpreted this finding as consistent with a buffering effect. However, closer examination of their results reveals that the severity of medical illness did not affect the relationship between depression and intimacy. The presence of the same relationship between depression and intimacy at different degrees of physical health actually supports the main-effect model of social support. This finding is consistent with studies in nonmedical samples that have found a strong relationship between marital adjustment and depression (cf., Barnett & Gotlib, 1988). However, such findings do not rule out the possibility that marital difficulties may result from, rather than cause, depression. Medically ill patients who become depressed may withdraw emotionally from their spouses. Depression in this context could be the cause of decreased intimacy, rather than the result of it.

In the second study, Fitzpatrick et al. (1988) examined the relationship between social support and psychological well-being in 158 patients with rheumatoid arthritis. They found that depressive symptoms were related to poorer social support and to lower self-esteem. They tested for the buffering effect by examining the impact on depression of the interaction between social support and level of functional physical disability. They found no evidence that social support moderated depressive symptoms, although social support was assessed only in terms of the availability of, and satisfaction with, emotional relationships. However, other aspects of social support, such as practical assistance with illness-related tasks, may be equally important in the medically ill and may protect against feelings of helplessness and depression (Thoits, 1986).

We tested the buffering hypothesis in a sample of 158 persons with insulin dependent diabetes mellitus (Littlefield et al., 1990). We found that patients' perceptions that they were not getting as much help and support as they needed on a number of dimensions (including illness-related tasks, domestic responsibilities, financial commitments, and emotional support) were related to higher levels of depressive symptoms. In addition, social support was found to buffer the depressive effect of more severe illness. Among patients with more severe illness-related impairment, those who reported that they received as much or more help as they needed, were less depressed than those who said they did not get as much help as they needed. Also, patients with less physical impairment reported less depressive symptomatology regardless of how supported they felt. This provides preliminary support for the buffering model among patients with a medical illness.

The buffering model suggests that support will be most protective at times of particular illness-related stress. Such times might include the initial diagnosis of a serious illness, the worsening or relapse of a medical condition, the discovery of a serious complication, or the institution of a demanding treatment. However, evidence to support the value of social interventions at such times is sparse. In addition, it is not known whether there are differences between the effects of naturally occurring versus professionally provided social support. Controlled studies of social support interventions are needed to determine whether support can alleviate or prevent depression. The treatment of depression in medical patients is further discussed in Chapter 9.

THE PROVISION OF SOCIAL SUPPORT

Sources of Support

A secure attachment to significant others has been described as "a basic component of humans nature" (Bowlby, 1988, p. 3). Furthermore, medical patients have preferences regarding the type and source of support they get. The most important sources of support for most patients in terms of preserving general well-being tend to be family and friends (cf., Wortman & Conway, 1985; Neuling & Winefield, 1988). A physical illness can cause distress in patients and, secondarily, in members of their social network by causing discomfort and pain, interference with abilities, roles, relationships, or appearance, or by other adverse effects. Such stressors may cause medical patients to feel especially vulnerable to rejection by others, thereby increasing the importance of emotional support and reassurance from loved ones (West et al., 1986).

Medical patients may receive support from other individuals with the same or a similar condition. Based on the assumption that support from peers is beneficial, self-help groups of medical patients are common. However, other patients are not always optimal companions. Social comparison theories predict that patients would prefer to receive emotional support and understanding from other patients (Schachter, 1959), or to enhance their subjective well-being through comparisons with others who are more severely affected (Wills, 1981). By contrast, utility theory (Rofe, 1984) proposes that patients choose companions based not on similarity, but on the companion's capacity to provide help in coping with the difficulties and distress associated with the illness. This is consistent with the person-environment fit model proposed by Broadhead et al. (1983). Other patients may be less able to provide support because they are themselves burdened with illness. Further, they may add to the patients' difficulties by focusing them on problems they may prefer to avoid or deny.

Rofe, Lewin, and Hoffman (1987) examined patient preferences regarding support in a hospital waiting room. They found that only 16 percent of 150 patients said they preferred to be with fellow patients while awaiting an examination in the hospital clinic. Only 6 percent of patients reported preferring the company of other patients on general occasions, while 67 percent said they preferred to be with healthy ones. Twenty-seven percent said they preferred to be alone. Patients who expressed a desire to spend their time in the company of healthy others had significantly higher negative emotion scores than patients who preferred to be alone. In addition, both in the waiting room and at other times, patients expressed a strong wish to avoid the discussion of illness.

These findings have implications for the types of interventions that may benefit patients at different times in the course of their illness. As Folkman and Lazarus (1988) suggested, when all necessary illness-related tasks have been carried out, little may be gained by remaining focused on the illness. Distraction or distancing from the emotional significance of the situation by talking about other things with persons not in the same position may be most beneficial to the well-being of many patients at this time. However, the need for new information or for emotional support may change with changing medical circumstances. For example, by virtue of their presence and importance when illness-related events occur, physicians have been reported to be both the greatest source of stress and the most important source of support to patients at certain times (Bloom, 1981).

What's Helpful and What's Not

Several other aspects of social support have been found to be more or less helpful. Wortman and Conway (1985) noted that it is not helpful to prevent patients from discussing their illness when they wish to do so. On the other hand, the findings of Rofe, Lewin, and Hoffman (1987) suggest that, in certain circumstances, patients prefer to avoid talking about their illness altogether, and perhaps even to be left alone. It is evident that caregivers should take their cues from their patients with respect to how much or how little to discuss the illness. In addition, several researchers have found that the negative aspects of social interactions are more related to negative mental health outcomes than are the positive aspects (cf., Wortman & Conway, 1985). For example, minimizing comments (e.g., "It could be worse.") and unrealistic optimism (e.g., "It will get better.") may be experienced by patients as dismissive and invalidating. Also, advice and suggestions from others who are unfamiliar with the illness can be both annoying and confusing. Thus, among women recovering from breast cancer surgery, informational support was found to be desired from the surgeon, but not from family and friends (Neuling & Winefield, 1988). Family and friends were more likely to be seen as providing unwanted advice than were professional caregivers, who were often seen as providing inadequate support.

Limitations of Social Support

Several investigators have discussed some of the limitations of social support. Thoits (1986) suggested that for the behavior of another to be experienced as supportive, the provider must be considered to be empathic. Help that is offered in a condescending or judgmental way is unlikely to be perceived as supportive. Others who have faced the same situation and reacted well to it may be regarded as particularly compassionate providers of support. This may help to explain the popularity of mutual help groups organized by former patients. The benefit of empathy based on personal experience may be superseded, however, by support from higher status helpers, such as doctors or therapists, whose presumed expertise overrides the need for similarity.

The social support literature tends to assume a positive and linear relationship between social support and well-being. By contrast, the literature on family functioning has paid more attention to maladaptive interactions such as overinvolvement among family members, and the failure to acknowledge the separate needs of individuals within the family. These family difficulties may help to explain the perception of some patients that they would be better able to manage their illness with less involvement from significant others. Support that is perceived as prying or nagging may undermine the self-esteem of the recipient, particularly if it conveys the message that the person is incompetent.

The following case report illustrates these and other aspects of the intricate relationship between the provider and recipient of social support.

Case Example

■ Following several years of progressive disability, Mr. J., a 42-year-old married man with alpha-1 antitrypsin deficiency, moved from his home to await lung transplantation. The wait for a lung transplant at this center may be six to 12 months or longer, and candidates are required to take up residence within a short radius of the hospital. Candidates are also expected to have a support person available continuously to assist them during their wait for, and recovery from, the lung transplant (Bright, Craven, & Kelly, 1990). These patients with severe pulmonary disability require substantial assistance with mobility, transportation to and from the hospital, household duties, and physical care during frequent exacerbations of illness. Mr. J. decided to move to the site of transplant with his mother, and to leave his wife at home with the children. He selected this arrangement both for financial reasons, and so as not to disrupt the schooling and other activities of his three children. It was intended that his wife would come to be with him at the time of the surgery.

Within one month of leaving home, Mr. J. appeared anxious, withdrawn, tearful, and demoralized. During a preliminary assessment, he confided that he could not believe how much he missed his wife and children, and that he did not know how he could remain in the city without them. In their absence, he realized how much he had come to depend upon them for emotional support and companionship. He expressed fears of dying away from home, without his family present. He felt depressed, largely due to the separation from his family, but he felt powerless to make alternative arrangements. He also did not wish to communicate his feelings to his wife by telephone because he believed that she would then fly to be with him, regardless of the financial hardship.

Mr. J. stated that he derived some comfort and reassurance from the weekly self-help/support meeting which most of the lung transplant candidates and recent recipients attend. He found that listening to the experiences of others helped him to prepare for what lay ahead. However, he feared that discussing his feelings in the group would result in uncontrollable tears and humiliation. The presence of his mother, who was now residing with him as his identified support person, proved to be a mixed blessing. He cared for her deeply and appreciated the sacrifices that she had made by moving to reside with him. However, he felt that she tried to do much more for him than he needed, and that this made him feel like "more of an invalid than I am." His mother seemed to him not to be attuned to his needs, and he said that she tried to "make me eat when *she* is hungry and go to bed when *she* is tired." By contrast, Mr. J. felt that his wife understood what he needed and when, and that he enjoyed her assistance and reassuring presence.

Several events helped to ameliorate temporarily Mr. J.'s depressed mood. He responded well to discussing his situation with the consulting psychiatrist individually, and in two joint sessions that included his mother. The latter facilitated more direct communication between them. A surprise visit by his wife also provided great relief, and he now felt able to discuss his feelings with her, although he insisted that she remain at home until the time of transplant. Fortunately, this patient received a successful transplant after only four months of waiting, after which both his physical health and emotional well-being improved. ■

This case illustrates the complicated relationship between social support and depressive symptoms. An unavoidable circumstance that required a severely ill patient to be isolated from his family contributed directly to demoralization and despondency. The loss of the preferred support person was only partly tempered by the presence of another family member and professional support persons. In fact, the poor fit, from his point of view, between his mother's supportive offerings and his needs, initially aggravated his sense of helplessness and loneliness. Both practical circumstances and his self-denying personality traits interfered with Mr. J. taking independent steps to alter his circumstance. In this case, the extreme demands of the treatment situation brought the role of social support into bold relief. Undoubtedly his needs for support were heightened not only by his isolation from his family, but because he faced an unavoidable life-threatening illness with uncertain treatment in a situation in which he could neither comfort nor distract himself in his usual ways.

CONCLUSIONS

There is now considerable evidence in the research literature that social support is related to depression. As Barnett and Gotlib (1988) concluded, the literature provides "consistent evidence of a negative relationship between many facets of social support and concurrent depression" (p. 111). Smaller networks, lower perceived adequacy of social support, and fewer close relationships all have been found to be related to the experience of depression. Billings and Moos (1985) concluded that low social integration, measured variously by self-report, social participation, or number of important relationships, may be characteristic of individuals prone to depression. Prospective studies suggest that marital dysfunction may be involved in the etiology of depression as well. The causal significance of these factors in the development of depression needs to be explored further with attention to the potential confounding of social support measures with those of depression.

In their influential review, House, Landis, and Umberson (1988) concluded that social support is a risk factor for mortality and physical morbidity. Although the evidence is still sketchy, we suggest that low social support is also a risk factor for depression in patients with a medical illness. There is a need for further research on social support and depression in the medically ill to clarify a number of issues, including the mechanisms by which support acts to prevent depression, the specific kinds of support that are beneficial to particular individuals, when social interventions may be experienced as aversive, and which individual characteristics contribute to the ability to obtain support. However, there seems little doubt at present that involvement with others that are experienced as supportive helps to preserve emotional well-being, particularly when illness strikes.

REFERENCES

Alloway, R. & Bebbington, P. (1987). The buffer theory of social support: A review of the literature. *Psychological Medicine, 17,* 91–108.

Barnes, G.E. & Prosen, H. (1984). Depression in Canadian general practice attenders. *Canadian Journal of Psychiatry, 29,* 2–10.

Barnett, P.A. & Gotlib, I.H. (1988). Psychosocial functioning and depression: Distinguishing among antecedents, concomitants, and consequences. *Psychological Bulletin, 104,* 97–126.

Billings, A.G. & Moos, R.H. (1985). Life stressors and social resources affect posttreatment outcomes among depressed patients. *Journal of Abnormal Psychology, 94,* 140–153.

Bloom, J.R. (1981). Cancer care providers and the medical care system: Facilitators or inhibitors of patient coping responses? In P. Ahmed (Ed.), *Living and Dying with Cancer.* (pp. 253–272). New York: Elsevier North Holland, Inc.

Bloom, J.R. (1982). Social support, accommodation to stress and adjustment to breast cancer. *Social Science and Medicine, 16,* 1329–1338.

Bowlby, J. (1988). Developmental psychiatry comes of age. *American Journal of Psychiatry, 145,* 1–10.

Bright, J., Craven, J.L., & Kelly, P. (1990). Psychosocial stressors in lung transplant candidates. *Journal of Health and Social Work, 15,* 125–132.

Broadhead, W.E., Kaplan, B.H., James, S.A., Wagner, E.H., Schoenbach, V.J., Grimson, R., Heyden, S., Tibblin, G., & Gehlbach, S.H. (1983). The epidemiologic evidence for a relationship between social support and health. *American Journal of Epidemiology, 117,* 521–537.

Brown, G.W. & Harris, T. (1986). Stressor, vulnerability and depression: A question of replication. *Psychological Medicine, 16,* 739–744.

Bukberg, J., Penman, D., & Holland, J.C. (1984). Depression in hospitalized cancer patients. *Psychosomatic Medicine, 46,* 199–212.

Cohen, S. (1988). Psychosocial models of the role of social support in the etiology of physical disease. *Health Psychology, 7,* 269–297.

Cohen, S. & Wills, T.A. (1985). Stress, social support, and the buffering hypothesis. *Psychological Bulletin, 98,* 310–357.

Coyne, J.C. & DeLongis, A. (1986). Going beyond social support: The role of social relationships in adaptation. *Journal of Consulting and Clinical Psychology, 54,* 454–460.

Craven, J.L., Rodin, G.M., Johnson, L., & Kennedy, S.H. (1987). The diagnosis of major depression in renal dialysis patients. *Psychosomatic Medicine, 49,* 482–492.

Dean, C. (1987). Psychiatric morbidity following mastectomy: Preoperative predictors and types of illness. *Journal of Psychosomatic Research, 31,* 385–392.

Fitzpatrick, R., Newman, S., Lamb, R., & Shipley, M. (1988). Social relationships and psychological well-being in rheumatoid arthritis. *Social Science and Medicine, 27,* 399–403.

Folkman, S. & Lazarus, R.S. (1988). The relationship between coping and emotion: Implications for theory and research. *Social Science and Medicine, 26,* 309–317.

Funch, D.P. & Mettlin, C. (1982). The role of support in relation to recovery from breast surgery. *Social Science and Medicine, 16,* 91–98.

Ganellen, R.J. & Blaney, P.H. (1984). Hardiness and social support as moderators of the effects of life stress. *Journal of Personality and Social Psychology, 47,* 156–163.

Ganster, D.C. & Victor, B. (1988). The impact of social support on mental and physical health. *British Journal of Medical Psychology, 61,* 17–36.

Gottlieb, B.H. (1987). Marshalling social support for medical patients and their families. *Canadian Psychology, 28,* 201–217.

Hengeveld, M.W., Ancion, F.A.J., & Rooijmans, H.G.M. (1987). Prevalence and recognition of depressive disorders in general medical inpatients. *International Journal of Psychiatry in Medicine, 17,* 341–349.

Holahan, C.K. & Holahan, C.J. (1987). Self-efficacy, social support, and depression in aging: A longitudinal analysis. *Journal of Gerontology, 42,* 65–68.

Hong, B.A., Smith, M.D., Robson, A.M., & Wetzel, R.D. (1987). Depressive symptomatology and treatment in patients with end-stage renal disease. *Psychological Medicine, 17,* 185–190.

House, J.S., Kahn, R.L., McLeod, J.D., & Williams, D. (1985). Measures and concepts of social support. In S. Cohen & S.L. Syme (Eds.), *Social Support and Health.* (pp. 83–108). New York: Academic Press, Inc.

House, J.S., Landis, K.R., & Umberson, D. (1988). Social relationships and health. *Science, 241,* 540–545.

Kessler, R.C., Price, R.H., & Wortman, C.B. (1985). Social factors in psychopathology: Stress, social support, and coping processes. *Annual Review of Psychology, 36,* 531–572.

Lefcourt, H.M., Martin, R.A., & Saleh, W.E. (1984). Locus of control and social support: Interactive moderators of stress. *Journal of Personality and Social Psychology, 47,* 378–389.

Lieberman, M.A. (1986). Social supports: The consequences of psychologizing: A commentary. *Journal of Consulting and Clinical Psychology, 54,* 461–465.

Littlefield, C.H., Rodin, G.M., Murray, M.A., & Craven, J.L. (1990). The influence of functional impairment and social support on depressive symptoms in persons with diabetes. *Health Psychology, 9,* 737–749.

Martelli, M.F., Auerbach, S.M., Alexander, J., & Mercuri, L.G. (1987). Stress management in the health care setting: Matching interventions with patient coping styles. *Journal of Consulting and Clinical Psychology, 55,* 201–207.

Moffic, H.S. & Paykel, E.S. (1975). Depression in medical inpatients. *British Journal of Psychiatry, 126,* 346–353.

Neuling, S.J. & Winefield, H.R. (1988). Social support and recovery after surgery for breast cancer: Frequency and correlates of supportive behaviours by family, friends and surgeon. *Social Science and Medicine, 27,* 385–392.

Nielsen, A.C. & Williams, T.A. (1980). Depression in ambulatory medical patients. *Archives of General Psychiatry, 37,* 999–1004.

O'Reilly, P. (1988). Methodological issues in social support and social network research. *Social Science and Medicine, 26,* 863–873.

Orth-Gomer, K. & Unden, A.L. (1987). The measurement of social support in population surveys. *Social Science and Medicine, 24,* 83–94.

Rodin, G. & Voshart, K. (1987). Depressive symptoms and functional impairment in the medically ill. *General Hospital Psychiatry, 9,* 251–258.

Rofe, Y. (1984). Stress and affiliation: A utility theory. *Psychology Review, 91*, 235–250.

Rofe, Y., Lewin, I., & Hoffman, M. (1987). Affiliation patterns among cancer patients. *Psychological Medicine, 17*, 419–424.

Rosen, D.H., Gregory, R.J., Pollock, D., & Schiffmann, A. (1987). Depression in patients referred for psychiatric consultation: A need for a new diagnosis. *General Hospital Psychiatry, 9*, 391–397.

Sandler, I.N. & Lakey, B. (1982). Locus of control as a stress moderator: The role of control perceptions and social support. *American Journal of Community Psychology, 10*, 65–80.

Sarason, I.G., Sarason, B.R., & Shearin, E.N. (1986). Social support as an individual difference variable: Its stability, origins, and relational aspects. *Journal of Personality and Social Psychology, 50*, 845–855.

Schachter, S. (1959). *The Psychology of Affiliation: Experimental Studies of the Sources of Gregariousness.* California: Stanford University Press.

Schulz, R. & Decker, S. (1985). Long-term adjustment to physical disability: The role of social support, perceived control, and self-blame. *Journal of Personality and Social Psychology, 48*, 1162–1172.

Schwab, J.J., Bialow, M., Brown, J.M., & Holzer, C.E. (1967). Diagnosing depression in medical inpatients. *Annals of Internal Medicine, 67*, 695–707.

Siegal, B.R., Calsyn, R.J., & Cuddihee, R.M. (1987). The relationship of social support to psychological adjustment in end-stage renal disease patients. *Journal of Chronic Diseases, 40*, 337–344.

Stephens, M.A.P., Kinney, J.M., Norris, V.K., & Ritchie, S.W. (1987). Social networks as assets and liabilities in recovery from stroke by geriatric patients. *Psychology and Aging, 2*, 125–129.

Thoits, P.A. (1986). Social support as coping assistance. *Journal of Consulting and Clinical Psychology, 54*, 416–423.

Wallston, B.S., Alagna, S.W., DeVellis, B.M., & DeVellis, R.F. (1983). Social support and physical health. *Health Psychology, 2*, 367–391.

Waltz, M., Badura, B., Pfaff, H., & Schott, T. (1988). Marriage and the psychological consequences of a heart attack: A longitudinal study of adaptation to chronic illness after 3 years. *Social Science and Medicine, 27*, 149–158.

West, M., Livesley, W.J., Reiffer, L., & Sheldon, A. (1986). The place of attachment in the life events model of stress and illness. *Canadian Journal of Psychiatry, 31*, 202–207.

Wethington, E. & Kessler, R.C. (1986). Perceived support, received support, and adjustment to stressful life events. *Journal of Health and Social Behavior, 27*, 78–89.

Wills, T.A. (1981). Downward comparison principles in social psychology. *Psychological Bulletin, 90*, 245–271.

Wortman, C.B. & Conway, T.L. (1985). The role of social support in adaptation and recovery from physical illness. In S. Cohen & S.L. Syme (Eds.), *Social Support and Health.* (pp. 281–301). New York: Academic Press, Inc.

234 /

DEPRESSION IN THE MEDICALLY ILL

Wright, J.H., Bell, R.A., Kuhn, C.C., Rush, E.A., Patel, N., & Redmon, J.E. (1980). Depression in family practice patients. *Southern Medical Journal, 73,* 1031–1034.

Yang, L., Zuo, C., Su, L., & Eaton, M.T. (1987). Depression in Chinese medical inpatients. *American Journal of Psychiatry, 144,* 226–228.

Zung, W.W.K., Magill, M., Moore, J., & George, D.T. (1983). Recognition and treatment of depression in a family medicine practice. *Journal of Clinical Psychiatry, 44,* 3–6.

8

Biological Factors

The two previous chapters in this section review the psychological and social mechanisms that may contribute to the development of depression in persons with a physical illness. This chapter focuses on a variety of biological mechanisms that have also been implicated in the production of depression in some patients. To a large extent, systematic research into the role of biological mechanisms in the development of depression in medical patients is still in its infancy. A decade after research in this area began, there is still need for the type of coordinated, disorder-by-disorder investigation called for by Klerman in 1981. Such research might help to elucidate the etiology of depression, not only in the medically ill, but also in the general population. For example, identifying the mechanisms by which viral diseases produce depression may provide valuable clues to the pathways and biochemistry involved in the production of depressive disorders in other circumstances.

In the first section of this chapter, we focus on the difficulties involved in isolating biological from other depressogenic mechanisms. Following this, we summarize the evidence to support a direct relationship between specific physical illnesses and depression and consider the biological mechanisms that have been implicated. We do not provide a comprehensive list of all physical conditions that have been postulated to cause depression. The interested reader is referred to reviews of this topic for a more detailed listing (e.g., Hall, 1980). We emphasize those illnesses in which specific mechanisms have been postulated to account for their association with depression. Biological mechanisms that have been implicated in the production of depression in the medically ill include the effects of pharmacologic agents (e.g., the antihypertensive agent reserpine) and metabolic disturbances associated with specific medical disorders (e.g., depressive symptoms with Cushing's syndrome). The term organic mood disorder is most applicable in these cases. It may be argued that symptoms of depression that are an inherent component of a medical disease should not be assigned a distinct psychiatric diagnosis. However, identifying the factors involved in the development of depression in these conditions may help to elucidate biological mechanisms responsible for depression generally. We do not assume that psychological factors are necessarily inconsequential when depression can be linked to a direct physical cause.

BIOLOGICAL MECHANISMS AND DEPRESSION IN THE PHYSICALLY ILL

Prevalence

It is often difficult to determine whether biological disturbances associated with a medical illness are specifically linked to depression. There have been some attempts to assess retrospectively the extent to which medically-related biological factors influenced the development of a depressive episode. A preliminary study in this vein by Kinzie et al. (1986) concluded that major depression resulted from a biological mechanism associated with a physical illness in 38 percent of a sample of 50 clinically depressed patients. In 14 percent of the sample, it was considered to be secondary to the combined effect of a physical illness and depressogenic medication; in 8 percent, an organic mood disorder was regarded as a direct complication of a medication. However, the method used to determine whether a biological mechanism was responsible for depression was not clearly specified. Others have reported that a medical condition either caused or contributed to a mental disturbance in from 5 percent to 42 percent of psychiatric patients, including those with mood disorders (Herridge, 1960; Davies, 1965; Koranyi, 1972; Hall et al., 1980; Summers et al., 1981). However, these studies also failed to specify the biological mechanisms purported to be involved in the association. This methodological problem plagues all research efforts in this area because criteria to establish a causal link between depression and a particular biological disturbance are extremely difficult to determine. As a result, current knowledge is limited in terms of the biological mechanisms involved in depressive illness that occurs concurrently with physical disease.

Although our understanding of the biological underpinnings of depression has expanded rapidly during the past two decades, we still lack a comprehensive biological theory that delineates direct mechanisms by which depression is produced or the interplay between biological and psychological factors in the etiology of depression. In the absence of such a theory, biological mechanisms to explain depression associated with any given disease are most compelling when psychological explanations can be ruled out. For example, when symptoms of depression begin prior to other manifestations of the illness (e.g., depression preceding the onset of pancreatic carcinoma), the cause of the depression is more likely to be an early biological manifestation of the illness. However, in such cases it is still possible that a psychological response to physical alterations, not necessarily with conscious awareness, contributes to depression. Biological mechanisms again may be suspected when depression is more prevalent in one illness than in others with a similar prognosis, severity, or level of disability. For example, Schiffer and Babigan (1984) supported their proposition that biological mechanisms act to produce depression in multiple sclerosis (MS) by demonstrating that depression rates in MS are higher than rates in amyotrophic lateral sclerosis, a disease with similar physical features. Similarly, Robinson et al. (1984a) argued that biological mechanisms were implicated in the etiology of poststroke depression because depression did not appear to be related to the extent of disability or to stroke severity.

Drug Effects

Depression has been reported to follow the administration of a wide range of physical agents. Unfortunately, most of the literature in this area is methodologically weak and/or consists of single case reports or small case series (Pascualy & Veith, 1989). Many studies in this field do not adequately define cases of depression (Zelnick, 1978). Systematic research is needed to conclude that an etiological relationship necessarily exists between a given drug and depression. Conclusions based on case reports require corroboration by controlled studies with adequate sample sizes before firm conclusions can be drawn. Physical illness, depressive disorders, and the prescription of drugs are each common enough that their co-occurrence may be coincidental. The credibility of specific associations based on single case studies is improved dramatically if the report includes observations about the response when the drug is administered, withdrawn, then readministered. If the postulated effects of the drug follow the pattern of administration, then stronger evidence for a causative association is provided. Other clinical features may also strengthen hypotheses about the association of depression with a particular drug. To be viewed as a side effect or a complication, depression must be absent prior to the initiation of the drug and begin following its administration, and preferably, but not necessarily, worsen with increased dosage.

It must be remembered that, for some drugs (e.g., reserpine), a prolonged latency period exists between the initiation of the drug and the onset of depression. However, a drug may still be responsible for initiating the depressed state even after it is discontinued. With L-asparaginase, depressive and other organic mental symptoms may occur several weeks after the agent is administered and discontinued. Further evidence for a causal association is provided if the depressed state remits with discontinuation of the proposed offending agent. When possible, a target drug with purported depressogenic effects should be compared to similar ones that do not cross the blood-brain barrier.

Preexisting vulnerability based on genetic loading or a history of major depression also confounds the association between a drug and a new episode of depression. An individual vulnerable to depression is more likely to become depressed when given a potentially depressogenic agent. For example, patients with a history of depression have been found to be at high risk for a recurrence if given reserpine (Quetsch et al., 1959; Pascualy & Veith, 1989). Similarly, Mindham, Marsden, and Parkes (1976) reported that over 50 percent of Parkinson's patients who developed depression during treatment with L-dopa had a history of depression, suggesting that these patients appear to be in double jeopardy. However, to substantiate a causative relationship with depression, pharmacologic agents should also produce changes in mental state in patients without any known psychiatric vulnerability, even if at a lower rate of occurrence. In fact, the strongest epidemiological evidence for a suspected pathogen would be the demonstration of an increased prevalence of depression in persons with no known preexisting vulnerability. Pascualy and Veith (1989) suggested that a history of mood disorders at least be documented in any study attempting to demonstrate that a drug is etiologically related to depression.

SPECIFIC ETIOLOGIC FACTORS

Cancer

Depressive disorders occur in approximately 20 to 30 percent of oncology patients, a prevalence rate similar to that in other serious physical illnesses. Depressive symptoms in cancer patients appear to be more likely with increased severity of illness (Massie & Holland, 1987). There are obvious psychological factors that contribute to an increased likelihood of depression in patients with this group of diseases. However, there are also indications that biological mechanisms also produce depression, at least in some oncology patients.

Brown and Paraskevas (1982) summarized several clinical reports in which depression was thought to be an early manifestation of cancer, well before either the diagnosis of the disease or the occurrence of physical discomfort or disability. A proposed etiologic mechanism for depression in this context was cancer-related immunologic interference with serotonergic pathways. Unfortunately, the absence of standardized criteria to diagnose depressive disorders in the studies reviewed, and the possibility that early symptoms of depression were coincidental, rather than presenting features of the cancer, make such a conclusion impossible to substantiate.

Cancer-related events may also account for the co-occurrence of depression and cancer. These include: brain metastases, central nervous system infection, chemotherapeutic agents, nutritional impairment, and/ or neoplastic cachexia. Other mechanisms by which cancer could be associated with depressive symptoms or disorders include: metabolic (e.g., hypercalcemia) and endocrine (e.g., hypercholesterolemia) disturbances, and the effects of ectopically produced psychoactive substances (e.g., parathormone, vasopressin, and methionine enkephalin) (Goldberg, 1981). Mitchell (1967) noted that certain cancers, especially bronchogenic, thymic, pancreatic, and renal, secrete ACTH-like material that causes Cushing's syndrome and, at least potentially, its associated depressive features.

Bruera et al. (1984) found that 59 percent of their malnourished cancer patients scored >20 on the Hamilton Rating Scale for Depression (HAM-D), while only 20 percent of the adequately nourished cancer patients scored in this range. Similarly, in a study of patients with head and neck cancer, depression was most frequent in those who were malnourished and underweight (Westin et al., 1988). Although Schmale (1979) suggested that anorexia and weight loss may result from a state of hopelessness in some persons with cancer, severe cachexia is more likely a cause of depression in these patients. Others have emphasized that tumors involving the central nervous system may be associated with depression. Fifty-eight percent of 326 patients with supratentorial neoplasms were found to have symptoms of depression and anxiety as early manifestations of illness (Guvener et al., 1964). Whitlock (1982) reviewed the case reports of depression associated with these tumors and concluded that mood disturbances are common with tumors of the frontal and the temporal lobes, and that meningiomas, in particular, appear to be associated with depressive symptoms. Noyes and Kathol

(1986) suggested that primary tumors of the lung, breast, gastrointestinal tract, and kidney often metastasize to the brain and may be associated with depression.

Prescribed treatments may also be responsible for depressive symptoms in some cancer patients. For example, mood symptoms may occur following radiotherapy (Forester, Kornfeld, & Fleiss, 1978). This effect depends on the field of treatment and appears to be most frequent with cranial irradiation (Proctor, Kernahan, & Taylor, 1981). Peck and Boland (1977) found that 24 percent of cancer patients reported at least moderate depressive symptoms following cancer chemotherapy, whereas only 12 percent reported such symptoms prior to treatment. This finding does not necessarily mean that all chemotherapeutic agents directly produce organic mood disorders. Rather, physical side effects of the treatment (e.g., anorexia) and psychological reactions to it are more likely responsible for the depressive symptoms. However, certain agents have been more specifically associated with depressive symptoms. For example, vincristine has been shown to produce dysphoria when used in a regimen for oat cell carcinoma (Silberfarb et al., 1983). L-asparaginase produces a depressive syndrome that may develop several weeks following treatment (Young, 1982). This agent may also produce other neurotoxic complications including delirium and seizures (Young, 1982). As the following case example illustrates, depressive symptoms may be part of a neurotoxic spectrum caused by the administration of this physical agent.

Case Example

■ Ms. W. was an 18-year-old woman with acute myelogenous leukemia of recent onset who was referred to psychiatry for assessment of depression. Although the initial diagnosis of leukemia was made one month prior to referral, she had initially maintained an optimistic and hopeful outlook. She tolerated her first course of chemotherapy well and was readmitted to hospital the following week to resume the second course of treatment. However, for several days prior to referral, Ms. W. was uncharacteristically withdrawn, lying still in bed for most of the day, not eating, and disinterested in any activity or social interaction. It appeared that this change in her emotional state had occurred abruptly. She had no history of depression or other psychiatric disturbance, of substance abuse, or of self-harm activity. For obvious reasons, staff initially presumed that the personal impact and meaning of her diagnosis had precipitated her depression. Referrals both to the clinical nurse specialist and to psychiatry were instituted to assess the situation fully and to assist her with adjustment.

On examination, the patient was cooperative throughout the interview and seemed to try to maintain interest in the process. However she was somnolent, remarkably slowed in her movements and her speech, and she responded to most questions with monosyllabic answers and with little fluctuation of speech intonation. She reported apathy and anergy, but denied intense feelings of depression and/or hopelessness. She was not tearful, and she strongly felt that her life was worth fighting for. No disturbances in orientation, memory, or other cognitive functions were found.

Although psychological reasons could easily be found to explain this patient's symptoms, several features of her presentation raised suspicion of an organic mental syndrome. In particular, psychomotor retardation was prominent and abrupt in onset, and anergy and somnolence in the absence of a severely depressed mood or feelings of hopelessness were out of keeping with a psychologically-mediated adjustment disorder. This patient had received L-asparaginase during her first course of chemotherapy. Over the few days subsequent to psychiatric evaluation, her level of consciousness deteriorated and she suffered from several generalized motor seizures. Investigations, including a metabolic screen, CAT scan of the head, and magnetic resonance imaging, revealed no other specific etiological factor. The patient gradually and fully recovered over one week's time and L-asparaginase was subsequently eliminated from her chemotherapeutic regimen. ∎

Cancer of the Pancreas

Depression in association with malignancy has been most closely linked with cancer of the pancreas. As early as 1923, Scholz and Pfeiffer reported "nervousness" preceding the diagnosis of carcinoma of the pancreas. Yaskin (1931) first reported that mental symptoms may be the earliest manifestation of this type of cancer. He observed depression with crying spells, insomnia, anxiety, and worry in patients with pancreatic cancer, all without obvious physical manifestations or signs of organic brain syndrome. Several studies subsequently examined the prevalence of psychiatric symptoms in patients with pancreatic carcinoma (Eusterman & Wilbur, 1933; Savage, Butcher, & Noble, 1952; Birnbaum & Kleeberg, 1958). In their review of this early literature, Fras, Litin, and Pearson (1967) concluded that depressive symptoms were the most common mental state changes observed with this tumor.

Several later studies further examined the association of depression with carcinoma of the pancreas. Fras, Litin, and Pearson (1967) compared 46 patients with pancreatic cancer to 64 patients with colonic cancer, all prior to surgery. Based on clinical interviews, they found at least mild depressive symptoms in 50 percent of those with cancer of the pancreas, whereas these symptoms were reported by only 13 percent of patients with colonic cancer. Depressive symptoms were often the presenting features with cancer of the pancreas. Based on data obtained retrospectively from living relatives of patients, Jacobsson and Ottosson (1971) compared 50 patients with carcinoma of the pancreas to 50 patients with gastric carcinoma. They found that the prevalence of depressive symptoms based on the relatives' estimates was similar in both groups. These authors suggested that pancreatic and gastric carcinomas both produce an "organic psychosyndrome" with prominent depressive features that are similar both in frequency and symptom profile. However, a significantly greater proportion of the patients with cancer of the pancreas reported psychological symptoms prior to the somatic manifestations of the carcinoma. Holland et al. (1986) found higher self-ratings of depression and other mental status changes, according to the Profile of Mood States (POMS), in 107 patients with advanced pancreatic carcinoma compared with 111 patients with gastric cancer.

Joffe et al. (1986) greatly improved upon previous methodology, in their study of 12 subjects with carcinoma of the pancreas and nine subjects with gastric carcinoma. Each patient was interviewed with the Schedule for Affective Disorders and Schizophrenia and was diagnosed according to Research Diagnostic Criteria. In addition, each subject completed the Beck Depression Inventory, the Spielberger State-Trait Anxiety Inventory, the SCL-90, and tests of cognitive functioning. Fifty percent of subjects with carcinoma of the pancreas fulfilled RDC criteria for major depression during the one year prior to diagnosis, while none of those with carcinoma of the stomach received this psychiatric diagnosis. A family history of mood disorder was the only feature which distinguished the depressed patients with pancreatic carcinoma.

A plethora of physical mechanisms, none substantiated, have been proposed to account for depression with pancreatic carcinoma. Many of these postulated mechanisms are based on etiological theories of depression that are now outdated including: interference with afferent inflow from the retroperitoneal autonomic nervous system (Latter & Wilbur, 1937; Drapiewski, 1944); disturbed carbohydrate metabolism (Drury & Farran-Ridge, 1925); nicotinic acid deficiency due to anorexia (Rothermich & von Haam, 1941); and changes in blood serum surface tension (Lovell, 1923, 1937). The more recent finding of increased urinary excretion of 5-hydroxy-indoleacetic acid (5-HIAA) in patients with pancreatic carcinoma (McMullen & Hanson, 1958) has prompted new etiologic formulations. Jacobsson and Ottosson (1971) suggested that a pancreatic tumor may metabolize tryptophan and thereby compete peripherally for this serotonin precursor, diminishing the supply available to the central nervous system. Brown and Paraskevas (1982) proposed that a protein released by the cancer cells could induce antibodies which, based on cross-reactivity with central nervous system tissue, could bind to serotonin receptors and thereby inhibit activity in pathways that utilize this neurotransmitter. Finally, Brown and Paraskevas (1982) also suggested that antibodies could stimulate the production of anti-idiotypic antibodies that would act as alternative receptors for serotonin and thus reduce its synaptic availability. Each of these mechanisms is compatible with the finding of increased 5-HIAA in the urine of patients with pancreatic cancer.

Poststroke Depression

Both major and minor depression have been shown to occur in a sizable proportion of poststroke patients (Robinson et al., 1983). A series of studies by Robinson and co-workers has shown that depression in these patients may begin as early as two weeks following brain injury and that severe depression is most common from six to 24 months following stroke (Robinson & Price, 1982). The occurrence of depression may substantially impair the functional rehabilitation and outcome of stroke patients (Parikh et al., 1988).

Stroke is an unfortunate and potentially disabling event that occurs most frequently in the elderly. Multiple mechanisms may be involved in the production of poststroke depression. It is obvious that depression may arise as a psychological response to this event and to the possibility of long-term physical and cognitive impairment. However, some evidence suggests that biological mechanisms are also involved in many patients. Folstein, Maiberger, and McHugh (1977) found that moderate depressive symptoms were reported by 45 percent of poststroke patients whereas only 10 percent of orthopaedic patients with similar levels of disability reported such symptoms. Robinson et al. (1984b, 1984c) concluded that the degree of disability accounted for only a small proportion of the depression found in a sample of 103 consecutive poststroke patients. These findings do not rule out psychological factors, but do invite speculation about biological mechanisms to account for poststroke depression. Subsequent studies have found a strong relationship between poststroke depressive disorder and the location of the stroke in the central nervous system (Robinson et al., 1984a; Lipsey et al., 1983; Robinson & Lipsey, 1985). Specifically, left anterior hemispheric lesions were often associated with major or minor depression, whereas lesions in other locations were significantly less likely to be complicated by depression. The closer a left-sided lesion was to the frontal pole, the greater was the likelihood of depression.

According to the biogenic amine hypothesis, major depression arises due to depletion of central nervous system biogenic amine neurotransmitters. Robinson (1979) has suggested that a stroke may cause depletion of these amines, secondary to disruption of ascending biogenic pathways, and that depression may result. Robinson (1979) and Robinson and Price (1982) argued that because of differential sensitivities to destruction, and because of asymmetrical lateralization of noradrenergic pathways in the central nervous system, left frontal lesions are most likely to disrupt this system. Such disruption of the central noradrenergic system may account for the association of left frontal lesions with poststroke depression. Supportive evidence for this theory is provided in a comprehensive conceptual article by Otto, Yeo, and Dougher (1987). These authors cite a large body of evidence which suggests that depression is associated with hemispheric activity that is relatively greater on the right than on the left side. This net effect may result either from lesions that produce decreased left-sided activity (i.e., left-sided stroke) or those that increase right-sided activity. Right-sided lesions are more commonly associated with apathy, agnosia, or euphoria, but less commonly associated with depressed mood. Similar findings have resulted from studies in which central nervous system depressants (e.g., sodium amytal) were applied to either the left or right hemisphere (Gainotti, 1972).

Parkinson's Disease

Parkinson's disease (PD) is a chronic neurological disorder characterized by tremor, rigidity, involuntary movements, and generalized disturbance in motor functioning. This disease of the basal ganglia is progressive and may be severely disabling or lethal. Depression was recognized as a complication of PD by Patrick & Levy (1922), who reported depressive reactions in 34 percent of clinic patients with this disease. Later studies substantiated this finding, with reports of 30 to 50 percent of PD patients demonstrating at least mild depressive symptoms. Starkstein and Robinson (1989) recently reviewed the literature on depression in PD and also reported preliminary findings from their own study of depressive disorders in these patients. They concluded that the diagnosis of major depression (MDE), based on

DSM-III criteria, could be made in 21 percent of PD patients, and dysthymic disorder in an additional 20 percent. There have been a small number of reports that levo-dopa, a common treatment for PD, is associated with depression (Goodwin, 1971). More commonly, however, depression is regarded as a symptom or complication of PD, which sometimes improves with levo-dopa treatment (Starkstein & Robinson, 1989). Other depressed PD patients require specific antidepressant treatment (Andersen et al., 1980).

The psychological impact of the profound physical, social, and occupational complications of PD are commonly thought to lead to depression in these patients. However, Starkstein and Robinson (1989) cite several lines of evidence which support the role of biological mechanisms in the etiology of depression in PD. Santamaria, Tolosa, and. Valles (1986) reported that most of the depressed patients in their sample with PD became depressed prior to the onset of motor symptoms. They suggested that these patients may be a distinct subset of patients with PD who are characterized by a younger age of onset, less severe physical symptoms, and a greater likelihood of a family history of mood disorder. Starkstein and Robinson (1989) further reported that the frequency of depression in patients with stage I PD (mild) was similar to that in patients with stages IV or V (severely disabling). Furthermore, treatment with levo-dopa alleviates the emotional symptoms in some PD patients. Together, these findings suggest at least that the psychological reaction to the illness or disability is not the sole mechanism responsible for producing depression in patients with PD.

Dopaminergic depletion in the nigrostriatal system is the hallmark of PD. Depletion of this amine in PD has also been demonstrated in the mesocorticolimbic dopaminergic system, but this abnormality does not appear to be involved in motor function. This disturbance may have importance in the production of psychological and/or behavioral symptoms by means of limbic connections (Fibiger, 1984). In addition, disruption of the ascending noradrenergic system as it arises from the locus ceruleus may occur in PD (Folstein et al., 1985). Two studies have now found that PD patients with predominantly right-sided symptoms (indicating left hemispheric pathology) report more severe depression than patients with opposite-sided symptoms (Direnfeld et al., 1984; Starkstein & Robinson, 1989). These preliminary findings suggest that, for some PD patients, asymmetric disturbances in biogenic amine systems may be important in the production of depression.

Others who have investigated the relationship between depression and PD have found evidence for the role of serotonin (Mayeux et al.,

1986, 1988). Levels of serotonin in the cerebrospinal fluid were found to be significantly lower in PD patients with major depression compared to euthymic PD patients (Mayeux et al., 1986). Further, low serotonin was associated with prominent psychomotor retardation and loss of self-esteem. In a later replication study with a new cohort of patients, the same investigators again found that serotonin was low in the cerebrospinal fluid of PD patients with major depression compared with that of euthymic patients with PD and of normal controls (Mayeux et al., 1988). Following treatment with the serotonin precursor 5-hydroxytryptophan, depression improved in six of the seven PD patients with major depression. Mayeux et al. (1988) suggested that their findings support the hypothesis that depression in PD is associated with a reduction in brain serotonin, although other biological or environmental factors may also be involved.

Multiple Sclerosis

Multiple sclerosis (MS) is a demyelinating condition characterized by lesions spread throughout the central nervous system. The course is variable, with prolonged remissions between episodes in some cases, and progressive, severe disability in others. Mood changes including euphoria (Cottrell & Wilson, 1926), depression (Surridge, 1969), and bipolar affective disorder (Joffe et al., 1987) have been described with MS. Joffe et al. (1987) found that 14 percent of a sample of 100 MS clinic patients could be diagnosed with a current major depressive episode, and that 47 percent met criteria for a past episode. A striking finding of this study was that 13 percent of MS patients reported a history which met criteria for a bipolar affective disorder. Other prevalence studies of depression in multiple sclerosis are listed in Chapter 1.

As with the other neurological conditions discussed, some evidence suggests that depression associated with MS is not due entirely to the patient's psychological reaction to illness and/or disability. For example, Schiffer and Babigan (1984) found that patients with MS experienced more episodes of depression than patients with amyotrophic lateral sclerosis, a progressive neurological condition also associated with substantial disability. Also, Joffe et al. (1987) reported no association between functional disability and mood disorder in MS. Schiffer et al. (1983) found that MS patients with cerebral involvement were more frequently depressed than patients without cerebral involvement. Rabins et al. (1986) have since replicated this finding. Whitlock and Siskind (1980) assessed the prevalence of depressive symptoms in 30 MS patients compared with 30 patients having other neurological conditions. Although the degree of disability was similar in both groups, 27 percent of the MS patients scored >14 on the Beck Depression Inventory whereas only 3 percent of the control group scored above this level. Though depression may sometimes be a psychological response to disability in MS, these preliminary findings suggest that depression in MS may arise as a result of central nervous system (CNS) dysfunction. This association may be due to demyelinating lesions that interrupt biogenic amine pathways. Honer et al. (1987) found predominant temporal lobe involvement, based on magnetic resonance testing, in eight MS subjects with psychiatric disorder, including five subjects with depression. To our knowledge, no controlled study has yet correlated the site of the CNS lesions with depression in these patients. Although the evidence remains scant and conflicting, Berrios and Quemada (1990) suggest the possibility that genetic factors (e.g., the human leukocyte system A) may in part account for the association of MS and depressive disorders.

Systemic Lupus Erythematosus

Psychosis, personality changes, and depression have all been reported in association with the autoimmune disease, systemic lupus erythematosus (SLE). When depression occurs in patients with this condition, determination of the exact mechanism is complicated, but necessary, to guide treatment. In a review of the historical literature on the association of mental disorders with SLE, Heine (1969) discussed four mechanisms by which depression and other mental disorders may occur with this disease—organic mood disorder secondary to central nervous system vascular lesions, mental syndromes secondary to other medical complications of SLE (e.g., renal failure), "functional" depression as a psychological reaction to the illness, and organic mood disorder secondary to corticosteroid treatment. Heine (1969) found depression in 18 percent of his sample of 38 SLE patients, based on clinical interviews and unspecified diagnostic criteria.

Rimon, Kronqvist, and Helve (1988) interviewed 30 patients with SLE and diagnosed psychiatric illness in 63 percent, of which almost one-half were a depressive illness, based on ICD-9 criteria. They concluded that corticosteroids were likely not responsible for the most severe episodes of psychiatric illness in their sample, and, in fact, suggested that a therapeutic trial of increased immunosuppression is indicated to treat this complication of SLE. These authors stated that the majority of depressed patients in their sample suffered from "protracted adjustment disorders," that could be understood in terms of a psychosocial reaction to chronic illness. Unfortunately, they provided no evidence to support this formulation, nor how depression of this kind was differentiated from that due to central nervous system lesions. As this study illustrates, further research is needed into the mechanisms by which depression is associated with SLE.

Infection

Viral illnesses are commonly followed by depressed mood, weakness, inactivity, and apathy (Himmelhoch et al., 1970). Hall (1980) stated that the most frequent postinfectious psychiatric complication is a depressive syndrome characterized by sadness and lability of mood, loss of energy, restless sleep, early morning wakening, and irritability. Depression occurred so frequently following an epidemic of St. Louis encephalitis that Azar, Bond, and Lawton (1966) recommended, at that time, that patients be monitored and informed of this potential complication. Other infections associated with depression include infectious mononucleosis, which infrequently may present as a depressive disorder with psychotic features (Schnell et al., 1966; Holmes et al., 1988), chronic brucellosis and tuberculosis (Schwab, 1969), and tertiary syphilis (Hall, 1980). The term posthepatitis syndrome has been applied to patients recovering from hepatitis who frequently complain of severe depressed mood, lethargy, irritability, and weakness (Hall, 1980). The mechanism by which many of these infections produce depressive symptoms and mood disorders is not presently known. However, interference with central nervous system biogenic amine pathways, due to clinical or subclinical viral encephalitis, may be responsible.

Human Immunodeficiency Virus

Human immunodeficiency virus (HIV) may produce a wide spectrum of disease, ranging from asymptomatic infection to acquired immunodeficiency syndrome (AIDS). Mood disorders are common in these patients, most often major depression or adjustment disorder with depressed, anxious, or mixed features (Atkinson et al., 1988). However, human immunodeficiency virus also produces a broad range of neuropsychiatric disorders. Thus, when the syndrome of depressed mood, anhedonia, social withdrawal, apathy, and psychomotor retardation occurs in patients with HIV infection, the differential diagnosis includes not only adjustment disorder and major depressive episode, but also delirium or AIDS dementia, the latter being a rapidly progressive dementia (Navia, Jordan, & Price, 1986; Price, Sidtis, & Rosenblum, 1988). AIDS dementia can often be distinguished from major depression by bedside cognitive testing. Further investigations that may be of help include neuropsychological testing, computerized axial tomography, or magnetic resonance imaging of the head. Schaerf and Miller (1989) also suggested that organic affective disorders may be common in these patients because the use of drugs with central nervous system activity is frequent among AIDS patients.

HIV infection is a good example of a physical illness that may be associated with depression mediated either by psychosocial or biological mechanisms. The psychological impact of the diagnosis of this lethal disease, the associated social isolation, and the presence of preexisting psychiatric vulnerabilities may all contribute to the occurrence of an adjustment disorder or major depression in these patients (Atkinson et al., 1988). However, DiGiovanni (1987) cautioned that such new psychiatric signs and symptoms should not be dismissed automatically as an "understandable" psychological reaction to a disease, because they may represent an early warning of AIDS dementia and HIV disease progression. Prompt and thorough medical/neurological and psychiatric evaluations are indicated in such cases to detect AIDS dementia complex. It is not known why AIDS dementia, in particular, commonly presents with prominent features of lethargy, apathy, and psychomotor retardation. However, HIV may have a predilection for CNS neuronal pathways involved in the regulation of motivation and movement.

Endocrine and Metabolic Abnormalities

Over the past two decades, a strong link between major depression and the endocrine system has been demonstrated. Extensive research followed the discovery of the association of major depression with changes in the hypothalamic-pituitary-adrenal axis (Sachar et al., 1970) and in the hypothalamic-pituitary-thyroid axis (Prange et al., 1972). These investigations documented the alterations that occur in these systems, with depression, and facilitated the development of diagnostic tools based on endocrine changes. The most well known of the latter is the dexamethasone suppression test, which has become a controversial but important research tool. Its potential for use in depressed medical patients was discussed further in Chapter 2.

Endocrine and other metabolic abnormalities have been regarded not only as correlates of major depression, but also as an etiologic mechanism. In support of the latter, changes in a variety of hormones and minerals have been observed to affect the central nervous system and to lead to depression and other mental state abnormalities. Sawin et al. (1979) found endocrine and metabolic disorders in more than one-fifth of psychiatric patients whose mental disorder was thought to be caused by a physical illness. Among the metabolic abnormalities cited were hypothyroidism, altered glucose metabolism, hypercortisolemia, and hypocalcemia. Each of these disturbances may be associated with or produce symptoms which mimic depression.

Thyroid Dysfunction

Overt hypothyroidism (low T3 and T4) is frequently associated with characteristic mental state changes including depressed mood, psychomotor slowing, low energy, decreased appetite and sexual drive, and poor concentration (Smith et al., 1972). Cognitive impairment or psychotic symptoms are also frequent in hypothyroidism and may occur in conjunction with depressive features. Subclinical hypothyroidism (i.e., manifest by increased TSH only) may present with sadness, disinterest, and sleep disturbance prior to the onset of other physical changes. In a series of 100 psychiatric inpatients admitted for major depression, Gold, Herridge, and Hapworth (1987) found subclinical, mild, or overt hypothyroidism in 15 percent. Pituitary supersensitivity to stimulation by exogenous administration of thyrotropin releasing hormone has been found in up to 5 percent of outpatients with major depression (Extein & Gold, 1986). However, the clinical significance of this laboratory abnormality is unclear in the absence of other manifestations of hypothyroidism. Hypothyroidism with depressive features may also occur following treatment with lithium carbonate (Extein & Gold, 1986). Discontinuation of lithium or thyroid replacement may be required in such cases.

Depressive features will improve with thyroid replacement in approximately half of depressed patients with overt hypothyroidism (Smith et al., 1972). The balance of patients will require a combination of thyroid replacement and either antidepressant drugs or electroconvulsive therapy to treat their depression (Extein & Gold, 1986). The value of thyroid replacement is less clear for patients with mildly elevated levels of thyroid stimulating hormone or an abnormal thyrotropin releasing hormone test, in the absence of other manifestations of thyroid disease (Gottlieb & Greenspan, 1989). When major depression occurs with these abnormalities, a combination of thyroid supplementation and a somatic therapy for depression is often required.

Abnormalities of Cortisol Metabolism

Hypocortisolism (or Addison's disease) is uncommon but may present with symptoms characteristic of depression. Depressed mood, loss of interest, loss of energy, psychomotor slowing, and social withdrawal have all been described in patients with this condition (Gottlieb & Greenspan, 1989). In fact, together with other mental status changes, these symptoms may occur in over half of all patients with Addison's disease (Smith et al., 1972). Also, physical symptoms such as fatigue and anorexia are common in this condition and may mimic depression. Most commonly, treatment of the underlying condition results in recovery from depression (Gottlieb & Greenspan, 1989).

Hypercortisolism may result from either the administration of exogenous corticosteroids (e.g., prednisone) or from the overproduction of adrenocorticotrophic hormone (ACTH) by the pituitary gland (i.e., Cushing's disease). ACTH levels, which are known to influence mood (Ettigi & Brown, 1978), are low with the administration of corticosteroids and elevated with Cushing's disease. Although depression may follow long-term prednisone use, organic hypomania and generalized anxiety syndrome are more common with exogenous corticosteroid administration. Psychological manifestations occur in over one-half of persons with Cushing's disease, and are often the earliest manifestations of the illness (Smith et al., 1972). Depressive symptoms commonly include lowered mood, insomnia, irritability, and suicidal ideation (Starkman, Schteingart, & Schork, 1981). Treatment of Cushing's disease is usually associated with gradual alleviation of the psychological manifestations (Smith et al., 1972). However, the literature is inconsistent and inconclusive regarding the use of somatic treatment for depression in patients with Cushing's disease (Gottlieb & Greenspan, 1989).

Vitamin Deficiencies

Deficiencies of vitamin B12 (Carney, 1979; Shovron et al., 1980) and folate (Reynolds et al., 1970; Coppen & Abou-Saleh, 1982) have each been implicated in the production of depressive disorders. It has been suggested that low folate levels in some patients with depression may result from decreased appetite and oral intake, but evidence to support this contention has not been forthcoming (Levitt & Joffe, 1989). Others have continued to search for a mechanism by which these vitamin deficiencies may produce depression. Reynolds, Carney, and Toone (1984) have proposed a methylation deficit to account for the association of folate and vitamin B12 deficiency with depression. Folate is required

252 /   DEPRESSION IN THE MEDICALLY ILL

for the production of S-adenosylmethionine which, along with vitamin B12, is required for the production of methionine and the methylation of neuronal membrane phospholipids. Reynolds and Stramentinoli (1983) have suggested that changes in neurotransmitter function, receptor sensitivity, or endocrine function in depression may be mediated by disturbances in membrane function resulting from a deficit of these precursors. The administration of S-adenosylmethionine, which rectifies these disturbances, has been demonstrated to have some antidepressant effects (Reynolds & Stramentinoli, 1983).

Other Metabolic Abnormalities

Hypocalcemia may result from a variety of conditions, the most common of which is hypoparathyroidism. Psychiatric manifestations occur in over one-half of patients with low calcium (Smith et al., 1972). The mental status changes most often found with hypocalcemia are confusional states and delirium, although depression and anxiety occur with some regularity. Dementia may occur secondary to longstanding hypocalcemia, but depressive symptoms and other mental state changes are often reversible with normalization of serum calcium (Smith et al., 1972). Hypercalcemia may also be associated with somatic and other symptoms of depression (Weizman et al., 1979). Low energy, loss of appetite, and apathy may occur with moderate elevations in this mineral (Ettigi & Brown, 1978). Hypercalcemia has been proposed as one mechanism by which certain malignancies may produce systemic symptoms of depression (Goldberg, 1981).

Medications

Major depression has been reported to be a potential complication of treatment with numerous drugs (Zelnick, 1978). Medications that produce central nervous system effects are among the most likely to produce mental side effects. These include both medications that exert their therapeutic action via the central nervous system, and neuroactive drugs that act peripherally, but still cross the blood-brain barrier. Presumably, any patient administered a "depressogenic" drug is at some risk. However, evidence suggests that patients with a genetic predisposition toward depression, or those with a history of depression, are at greatest risk for an organic mood disorder when administered a drug capable of producing this syndrome (Pascualy & Veith, 1989).

The extensive literature investigating depression as an adverse drug reaction is summarized in two excellent reviews by Zelnick (1978) and

Pascualy and Veith (1989). They cite common methodological problems which limit the reliability and generalizability of the findings reported in many of these studies. For instance, the bulk of this literature consists of case reports or uncontrolled clinical studies. In addition, case definition is often not adequately specified. In many reports, it is unclear whether the subject experienced a major depressive episode or only transient symptoms of depression. Alternatively, other side effects may be misinterpreted and reported as depression. This is most likely to occur with drugs that produce fatigue (e.g., guanethidine) or sedation (e.g., benzodiazepines). Furthermore, many reports do not indicate whether a careful evaluation has been undertaken to rule out other common contributions to depression in the medically ill including organic complications of the illness, other medications, psychological or social factors, predisposing vulnerability, or simply coincidence. Therefore, it is often problematic to determine which drugs produce depression and with what frequency. Zelnick (1978) points out that over 100 drugs have been reported to cause depression, but few of these reports satisfy even minimal criteria to demonstrate a cause and effect relationship.

Antihypertensives

To demonstrate the complexities involved in establishing whether a drug causes depression, we briefly summarize the literature on the depressogenic effect of certain antihypertensives. Several antihypertensive drugs, including alpha-methyl-dopa, propranolol, and reserpine, have been implicated as causes of depression. These drugs exert complex inhibitory effects on central nervous system pathways that utilize biogenic amines as neurotransmitters. Depletion and/or underactivity of central norepinephrine or serotonergic pathways with these drugs have been postulated to produce depression. However, despite a plethora of case reports, there is little evidence that any of these drugs consistently cause depression (Pascualy & Veith, 1989). For example, in an early study, depression was reported in up to 50 percent of patients treated with the beta-blocker propranolol (Waal, 1967). Similarly, Henningsen and Mattiasson (1979) described nightmares, insomnia, and depressive symptoms in a sample of patients receiving beta-blockers including propranolol. Amelioration of these symptoms occurred in three-quarters of their sample when they were switched to atenolol, a selective beta-1 antagonist with less central nervous system concentration than occurs with an equivalent dose of propranolol. On the other hand, Paykel, Flemingero, and Watson (1982) carefully reviewed 31 studies of propranolol use and found depression in only 1.1 percent of patients treated. Not surprisingly, these authors concluded that there is little evidence to prove that propranolol causes depression.

Alpha-methyl-dopa, which acts by suppressing sympathetic nervous system outflow, is another antihypertensive implicated in the development of depression. Johnson et al. (1966) found depression in 4 percent of a sample of 100 patients receiving methyldopa, while others subsequently reported depression in 5.7 percent (Granville-Grossman, 1971) and 3.6 percent (Paykel, Flemingero, & Watson, 1982). However, after reviewing a large number of studies, Demuth and Ackerman (1983) concluded that depressive symptoms associated with alpha-methyldopa rarely meet DSM-III criteria for major depressive episode.

Guanethidine, an antihypertensive agent that blocks the release of norepinephrine at postganglionic sympathetic neurons, has also been thought to lead to depression (Bauer et al., 1961; Prichard et al., 1968). However, in a major retrospective review, Paykel, Flemingero, and Watson (1982) concluded that the incidence of depression with this drug is likely no more than would be expected in the general population. Others have suggested that the generalized weakness and fatigue that this drug may cause have, in some reports, been misinterpreted as depression (Dollery, Emslie-Smith, & Milne, 1960; Pascualy & Veith, 1989).

Reserpine, an antihypertensive that depletes dopamine, norepinephrine, and serotonin in the peripheral and central nervous system, appears to have the strongest association with depression. An early study found depression in 26 percent of 387 patients on reserpine, and in over one-half of those patients with a previous history of depression (Quetsch et al., 1959). Goodwin and Bunney (1971) reviewed 16 studies of depression with reserpine and found an average incidence of 20 percent.

In conclusion, then, it seems that although there are numerous case observations of depression occurring in patients treated with antihypertensives, systematic research does not, for the most part, support a causal association. With the exception of reserpine, the prevalence of depression in patients taking antihypertensives is not greater than in the general population.

Cyclosporine

The decapeptide cyclosporine is widely used following organ transplantation and in other clinical situations which require immunosuppression. Cyclosporine is a highly lipophilic drug that appears to exert its action via a specific binding protein called 'cyclophilin.' Interestingly, this protein has been found in the highest concentrations in lymphoid tissue, the kidneys, and the central nervous system, the sites of the drug's intended action and most common side effects. There is some evidence that the lymphocyte surface binding site is identical to the prolactin receptor (Russell et al., 1985, 1987). From the beginning, the potential of cyclosporine for neurotoxicity has been reported but not widely recognized or well understood. More recently, it has become apparent that cyclosporine may produce a wide spectrum of neurological and psychiatric complications (de Groen et al., 1987). In some patients, depressed mood, lethargy, inactivity, apathy, poor concentration, and social withdrawal may occur during the first few weeks following the initiation of this drug (Powles et al., 1980; Hows, Palmer, & Gordon-Smith, 1982; de Groen et al., 1987). Neurological symptoms such as tremulousness, headache, cortical blindness, or seizures in patients recently started on cyclosporine suggest that an organic neurobehavioral syndrome has been produced by this drug. Because patients receiving cyclosporine commonly suffer from serious physical illnesses which are emotionally distressing, there is great risk that organic mood disturbances will be missed and that the depressive features will be regarded as a psychological reaction to illness. Craven (1989) reported a case of cyclosporine-associated organic mood syndrome that responded well to treatment with methylphenidate. An improved understanding of the central nervous system actions of this drug may produce insights into the production of organic mood and other mental disorders. Other factors clearly contribute to the likelihood of cyclosporine-associated organic mental syndromes. Liver transplant recipients appear particularly prone to these complications, possibly due to a higher prevalence of preexisting central nervous system vulnerability (e.g., presurgical hepatic encephalopathy, alcohol abuse) compared with other transplant recipients (Craven, 1991).

Other Drugs

In high doses, other drugs can also produce symptoms that may be misinterpreted as depression. Digitalis intoxication is a common clinical problem that may present with sadness, fatigue, general malaise, loss of energy, and drowsiness. Wamboldt, Jefferson, and Wamboldt (1986) reported on three patients referred for psychiatric consultation who were subsequently found to have digitalis intoxication. In a similar vein, Pascualy and Veith (1989) suggested that at least some patients who have been reported as depressed while on high doses of benzodiazepines, may, in fact, have been sedated. These observations underscore the importance of careful evaluation and documentation of case reports, rather than simply recording the finding of depression.

CONCLUSIONS

Depression has been reported in association with a large number of medications. However, methodological limitations and inconsistent findings are common in this literature. Prospective studies are needed in which symptoms are appropriately documented and other potential causes of the suspected depression are systematically eliminated. Only then will it be clear which drugs actually produce depression. The mechanisms by which depression occurs require clarification. Improved understanding of the medications most likely to cause depression will help focus research on the biological mechanisms involved in depression.

REFERENCES

Andersen, J., Aabro, E., Gulmann, N., Hjelmsted, A., & Pedersen, H.E. (1980). Anti-depressive treatment in Parkinson's disease: A controlled trial of the effect of nortriptyline in patients with Parkinson's disease treated with L-DOPA. *Acta Neurologica Scandinavica, 62,* 210–219.

Atkinson Jr., J.H., Grant, I., Kennedy, C.J., Richman, D.D., Spector, S.A., & McCutchan, J.A. (1988). Prevalence of psychiatric disorders among men infected with human immunodeficiency virus: A controlled study. *Archives of General Psychiatry, 45,* 859–864.

Azar, G.J., Bond, J.O., & Lawton, A.H. (1966). St. Louis encephalitis: Age aspects of 1962 epidemic in Pinellas County, Florida. *Journal of the American Geriatrics Society, 14,* 326–333.

Bauer, G.E., Croll, F.J.T., Goldrick, R.B., Jeremy, D., Raftos, J., Whyte, H.M., & Young, A.A. (1961). Guanethidine in treatment of hypertension. *British Medical Journal, 2,* 410–415.

Berrios, G.E. & Quemada, J.I. (1990). Depressive illness in multiple sclerosis: Clinical and theoretical aspects of the association. *British Journal of Psychiatry, 156,* 10–16.

Birnbaum, D. & Kleeberg, J. (1958). Carcinoma of the pancreas: A clinical study based on 84 cases. *Annals of Internal Medicine, 48,* 1171–1184.

Brown, J.H. & Paraskevas, F. (1982). Cancer and depression: Cancer presenting with depressive illness: An autoimmune disease? *British Journal of Psychiatry, 141,* 227–232.

Bruera, E., Carraro, S., Roca, E., Cedaro, L., & Chacon, R. (1984). Association between malnutrition and calorie intake, emesis, psychological depression, glucose taste, and tumor mass. *Cancer Treatment Reports, 68,* 873–875.

Carney, M.W.P. (1979). Psychiatric aspects of folate deficiency. In M.I. Boetz & E.H. Reynolds (Eds.), *Folic Acid in Neurology, Psychiatry and Internal Medicine.* (pp. 475–482). New York: Raven Press.

Coppen, A. & Abou-Saleh, M.T. (1982). Plasma folate and affective morbidity during long-term lithium therapy. *British Journal of Psychiatry, 141,* 87–89.

Cottrell, S.S. & Wilson, S.A.K. (1926). The affective symptomatology of disseminated sclerosis: A study of 100 cases. *Journal of Neurology and Psychopathology, 7,* 1–30.

Craven, J.L. (1989). Methylphenidate for cyclosporine-associated organic mood disorder. *American Journal of Psychiatry, 146,* 553.

Craven, J., (1991). Cyclosporine-associated organic mental syndromes in liver transplant recipients. *Psychosomatics, 32,* 94–102.

Davies, D.W. (1965). Physical illness in psychiatric outpatients. *British Journal of Psychiatry, 111,* 27–33.

de Groen, P.C., Akasmit, A.J., Rakela, J., Forbes, G.S., & Krom, R.A.F. (1987). Central nervous system toxicity after liver transplantation: The role of cyclosporine and cholesterol. *New England Journal of Medicine, 317,* 861–866.

Demuth, G.W. & Ackerman, S.H. (1983). Alpha-methyldopa and depression: A clinical study and review of the literature. *American Journal of Psychiatry, 140,* 534–538.

DiGiovanni, C. (1987). Psychiatric aspects. *Maryland Medical Journal, 36,* 35–36.

Direnfeld, L.K., Albert, M.L., Volicer, L., Langlais, P.J., Marquis, J., & Kaplan, E. (1984). Parkinson's disease: The possible relationship of laterality to dementia and neurochemical findings. *Archives of Neurology, 41,* 935–941.

Dollery, C., Emslie-Smith, D., & Milne, M. (1960). Guanethidine in the treatment of hypertension. *Lancet, 2,* 381–389.

Drapiewski, J.F. (1944). Carcinoma of the pancreas: A study of neoplastic invasion of nerves and its possible clinical significance. *American Journal of Clinical Pathology, 14,* 549–556.

Drury, K.K. & Farran-Ridge, C. (1925). Some observations on the types of bloodsugar curve found in different forms of insanity. *Journal of Mental Science, 41,* 8–29.

Ettigi, P.G. & Brown, G.M. (1978). Brain disorders associated with endocrine dysfunction. *Psychiatric Clinics of North America, 1,* 117–136.

Eusterman, G.G. & Wilbur, K.L. (1933). Primary malignant neoplasm of pancreas: Clinical study of 88 verified cases without jaundice. *Southern Medical Journal, 26,* 875–883.

Extein, I. & Gold, M.S. (1986). Psychiatric application of thyroid tests. *Journal of Clinical Psychiatry, 47,* 13–16.

Fibiger, H.C. (1984). The neurobiological substrates of depression in Parkinson's disease: A hypothesis. *Canadian Journal of Neurological Sciences, 11,* 105–107.

Folstein, M.F., Maiberger, R., & McHugh, P.R. (1977). Mood disorder as a specific complication of stroke. *Journal of Neurology, Neurosurgery, and Psychiatry, 40,* 1018–1020.

Folstein, M.F., Robinson, R., Folstein, S., & McHugh, P.R. (1985). Depression and neurological disorders: New treatment opportunities for elderly depressed patients. *Journal of Affective Disorders, 1,* S11–S14.

Forester, B.M., Kornfeld, D.S., & Fleiss, J. (1978). Psychiatric aspects of radiotherapy. *American Journal of Psychiatry, 135,* 960–963.

Fras, I., Litin, E.M., & Pearson, J.S. (1967). Comparison of psychiatric symptoms in carcinoma of the pancreas with those in some other intra-abdominal neoplasms. *American Journal of Psychiatry, 123,* 1553–1562.

Gainotti, G. (1972). Emotional behavior and hemispheric side of the lesion. *Cortex, 8,* 41–55.

Gold, M.S., Herridge, P., & Hapworth, W.E. (1987). Depression and "symptomless" autoimmune thyroiditis. *Psychiatric Annals, 17,* 750–757.

Goldberg, R.J. (1981). Management of depression in the patient with advanced cancer. *Journal of the American Medical Association, 246,* 373–376.

Goodwin, F. (1971). Behavioral effects of L-dopa in man. *Seminars in Psychiatry, 3,* 477–492.

Goodwin, F.K. & Bunney, W.E. (1971). Depressions following reserpine: A reevaluation. *Seminars in Psychiatry, 3,* 435–448.

Gottlieb, G.L. & Greenspan, D. (1989). Depression and endocrine disorders. In R.G. Robinson & P.V. Rabins (Eds.), *Depression and Coexisting Disease.* (pp. 83–102). New York: Igaku-Shoin.

Granville-Grossman, K.L. (1971). Alpha-methyldopa. In K.L. Granville-Grossman (Ed.), *Recent Advances in Clinical Psychiatry.* (pp. 80–87). Edinburgh: Churchill Livingstone.

Guvener, A., Bagchi, B.K., Kooi, K.A., & Calhoun, H.D. (1964). Mental and seizure manifestations in relation to brain tumors: A statistical study. *Epilepsia, 5,* 166–167.

Hall, R.C., Gardner, E.R., Stickney, S.K., LeCann, A.F., & Popkin, M.K. (1980). Physical illness manifesting as psychiatric disease: II. Analysis of a state inpatient population. *Archives of General Psychiatry, 37,* 989–995.

Hall, R.C.W. (1980). Depression. In R.C. Hall (Ed.), *Psychiatric Presentations of Medical Illness: Somato Psychic Disorders.* (pp. 37–63). New York: Spectrum Publications, Inc.

Heine, B.E. (1969). Psychiatric aspects of systemic lupus erythematosus. *Acta Psychiatrica Scandinavica, 50,* 307–326.

Henningsen, N. & Mattiasson, I. (1979). Long-term clinical experience with atenolol: A new selective B-1-blocker with few side effects from the central nervous system. *Acta Medica Scandinavica, 205,* 61–66.

Herridge, C.F. (1960). Physical disorders in psychiatric illness: A study of 209 consecutive admissions. *Lancet, 2,* 949–951.

Himmelhoch, J., Pincus, J., Tucker, G., & Detre, T. (1970). Subacute encephalitis: Behavioral and neurological aspects. *British Journal of Psychiatry,* *116,* 531-538.

Holland, J.C., Korzun, A.H., Tross, S., Silberfarb, P., Perry, M., Comis, R., & Oster, M. (1986). Comparative psychological disturbance in patients with pancreatic and gastric cancer. *American Journal of Psychiatry, 143,* 982-986.

Holmes, G.P., Kaplan, J.E., Gantz, N.M., Komaroff, A.L., Schonberger, L.B., Straus, S.E., Jones, J.F., Dubois, R.E., Cunninghan-Rundles, C., Pahwa, S., Tosato, G., Zegans, L.S., Purtilo, D.T., Brown, N., Schooley, R.T., & Brus, I. (1988). Chronic fatigue syndrome: A working case definition. *Annals of Internal Medicine, 108,* 387-389.

Honer, W.G., Hurwitz, T., Li, D.K., Palmer, M., & Paty, D.W. (1987). Temporal lobe involvement in multiple sclerosis patients with psychiatric disorders. *Archives of Neurology, 44,* 187-190.

Hows, J.M., Palmer, S., & Gordon-Smith, E.C. (1982). Use of cyclosporin A in allogeneic bone marrow transplantation for severe aplastic anemia. *Transplantation, 33,* 382-386.

Jacobsson, L. & Ottosson, J.O. (1971). Initial mental disorders in carcinoma of pancreas and stomach. *Acta Psychiatrica Scandinavica [Suppl], 221,* 120-127.

Joffe, R.T., Lippert, G.P., Gray, T.A., Sawa, G., & Horvath, Z. (1987). Mood disorder and multiple sclerosis. *Archives of Neurology, 44,* 376-378.

Joffe, R.T., Rubinow, D.R., Denicoff, K.D., Maher, M., & Sindelar, W.F. (1986). Depression and carcinoma of the pancreas. *General Hospital Psychiatry,* *8,* 241-245.

Johnson, P., Kitchin, A.H., Lowther, C.P., & Turner, R.W. (1966). Treatment of hypertension with methyldopa. *British Medical Journal, 1,* 133-137.

Kinzie, J.D., Lewinsohn, P., Maricle, R., & Teri, L. (1986). The relationship of depression to medical illness in an older community population. *Comprehensive Psychiatry, 27,* 241-246.

Klerman, G.L. (1981). Depression in the medically ill. *Psychiatric Clinics of North America, 4,* 301-317.

Koranyi, E.K. (1972). Physical health and illness in a psychiatric outpatient department population. *Canadian Psychiatric Association Journal [Suppl],* *17,* 109-116.

Latter, K.A. & Wilbur, K.L. (1937). Psychic and neurologic manifestations of cancer of the pancreas. *Proceedings of the Mayo Clinic, 12,* 457-462.

Levitt, A.J. & Joffe, R.T. (1989). Folate, B12, and life course of depressive illness. *Biological Psychiatry, 25,* 867-872.

Lipsey, J.R., Robinson, R.G., Pearlson, G.D., Rao, K., & Price, T.R. (1983). Mood change following bilateral hemisphere brain injury. *British Journal of Psychiatry, 143,* 266-273.

Lovell, C. (1923). The surface tension of the serum in anxiety psychoses. *Journal of Mental Science, 69,* 497-501.

Lovell, C. (1937). Cerebral edema in certain mental disorders. *British Medical Journal, 2,* 656–659.

Massie, M.J. & Holland, J.C. (1987). The cancer patient with pain: Psychiatric complications and their management. *Medical Clinics of North America, 71,* 243–258.

Mayeux, R., Stern, Y., Sano, M., Williams, J.B.W., & Cote, L.J. (1988). The relationship of serotonin to depression in Parkinson's disease. *Movement Disorders, 3,* 237–244.

Mayeux, R., Stern, Y., Williams, J.B.W., Cote, L., Frantz, A., & Dyrenfurth, I. (1986). Clinical and biochemical features of depression in Parkinson's disease. *American Journal of Psychiatry, 143,* 756–759.

McMullen, F.F. & Hanson, H.H. (1958). Excessive urinary 5-hydroxy 3-indoleacetic acid in the absence of metastatic carcinoid. *Circulation, 18,* 883–886.

Mindham, R.H.S., Marsden, C.D., & Parkes, J.D. (1976). Psychiatric symptoms during L-dopa therapy for Parkinson's disease and their relationship to physical disability. *Psychological Medicine, 6,* 23–33.

Mitchell, W.M. (1967). Etiological factors producing neuropsychiatric syndromes in patients with malignant disease. *International Journal of Neuropsychiatry, 3,* 464–468.

Navia, B.A., Jordan, B.D., & Price, R.W. (1986). The AIDS dementia complex: I. Clinical features. *Annals of Neurology, 19,* 517–524.

Noyes Jr., R. & Kathol, R.G. (1986). Depression and cancer. *Psychiatric Developments, 2,* 77–100.

Otto, M.W., Yeo, R.A., & Dougher, M.J. (1987). Right hemisphere involvement in depression: Toward a neuropsychological theory of negative affective experiences. *Biological Psychiatry, 22,* 1201–1215.

Parikh, R.M., Lipsey, J.R., Robinson, R.G., & Price, T.R. (1988). A two-year longitudinal study of poststroke mood disorders: Prognostic factors related to one and two year outcome. *International Journal of Psychiatry in Medicine, 18,* 45–56.

Pascualy, M. & Veith, R.C. (1989). Depression as an adverse drug reaction. In R.G. Robinson & P.V. Rabins (Eds.), *Depression and Coexisting Disease.* (pp. 132–151). New York: Igaku-Shoin.

Patrick, H.T. & Levy, D.M. (1922). Parkinson's disease: A clinical study of 146 patients. *AMA Archives of Neurology and Psychiatry, 7,* 711–720.

Paykel, E.S., Flemingero, R.F., & Watson, J.P. (1982). Psychiatric side effects of antihypertensive drugs other than reserpine. *Journal of Clinical Psychopharmacology, 2,* 14–39.

Peck, A., & Boland, J. (1977). Emotional reactions to radiation treatment. *Cancer, 40,* 180–184.

Powles, R.L., Clink, H.M., Spence, D., Morgenstern, G., Watson, J.G., Selby, P.J., Woods, M., Barrett, A., Jameson, B., Sloane, J., Lawler, S.D., Kay, H.E.M., Lawson, D., McElwain, T.J., & Alexander, P. (1980). Cyclosporin A to prevent graft-versus-host disease in man after allogenic bone-marrow transplantation. *Lancet, 1,* 327–329.

Prange Jr., A.J., Wilson, I.C., Lara, P.P., Alltop, L.B., & Breese, G.R. (1972). Effects of thyrotropin releasing hormone in depression. *Lancet, 2,* 999–1002.

Price, R.W., Sidtis, J., & Rosenblum, M.L. (1988). The AIDS dementia complex: Some current questions. *Annals of Neurology, 23,* 27–33.

Prichard, B.N.C., Johnston, A.W., Hill, I.D., & Rosenheim, M.L. (1968). Bethanidine, guanethidine, and methyldopa in treatment of hypertension: A within-patient comparison. *British Medical Journal, 1,* 135–144.

Proctor, S.J., Kernahan, J., & Taylor, P. (1981). Depression as a component of post-cranial irradiation somnolence syndrome. *Lancet, 1,* 1215–1216.

Quetsch, R., Achor, R., Litin, E., & Faucett, R.L. (1959). Depressive reactions in hypertensive patients: A comparison of those treated with rauwolfia and those receiving no specific antihypertensive treatment. *Circulation, 19,* 366–375.

Rabins, P.V., Brooks, B.R., O'Donnell, P., Pearlson, G.D., Moberg, P., Jubelt, B., Coyle, P., Dalos, N., & Folstein, M.F. (1986). Structural brain correlates of emotional disorder in multiple sclerosis. *Brain, 109,* 585–597.

Reynolds, E.H., Carney, M.W., & Toone, B.K. (1984). Methylation and mood. *Lancet, 2,* 196–198.

Reynolds, E.H., Preece, J.M., Bailey, J., & Coppen, A. (1970). Folate deficiency in depressive illness. *British Journal of Psychiatry, 117,* 287–292.

Reynolds, E.H. & Stramentinoli, G. (1983). Folic acid, S-adenosylmethionine and affective disorder. *Psychological Medicine, 13,* 705–710.

Rimon, R., Kronqvist, K., & Helve, T. (1988). Overt psychopathology in systemic lupus erythematosus. *Scandinavian Journal of Rheumatology, 17,* 143–146.

Robinson, R.G. (1979). Differential behavioral and biochemical effects of right and left hemispheric cerebral infarction in the rat. *Science, 205,* 707–710.

Robinson, R.G., Kubos, K.L., Starr, L.B., Rao, K., & Price, T.R. (1984a). Mood disorders in stroke patients: Importance of lesion location. *Brain, 107,* 81–93.

Robinson, R.G. & Lipsey, J.R. (1985). Cerebral localization of emotion based on clinical-neuropathological correlations: Methodological issues. *Psychiatric Developments, 4,* 335–347.

Robinson, R.G. & Price, T.R. (1982). Post-stroke depressive disorders: A follow-up study of 103 patients. *Stroke, 13,* 635–641.

Robinson, R.G., Starr, L.B., Kubos, K.L., & Price, T.R. (1983). A two-year longitudinal study of post-stroke mood disorders: Findings during the initial evaluation. *Stroke, 14,* 736–741.

Robinson, R.G., Starr, L.B., Lipsey, J.R., Rao, K., & Price, T.R. (1984b). A two-year longitudinal study of post-stroke mood disorders: Dynamic changes over the first six months of follow-up. *Stroke, 15,* 510–517.

Robinson, R.G., Starr, L.B., & Price, T.R. (1984c). A two-year longitudinal study of mood disorders following stroke: Prevalence and duration at six months follow-up. *British Journal of Psychiatry, 144,* 256–262.

Rothermich, N.O. & von Haam, E. (1941). Pancreatic encephalopathy. *Journal of Clinical Endocrinology, 1,* 872–881.

Russell, D.H., Buckley, A.R., Montgomery, D.W., Larson, N.A., Gout, P.W., Beer, C.T., Putnam, C.W., Zukoski, C.F., & Kibler, R. (1987). Prolactin-dependent mitogenesis in Nb2 node lymphoma cells: Effects of immunosuppressive cyclopeptides. *Journal of Immunology, 138,* 276–284.

Russell, D.H., Kibler, R., Matrisian, L., Larson, D.F., Poulos, B., & Magun, B.E. (1985). Prolactin receptors on human T and B lymphocytes: Antagonism of prolactin binding by cyclosporine. *Journal of Immunology, 134,* 3027–3031.

Sachar, E.J., Hellman, L., Fukushima, D.K., & Gallagher, T.F. (1970). Cortisol production in depressive illness: A clinical and biochemical clarification. *Archives of General Psychiatry, 23,* 289–298.

Santamaria, J., Tolosa, E., & Valles, A. (1986). Parkinson's disease with depression: A possible subgroup of idiopathic parkinsonism. *Neurology, 36,* 1130–1133.

Savage, C., Butcher, W., & Noble, D. (1952). Psychiatric manifestations in pancreatic disease. *Journal of Clinical and Experimental Psychopathology, 13,* 9–16.

Sawin, C.T., Chopra, D., Azizi, F., Mannix, J.E., & Bacharach, P. (1979). The aging thyroid. *Journal of the American Medical Association, 242,* 247–250.

Schaerf, F.W. & Miller, R.R. (1989). Depression and human immunodeficiency virus (HIV-1) infection. In R.G. Robinson & P.V. Rabins (Eds.), *Depression and Coexisting Disease.* (pp. 169–185). New York: Igaku-Shoin.

Schiffer, R.B. & Babigan, H.M. (1984). Behavioral disorders in multiple sclerosis, temporal lobe epilepsy, and amyotrophic lateral sclerosis: An epidemiologic study. *Archives of Neurology, 41,* 1067–1069.

Schiffer, R.B., Caine, E.D., Bamford, K.A., & Levy, S. (1983). Depressive episodes in patients with multiple sclerosis. *American Journal of Psychiatry, 140,* 1498–1500.

Schmale, A.H. (1979). Psychological aspects of anorexia: Areas for study. *Cancer, 43,* 2087–2092.

Schnell, R.G., Dyck, P.J., Bowie, E.J., Klass, D.W., & Taswell, H.F. (1966). Infectious mononucleosis: Neurologic and EEG findings. *Medicine, 45,* 51–63.

Scholz, T. & Pfeiffer, F. (1923). Roentgenologic diagnosis of carcinoma of tail of the pancreas. *Journal of the American Medical Association, 81,* 275–277.

Schwab, J.J. (1969). Psychiatric illness produced by infections. *Hospital Medicine, 5,* 98–108.

Shovron, S.D., Carney, M.W.P., Chanarin, I., & Reynolds, E.H. (1980). The neuropsychiatry of megaloblastic anemia. *British Medical Journal, 281,* 1036–1038.

Silberfarb, P.M., Holland, J.C.B., Anbar, D., Bahna, G., Maurer, H., Chahinian, A.P., & Comis, R. (1983). Psychological response of patients receiving two drug regimens for lung carcinoma. *American Journal of Psychiatry, 140,* 110–111.

Smith, C.K., Barish, J., Correa, J., & Williams, R.H. (1972). Psychiatric disturbance in endocrinologic disease. *Psychosomatic Medicine, 34,* 69–86.

Starkman, M.N., Schteingart, D.E., & Schork, M.A. (1981). Depressed mood and other psychiatric manifestations of Cushing's syndrome: Relationship to hormone levels. *Psychosomatic Medicine, 43*, 3–18.

Starkstein, S.E. & Robinson, R.G. (1989). Affective disorders and cerebral vascular disease. *British Journal of Psychiatry, 154*, 170–182.

Summers, W.K., Munoz, R.A., Read, M.R., & Marsh, G.M. (1981). The psychiatric physical examination: Part II: Findings in 75 unselected psychiatric patients. *Journal of Clinical Psychiatry, 42*, 99–102.

Surridge, D. (1969). An investigation into some psychiatric aspects of multiple sclerosis. *American Journal of Psychiatry, 115*, 749–764.

Waal, H.J. (1967). Propranolol-induced depression. *British Medical Journal, 2*, 50.

Wamboldt, F.S., Jefferson, J.W., & Wamboldt, M.Z. (1986). Digitalis intoxication misdiagnosed as depression by primary care physicians. *American Journal of Psychiatry, 143*, 219–221.

Weizman, A., Eldar, M., Shoenfeld, Y., Hirschorn, M., Wijsenbeek, H., & Pinkhas, J. (1979). Hypercalcemia-induced psychopathology in malignant disease. *British Journal of Psychiatry, 135*, 363–366.

Westin, T., Jansson, A., Zenckert, C., Hallstrom, T., & Edstrom, S. (1988). Mental depression is associated with malnutrition in patients with head and neck cancer. *Archives of Otolaryngology—Head and Neck Surgery, 114*, 1449–1453.

Whitlock, F.A. (1982). *Symptomatic Affective Disorders: A Study of Depression and Mania Associated with Physical Disease and Medication.* New York: Academic Press, Inc.

Whitlock, F.A. & Siskind, M.M. (1980). Depression as a major symptom of multiple sclerosis. *Journal of Neurology, Neurosurgery, and Psychiatry, 43*, 861–865.

Yaskin, J.C. (1931). Nervous symptoms as earliest manifestations of carcinoma of the pancreas. *Journal of the American Medical Association, 96*, 1664–1668.

Young, D.F. (1982). Neurological complications of cancer chemotherapy. In A. Silverstein (Ed.), *Neurological Complications of Therapy: Selected Topics.* (pp. 57–113). Mount Kisco, New York: Futura Publishing Co.

Zelnick, T. (1978). Depressive effects of drugs. In O. Cameron (Ed.), *Presentations of Depressions and Depressive Symptoms in Medical and Other Psychiatric Disorders, ed. 1.* (pp. 382–383). New York: Wiley Interscience Publication.

PART III

TREATMENT

9

Psychological Treatments

Considering the wide array of factors that may contribute to depression in persons with a physical illness, an eclectic and integrative approach is needed in the selection of optimal and appropriate treatment. Such treatment may include practical physical interventions, and pharmacologic, psychological, and social treatments. Additional interventions that may relieve depression include optimizing the medical status of the patient, restructuring the social environment, assisting with occupational functioning, and identifying and eliminating depressogenic drugs that are not essential to the medical treatment. Even when a broad range of factors can be identified that contribute to or perpetuate depression in a medical patient, attention to one specific underlying factor may alleviate the mood disturbance. For example, when major depression is associated with hypothyroidism, the gradual institution of thyroid replacement medication not only takes precedence over other specific antidepressant treatments, but may, by itself, relieve the depression. In other cases, medical treatments should be instituted concurrently with psychological and biological therapies for depression.

In the medical setting, the etiology of depression should usually be understood from multiple perspectives. Similarly, treatment selection often requires the consideration of diverse modalities. For the purpose of clarity, we have divided into separate chapters our discussion of biological and psychological treatments. However, this literary convenience should not be taken to imply that the use of one treatment modality in any way precludes the concurrent or sequential use of others. In this regard, although the efficacy of antidepressant medication for major depression has been substantiated in a variety of controlled studies (see Chapter 11), it has become evident that combining psychotherapeutic and pharmacologic treatments often results in greater benefits than with either approach alone (Elkin et al., 1988; Conte et al., 1986). These treatments may act differentially, such that medication ameliorates vegetative symptoms most effectively but that psychotherapy is more effective in improving psychological and social adjustment (Beckham & Leber, 1985). This differential effect may be particularly relevant in the physically ill, in whom major depression is often preceded by and associated with a relative inability to cope with the multiple tasks and stresses associated with the condition. Treatment that is directed solely toward the vegetative symptoms of depression without strengthening coping skills may leave the patient with a persistent vulnerability to subsequent adaptive failure and depressive episodes. By contrast, assisting the patient to develop more effective coping skills may minimize the risk of recurrent depression after the acute episode has resolved.

Not surprisingly, depression has been shown to persist when medical illness is unremitting (Mann, Jenkins, & Belsey, 1981; Schulberg, McClelland, & Gooding, 1987; Magruder-Habib et al., 1989). Treatments for depression also may be less effective in patients with active medical disease than in those whose illness is relatively inactive or asymptomatic. Unfortunately, some evidence suggests that depression associated with more severe medical illness tends to be treated less vigorously. In this regard, Broadhead et al. (1989) reported that more severe physical illness in depressed general practice patients is associated with a lower rate of treatment for depression with either tricyclics or follow-up visits. This lower rate of treatment prescribed by physicians may result either from their lack of awareness of appropriate treatment and/or from unduly pessimistic beliefs about the relative risks and benefits of antidepressant treatment in the medically ill.

Throughout this text, we are careful to distinguish clinical depression from milder forms of dysphoria. This distinction is particularly important in treatment selection. For example, psychotherapy may be the most appropriate modality for patients with mild depression associated not with an overt psychiatric disorder, but with a less clearly defined state that has been labelled "demoralization" (Frank, 1961). The boundaries of this state and its relationship to depression are not clear, although Frank (1961) suggested that it is common to all patients seeking psychotherapeutic help. He used the term demoralization in this context to refer to feelings of powerlessness, isolation, and hopelessness that result when individuals find that they can neither meet nor remove themselves from the demands of their environment. This state is not synonymous with clinical depression, but likely overlaps with it. Medical patients who are experiencing significant dysphoria or demoralization may benefit from psychotherapeutic interventions, not only to improve their emotional well-being, but also to forestall or prevent the development of a full-blown depressive disorder.

PSYCHOTHERAPY FOR DEPRESSION IN THE MEDICALLY ILL

The onset of a serious medical illness that alters profoundly the life trajectory of an individual may trigger feelings of depression and hopelessness. The implications of the illness and the feelings associated with it may seem too threatening for that person to tolerate. Psychotherapy in such cases can help to integrate these warded-off thoughts and feelings into the individual's awareness and to resolve some of the grief and sadness that may otherwise contribute to an overt depressive disorder. We focus in this chapter on the role of psychotherapy both as a treatment for existing depression and as a prophylactic measure to prevent this complication. There is little empirical data regarding the indications for or the efficacy of specific psychotherapeutic treatments for medical patients. Therefore, the discussion in this chapter is based on clinical observations and experience, and on extrapolations from nonmedical samples. Our emphasis here reflects our own clinical interests in two of the most common psychotherapeutic approaches to depression, namely cognitive therapy and psychodynamic psychotherapy. In addition, we briefly discuss the popular move toward group treatment of medical patients. We do not deal with psychoeducational approaches at length because they are not as directly related to the treatment of depression. However, such interventions may be of great practical and psychotherapeutic value to medical populations. Information presented in a therapeutic context may provide structure and a sense of mastery to individuals who may otherwise feel overwhelmed by their condition.

Nonspecific Therapeutic Factors in Psychotherapy

Although we emphasize the specific characteristics of psychodynamic and cognitive therapies for depression, we are aware that much of the benefit of such treatments may be due to nonspecific factors that are common to a variety of psychotherapeutic modalities. These nonspecific factors include the presence of an emotionally charged, confiding relationship, a therapeutic rationale that is accepted by the patient, the provision of new information, strengthened expectations of help, new success experiences, and emotional arousal (Frank, 1961). Karasu (1986) suggested that three therapeutic factors that can be identified in most forms of psychotherapy are affective experiencing, cognitive mastery, and behavioral regulation. Although the first of these is a sine qua non of psychodynamic therapy and the second of cognitive therapy, all three elements are present in both modalities.

It must also be emphasized that psychotherapeutic assistance may be provided not only through a formal process of psychotherapy, but also in the context of the ongoing doctor-patient relationship. For many medical patients, the relationship with a medical practitioner who is prepared to listen to their experience is the most important component of treatment. However, as Balint (1957) suggested in his treatise on psychotherapy in the medical setting, the practitioner may need to shift from a questioning, diagnosis-seeking mode to an empathic, listening one.

Psychotherapy with a therapist other than the medical practitioner is sometimes necessary because of the inability or unwillingness of the primary care physician to allow the patient to communicate. In a study of a primary care practice at a teaching hospital, Beckman and Frankel (1984) found that in less than a third of the visits to resident physicians were patients allowed to complete their opening statement of concerns. In more than two-thirds of the visits, the physician interrupted the patient's initial statement and directed questions toward a specific medical concern. In the majority of cases, patients were not given an opportunity to complete their opening statements, and communication shifted to physician-centered direct questioning, on average, after only 18 seconds. Ironically, it was not only personal information that was lost when the physicians interrupted the spontaneous flow of information in these ways, but also the communication of important medical information. Too often, physicians regard their role in terms of the narrow search for medical facts and the prescription of medical treatment. However, many patients look to their health care provider for emotional support related to their illness. Understanding the underlying meaning of statements from patients is obviously not possible when communications from the patient are ignored or blocked. The sense of despair and isolation experienced by many patients may be intensified when they feel cut off in this way from meaningful communication with their medical practitioner.

Although the therapeutic relationship may be one of the most powerful tools to preserve and protect emotional well-being, this factor is often underestimated by practicing physicians. The reasons for the current neglect of this traditional healing role of the physician are complex.

The problem may begin with modern medical school training which does not emphasize communicative skills and empathic listening. It may also be that clinical training often takes place in acute treatment settings in tertiary care centers which focus on the immediate medical condition rather than on the experience and emotional health of the individual. Although there has been a recent shift of medical training to ambulatory settings and to the community, the principal location of most medical training is still in tertiary care settings oriented toward biotechnology and superspecialization.

The relative neglect of therapeutic relationships with caregivers is unfortunate since medical patients with milder or more transient forms of depression may respond with improved mood simply to interested listening by a health care professional. Indeed, the responsiveness of the hospital environment to anxieties and concerns of patients may be particularly important in tertiary settings where patients are often far from home or have little contact with family or friends. Even when families are available, patients may not wish to burden them further with emotional complaints.

Technical Considerations in Psychotherapy of the Medically Ill

The principles of psychotherapy in the medically ill are, in most respects, similar to those in nonmedical patients. However, certain alterations in technique may be necessary. For example, the therapist must be prepared to shift to more supportive approaches with patients who develop acute medical complications or who have distressing physical symptoms (Rodin, 1984). Also, therapists who undertake regular therapy with medical patients must accept that periodic disruptions in treatment are likely. For these and other reasons, brief and/or intermittent forms of psychotherapy may be necessary. Some medical patients who might benefit from psychotherapy are reluctant to accept a treatment that implies that they are "damaged" in yet another way. Such patients, particularly those with milder manifestations of depression, may prefer brief or periodic interventions that emphasize psychoeducation. At times, therapy may need to be continued at the bedside, requiring flexibility not only with regard to scheduling and privacy, but also with respect to the maintenance by the therapist of the usual position of therapeutic neutrality. In other cases, it is appropriate when a patient is hospitalized to halt temporarily intensive psychotherapeutic work and to maintain the relationship by means of briefer and more supportive interactions at the bedside or by telephone. In such cases, the psychological significance of these changes in the parameters of treatment can often be fruitfully explored with the patient, particularly in the context of psychodynamic therapy. Nevertheless, considerable adjustment is often necessary for the therapist of the medically ill patient to feel comfortable in venturing from the relatively protected and familiar confines of the consulting office and the usual psychotherapeutic situation.

Medical illness frequently represents an emotional crisis that responds well to brief therapeutic interventions. Intermittent sessions (Castelnuovo-Tedesco, 1965) or even single interviews (Malan et al., 1975) can be beneficial to provide relief from and understanding of overwhelming feelings of anxiety or depression, morbid preoccupations about the future, and/or profound feelings of defectiveness triggered by the illness. Patients who present in a crisis, including one precipitated by medical illness, are often highly motivated for treatment. With mildly depressed patients, brief, focal interventions may help to prevent or forestall the development of more florid depressive symptoms. When based upon a well conceptualized formulation, such interventions may have particular applicability in the medical setting (Perry, Cooper, & Michels, 1987). In addition, the secondary gain related to dependence in long-term therapy can sometimes be avoided with brief therapy.

The presence of a severe physical illness may have significant implications for the content of ongoing psychotherapy. During times of acute medical illness and physical distress, interpretive work may be not only ineffective but undesirable. At such times, preoccupation with the immediate concerns of illness may temporarily interfere with the patient's capacity or willingness to explore his or her inner life. With patients already engaged in insight-oriented psychotherapy, a concurrent medical crisis may necessitate a shift away from approaches that result in emotional arousal. Unnecessary emotional arousal at times of acute medical illness may be undesirable not only because of generalized weakness and the stress of illness, but also because of specific adverse consequences that may result (e.g., the risk of arrhythmias with acute myocardial infarction). Supportive interventions and simple cognitive techniques may be preferable at such times to diminish feelings of isolation and to promote a sense of mastery.

Severe physical illness is frequently associated with metabolic, neurological, or systemic disorders that impair concentration and other aspects of cognitive functioning. Routine cognitive testing should be part of the evaluation for psychotherapy in medical patients. In some cases, the cognitive impairment will be the focus of psychotherapy. For example, in the early phases of a dementing process or with a condition such as endstage renal disease in which there may be subtle cognitive disturbances, the awareness of the impairment may be the most painful aspect of the patient's experience. This is most likely to be the case with individuals who have greatly valued or relied upon intellectual functioning to maintain self-esteem and/or to perform in a highly valued occupation. Brodsky and Brodsky (1984) suggested that, following the complete resolution of an organic mental syndrome, it may subsequently be therapeutic to discuss memories of these events. However, both expressive and cognitively oriented psychotherapy are often inappropriate or contraindicated when there is severe cognitive impairment, even though psychological meaning may be evident in the patient's symptoms.

PSYCHODYNAMIC PSYCHOTHERAPY

What is Psychodynamic Psychotherapy?

The term psychodynamic has been applied to a wide range of therapeutic approaches that are based upon an understanding of conscious and unconscious processes, and how they are manifested in the therapeutic relationship (Wallace, 1983). Psychodynamic psychotherapy, also referred to as supportive-expressive psychotherapy, includes both supportive approaches aimed at bolstering existing defenses and means of adaptation, and expressive ones, in which cognitive and affective understanding are emphasized. Supportive aspects of psychodynamic therapy include not only specific interventions such as reassurance but also, as Lüborsky (1984) noted, aspects of the treatment situation including the regularity of appointments, the joint establishment of treatment goals, and a positive experience of the therapist. However, supportive and interpretive approaches should be regarded as parts of a continuum rather than as distinct modalities. Indeed, as Holmes (1988) recently suggested, all therapy is or should be supportive; even therapy, the sole purpose of which is support, must include attention to the emotional, unconscious, and unexpressed aspects of the patient's story.

There has been ongoing debate about the relative importance of different factors in producing therapeutic change in psychodynamic therapy. Opinions about what is most therapeutic have often shifted as different models have evolved. Cooper (1989) recently reviewed the evolution of psychoanalytic concepts of treatment ranging from Freud's early emphasis on the therapeutic value of catharsis and making the unconscious conscious, to the emphasis of later psychoanalytic writers on the therapeutic value of the corrective emotional experience and of the empathic bond between patient and therapist. However, Michels (1986) suggests that apparently divergent views regarding the elements of change in psychoanalytic therapy actually emphasize one or more of three factors, namely, insight, an intense emotional experience, and the establishment of a new relationship. The indications and criteria for psychodynamic therapy, particularly of a brief nature (Malan, 1976), include the presence of an emotional crisis, motivation for insight, psychological mindedness, and evidence of the capacity to form a meaningful relationship. Other factors that determine suitability for psychodynamic therapy include frustration tolerance, impulse control, reality testing, and the availability of affect (Paolino, 1981).

Psychodynamic therapy is most commonly conducted within the context of regular (e.g., weekly) appointments over a circumscribed, although not necessarily predetermined, period of time. It is assumed that treatment will eventually stop and that the termination phase may, in itself, be growth-promoting (Firestein, 1978). With severe characterological defects or other less treatable conditions, long-term supportive therapy may be necessary. Chronic medical illness may be added to the list of criteria for longer or more open-ended treatment, because of the ongoing difficulties in adjustment and because of the sense of uncertainty and unpredictability associated with it.

Application of Psychodynamic Therapy to Depression

There has been little empirical research on the process or outcome of psychodynamic therapy for depression. Thus, any claims about its effectiveness must be cautious at present. However, the view that there have been no new developments in the psychodynamic understanding of depression (Kovacs, 1983; Strupp et al., 1982) no longer seems tenable. Of particular interest in this regard are recent clinical observations and theoretical formulations regarding the nature and function of affect (Stern, 1985; Emde, 1983; Lichtenberg, 1983; Demos, 1984). Some of these observations and their clinical and theoretical implications are noted in Chapters 3 and 7, and they are discussed briefly in the following section.

Freud emphasized the adaptive function of anxiety as a signal to mobilize defensive operations (Freud, 1926), but he did not regard depressive affect as central to the maintenance of intrapsychic homeostasis. More recently, however, depression and other affects have also come to be regarded as adaptive signals which are utilized to monitor and organize ongoing experience (Brenner, 1982; Stolorow, Brandchaft,

& Atwood, 1987). Psychodynamic approaches that have evolved from this stance place particular emphasis on the integration of affect into subjective experience (Stolorow, Brandchaft, & Atwood, 1987). From this perspective, clinical depression is seen to arise when depressive affect cannot be tolerated or integrated into ongoing subjective experience. Depressive symptoms that are biologically and psychologically autonomous may be regarded as more extreme manifestations of this phenomenon.

With regard to treatment and care, the traditional psychoanalytic position has emphasized the therapeutic value of the recovery and working through of repressed mental contents. More recent approaches suggest that what may be more important than the recovery of repressed memories is the creation of meaning, and an increase in the capacity to tolerate and organize subjective experience. More specifically, a primary goal of therapy may be to create with the patient a narrative that provides a meaningful framework within which to organize their personal world (Stolorow, Brandchaft, & Atwood, 1987; Spence, 1982; Gedo, 1979). This goal is often more acceptable and more achievable than uncovering unconscious material in medical patients with whom intensive psychoanalytic approaches would otherwise not be feasible.

Psychotherapeutic treatment in the medically ill is appropriately directed toward helping patients to understand the impact of medical illness in terms of their current conflicts and vulnerabilities. The effectiveness of so-called genetic interpretations that relate current difficulties to early life experience may depend not so much on their validity based upon external criteria (e.g., whether current feelings of depression are actually due to an experience of loss during an important developmental period), but upon the power of the interpretation to supply the patient with a new pattern for organizing information (Gedo, 1979) (e.g., the sadness associated with the illness resembles the sense of loss experienced when recalling your mother's death). Helping patients to integrate warded-off affects into their subjective experience may be essential not only to resolve depressive feelings but also to permit them to derive meaning from the subjective experience. This approach is consistent with the view of Stolorow, Brandchaft, and Atwood (1987) who emphasize that affects are the organizers of self-experience and that a central task of psychotherapy with the patient who has a disturbance in affect is to assist with integrating affects into the ongoing flow of subjective experience. Only then can affects serve their adaptive signal function, rather than triggering painful subjective states that cannot be understood or communicated. Indeed, Stolorow, Brandchaft, and Atwood (1987) assert that grief and mourning, a common accompaniment of serious medical illness, can proceed only if depressive affect can be identified, tolerated, and comprehended. This process may be blocked with medically ill patients who have cognitively understood the implications of their condition but who have warded-off all of the associated feelings. Without psychological treatment, such patients may be at risk for overt depression.

Application to the Medically Ill

Psychodynamic therapy emphasizes the therapeutic value of understanding and interpreting the patient's emotional experience as it is manifest in the therapeutic relationship. Indeed, interpretations that involve the transference relationship are considered by some to be the central therapeutic factor in psychodynamic therapy (Arlow, 1987). Transference is of particular value since it permits access to intrapsychic life via the immediacy of a current relationship. However, the necessary reliance of medical patients on multiple caregivers may dilute or otherwise alter the nature of the therapeutic relationship that can develop in psychotherapy. Complex medical conditions, or those associated with multisystem disease, often require collaborative management by many medical and nonmedical specialists. Indeed, negotiating the transactions with multiple practitioners and specialists is, for some patients, the most complicated illness-related task. Patients who are severely ill may be unwilling or unable to invest emotional energy into yet another therapeutic relationship. Formal psychotherapeutic interventions may need to be postponed in such circumstances. For other medical patients, the establishment of a psychotherapeutic relationship, distinct from their physical care helps not only to alleviate feelings of depression and hopelessness, but also to facilitate the complex task of negotiating relationships with numerous other caregivers.

A serious medical illness inevitably affects the emotional life of the individual affected. When there is an exacerbation of the disease, illness-related issues may dominate the psychotherapeutic treatment. Indeed, if the illness and its personal implications do not emerge in treatment, it may be assumed that emotionally significant issues related to this condition are being avoided. On the other hand, when the illness and its management remain in focus at all times, exploration of fantasy life may be limited. Attention to the physical reality of the illness may serve, in such cases, to protect or distract the patient from the emotional implications and personal meaning of the illness. Such distraction is sometimes necessary to diminish tension or distress that seems unbearable. At other times, preoccupation with details of the illness represents, either for the patient or the therapist, an avoidance of the underlying emotional significance of the illness. It is a delicate matter of clinical judgment to determine whether and when it may be therapeutic to interpret such defenses.

The therapist who treats a medically ill patient must be prepared to help the patient deal with immediate and often life-threatening concerns related to the medical condition. At such times, the therapist must be ready to shift with the patient away from the inner world of fantasy life toward the physical reality of the illness and the concrete decisions which must be made regarding medical treatment. However, when the therapist becomes too preoccupied with the physical or external reality of the condition, an imbalance in the mode of listening may then result, such that the intrapsychic or personal reality of the individual is neglected (Schafer, 1985). When such an imbalance occurs with the medically ill, the therapist or other caregiver may tend to ignore the psychological basis for depression and other psychological symptoms, attributing them solely to the obvious physical reality. Psychological experiences such as feeling hopeless or defective may then be dismissed as generic accompaniments of illness, rather than understood as a more individual, personal psychological experience (Coen, 1986). When therapists do not appreciate that there are symbolic implications of an illness, psychological symptoms may be regarded solely as expectable reactions to external reality rather than as subjective truths that have been concretized by the illness (Stolorow, Brandchaft, & Atwood, 1987). For example, the physical reality of the illness may be experienced as a confirmation or illustration of a psychological sense of defectiveness, although the latter preceded the occurrence of the medical condition. The dynamically oriented therapist must attend both to the concrete concerns of medical patients and to the underlying meaning of these concerns. Reports of depression in medical patients, like feelings of emptiness or nonhumanness reported by borderline patients (Singer, 1988), may represent not only a direct perception or a symptom of a psychiatric disorder, but also a subjective experience that may include wishes, fears, and defenses.

Physical illness in a patient may affect the neutrality of the therapist in various ways. Therapists may feel inclined to collude with maladaptive denial or to gratify directly wishes for support, because of discomfort and feelings of helplessness that the illness generates in the therapist. Of course, it is often appropriate and necessary for therapists of the medically ill to assume a more directly supportive role, particularly with more severely depressed or ill patients. However, therapists of such patients may also be susceptible to a "rescue fantasy" in which the therapist harbors unrealistic expectations that his or her involvement will protect the patient from suffering (Sourkes, 1982). Such an approach may not only encroach upon the family's role with the patient, but it may also underestimate and interfere with the emerging capacity of the patient to function more autonomously and to tolerate feelings related to the illness. Therapists of the medically ill must be prepared to tolerate feelings of helplessness and despair that are, to some extent, inevitable under such conditions. Empathic listening is often more helpful than reassurance, which may seal off the patient's experience.

The therapeutic position that has been considered to be optimal in psychoanalytic treatment is midway between the polarities of curative zeal and therapeutic nihilism (Cooper, 1986). This position may be difficult for therapists to maintain in the face of an irreversible or terminal medical condition. Therapists may protect themselves from the enormity of the patient's dilemma by colluding with patients who deny the implications of illness or by detaching themselves emotionally from those patients who are seriously ill. Although the adaptive function of denial to deal with acute medical illness has been empirically demonstrated (Lazarus, 1979; Levenson et al., 1989), therapists who do not address extreme denial of a serious medical condition may leave patients feeling alone with the emotional burden of the condition.

PSYCHODYNAMIC TREATMENT OF DEPRESSION IN MEDICAL PATIENTS

For the purposes of discussion, we have identified three phases in the psychodynamic treatment of depression in the medically ill. These phases, which are not always or necessarily sequential, are: (1) the facilitation of grief and mourning; (2) the provision of meaning; and (3) the achievement of a sense of mastery over the feelings associated with the illness. The extent to which these tasks can be accomplished depends upon a variety of factors including the severity and stability of the medical condition, the depth of depression, and the characteristics of the patient.

The Expression of Grief

With the onset of a serious medical illness or of a new complication related to a chronic illness, there may be a period of shock, disbelief, or numbness that is akin to grief following bereavement. The extent to which the feelings associated with this event can subsequently be integrated into the patient's subjective experience may be an important determinant of whether depressive feelings persist. Individuals who ward off depressive affect may be at risk subsequently to feel overwhelmed when such feelings, which have not previously been processed, are triggered by an illness-related event. The inability to identify or share such feelings because of the absence of emotional involvement with family, friends, or professional caregivers may also lead to a sense of isolation and alienation. As a result, individuals who are most in need of emotional assistance may be deprived of it.

Acute medical illness and chronic disease may trigger feelings of sadness and grief that cannot necessarily be identified or expressed. For patients who are burdened with such feelings, the first phase of therapy may involve bringing into awareness, in a gradual and tolerable fashion, thoughts and emotions connected with the illness. The following case illustrates how this process was facilitated in a patient who developed a serious medical illness during the course of intensive psychotherapy.

Case Example

■ A 35-year-old single woman who developed a malignancy was referred for psychotherapeutic treatment to treat severe symptoms of anxiety. These presenting symptoms subsided after several months of weekly psychotherapy. However, when signs of a recurrence of her malignancy appeared, she reported feelings of terror and panic. In a psychotherapy session shortly thereafter, she became agitated, paced the room, and eventually interrupted the session temporarily because she felt the need to vomit. In subsequent sessions, she reported feelings of "uncertainty" and "panic" that seemed to her to be similar to childhood experiences in which she would wake up at night feeling afraid that she would die, as if she were in a "black hole." After a particularly stressful medical procedure, she said, "I feel anxious all of the time. I feel overwhelmed, at the mercy of things. I feel shell-shocked. Like I am not part of the world. I have lost all sense of myself." ■

The therapeutic task in this phase was to calm her anxiety and to provide a secure environment in which her thoughts and feelings could be safely discussed. The provision of insight is not the most important therapeutic element at such times. Although a profound psychological reaction to the illness may be evident, the distress may be too great for the patient to feel able to engage in or to benefit from introspection or insight. The stabilizing effect of the therapeutic relationship in this phase is often more beneficial than specific interpretations. In fact, the process of understanding often cannot begin until the period of acute grief has passed and the patient feels less overwhelmed.

As noted in the psychodynamic treatment of stress response syndromes (Horowitz et al., 1984), these initial symptoms often subside once a firm therapeutic alliance is established. In the case described above, the patient reported that the relationship with the therapist gave her "a sense of safety" and "the courage to face things inside myself." It is only once such a relationship is established that patients are more able to focus on the meaning of events, to permit the unfolding of associations, and to allow a mourning process that has been stymied to proceed to completion (Horowitz et al., 1984).

Meaning and Mourning

Depressive symptoms are intimately tied, as we emphasized in Chapter 6, to the personal meaning of the illness. This meaning is determined by a complex interaction among the nature of the illness, the premorbid personality, and the life stage, life experience, intrapsychic conflicts, and vulnerabilities of the individual affected. For example, damage to the sense of self may be a common sequela of a serious illness (Muslin, 1984), but this effect will be most prominent in individuals whose sense of self has been less firmly established or who have particularly depended upon physical health, appearance, or integrity to bolster self-esteem. As with the elderly (Cooper, 1984), a sense of loss may be commonly associated with medical illness, but it will have particular significance for those who have experienced recurrent or traumatic losses at critical life phases.

Depression in the medically ill is often related to the lowered self-esteem and to the sense of helplessness that results when there is a sudden shift in an individual's perceived life trajectory (Viederman & Perry, 1980). Integration and working through of the personal meaning of the illness is an important component of the treatment process in the psychodynamic treatment of depression in the medically ill (Rodin, 1988). As already noted, feelings of sadness related to the illness can be expressed more safely in the presence of a firmly established therapeutic relationship. However, the provision of meaning and the organization of experience in this second phase may also help to diminish terrifying feelings of helplessness. Providing a coherent organization that helps the individual understand the impact of the illness in terms of his or her unique life experience and personality helps to diminish the state of disequilibrium that the illness has triggered.

In the case just described, the illness seemed to revive profound fears of disintegration associated with an unstable sense of self. It was possible to understand these fears in terms of this patient's own life-experience. During her childhood, she felt that neither of her parents recognized her own individuality nor responded to her particular needs. In order to receive approval or attention, she felt obliged to present herself in ways that she felt satisfied her parents. This situation, in which her own sense of self was not validated, left her with a veneer of self-sufficiency beneath which there was uncertainty about her identity and about her capacity to function autonomously. She said after the illness was diagnosed: "I feel sad. As if I'm losing everything. Everything is being ripped away from me. I have lost control over the way I look and feel, and over my ability to be attractive."

For this patient, the walling-off of inner feelings had been adaptive until she became medically ill. However, when profound fears were triggered by the diagnosis of malignancy, this means of adaptation was ineffective and isolating. She felt that no one could understand her fears or soothe her anxiety. She said: "My family and I are all going through hell. But there's a wall. We can't comfort each other. Their anxieties and fears just magnify my own. We're all whirling around, nobody is in control." Conveying to this patient an understanding of her current feelings in terms of their historical context helped to provide an observing perspective and an increased sense of mastery.

Many of this patient's fears became manifest in the transference relationship. She experienced, at times, the same sense of distance, nonrecognition, and nonengagement from her therapist and other care-givers as she had experienced with her parents. She said, "It bothers me that the doctors have so much power. You're so dependent on them. You're just a body." After a psychotherapy session in which she had revealed some personal feelings she said: "I felt stripped, depleted, treated like a bunch of component parts. I fear that if I expose everything, you will simply look at it like a surgeon and then close me up without anything being changed." On another occasion, she related: "I have a childish fear of you leaving me. When I am in that state, I feel tired, needy, and weak. I can't cope with my ill health. I feel that I have lost all control over my life. I feel victimized, paralyzed by the state of my health. My state of mind disconnects me from the world. I fear that I will never get better, that I will die."

The sense of disconnection from the therapist and the feeling that the therapist regarded her more as a patient than a person were recurrent themes to which the patient returned. Repeatedly when the patient doubted the therapist's empathic involvement based upon some per-

282 /   DEPRESSION IN THE MEDICALLY ILL

ceived action, inaction, or misunderstanding, the therapeutic relationship was derailed. In fact, the threat posed by a perceived disconnection from the therapist was a central focus of treatment. Only when this derailment was addressed and the patient again felt herself engaged with the therapist could other issues be explored.

The interpretive phase of therapy can fully begin only when the patient feels safe enough to verbalize emotional concerns and to be receptive to the therapist's response. Only when the patient experiences empathic involvement of the therapist is it possible for the process of self-understanding to proceed and for the meaning of the illness to be understood in terms of the patient's personal psychology. Illness-related fears that were previously regarded as overwhelming may now seem tolerable and understandable to the patient in terms of his or her personal psychology and life history. The empathic involvement of the therapist facilitates such communication and allows the process of self-understanding to proceed.

The Attainment of a Sense of Mastery

Medical illness often represents a major threat to the sense of competence and mastery that an individual has attained. A common denominator of successful psychotherapeutic treatment is the re-establishment of this sense of mastery. This change is often first evident in terms of the ability to tolerate a broader range of emotional experiences related to the illness. However, it may also be associated with a greater capacity in the patient to experience and tolerate affect of various kinds. Once feelings related to an illness can be more easily accepted, the process of working through and understanding meaning may proceed. Basch (1988) has suggested that an increase in the sense of mastery is the most important therapeutic factor in most forms of psychotherapy. With the medically ill, this may be a particularly important aspect of psychotherapeutic treatment.

In the case described above, the patient became more able to express her feelings and fears related to the illness, as treatment progressed. These feelings were often triggered by a new round of follow-up testing. At a later stage of treatment she said, "I don't have as much interest in falling apart as I did when I came. I don't have to respond to the physical symptoms with panic. At the beginning, it was a luxury I indulged in." Although her fears about her condition persisted, her capacity to tolerate them increased and the extent to which they triggered a psychological sense of disorganization diminished. This patient both demonstrated and experienced an increased sense of mastery over her illness-related fears, and an increased capacity to tolerate emotional experience.

In summary, an important focus of psychodynamic therapy in the medically ill is the understanding or organizing of affective experience. From this perspective, depressive states are seen to arise when affects cannot be tolerated or integrated into subjective experience. Psychodynamic therapy may increase the capacity of patients in this regard and may then help to resolve depressive symptoms or to prevent the occurrence of depressive states.

COGNITIVE THERAPY OF DEPRESSION

The modern cognitive theory and therapy for depression was developed by Beck and his colleagues (Beck et al., 1979; Beck & Young, 1985), building upon the work of Adler (1927), Kelly (1955), and Horney (1950). The cognitive model assumes that cognitive disturbances are core components of depression and that the characteristic mood, behavior, and biochemistry of depression are secondary to depressive cognitions. According to this model, depression is characterized by a "cognitive triad"—a negative view of self, the environment, and the future. The negative view of self is reflected in lowered self-esteem, and feelings of worthlessness, inadequacy, and deficiency. The environment is regarded as overwhelming, with insurmountable obstacles, and the future is seen as hopeless and unchangeable. The sense of an unchanging, negative future may lead to suicidal ideation and, in some cases, self-harm behavior. The negative triad may be activated by underlying negative schemas, i.e., maladaptive attitudes and beliefs about self, others, and the world that are formed early in life through interactions with the environment, and that remain out of awareness until activated by a negative life event, such as a physical illness.

Cognitive distortions related to events, interactions with others, and, most particularly, to self-worth, are thought to perpetuate the depressive outlook. Depressed persons may not only be unable to generate calming positive illusions about themselves and the world, but they may also selectively attend to the negative aspects of situations so that events are interpreted in a self-denigrating manner. Cognitive distortions employed by depressed patients in this way include arbitrary inferences, all-or-nothing thinking, overgeneralizing, selectively attending to negative aspects of a situation, and magnifying negative events out of proportion. By contrast, nondepressed individuals typically see themselves and their world in a positively biased light. They employ what

Taylor and Brown (1988) have termed "positive illusions" to filter their interpretation of events.

A core feature of the cognitive approach to therapy is the early establishment of a collaborative relationship between therapist and patient. Through the joint selection of the goals of treatment and through regular feedback, both patient and therapist participate in a process that has been called "collaborative empiricism" (Beck & Young, 1985).

Three main types of interventions are used in cognitive therapy (Kovacs, 1983):

1. *Didactic techniques.* These include teaching the patient about the cognitive theory of depression, using examples from the patient's own life as illustration. In addition, the rationale for all intervention strategies is explained as each is introduced during the course of therapy. This educative process encourages a working alliance between the client and therapist and ensures that the patient clearly understands the context and rationale of the therapeutic process. It also provides a framework for the individual to understand his or her disturbance, which may lead to an increased sense of mastery. With the medically ill, explanations provided take into account how depression can arise in this context.

2. *Self-monitoring and behavioral techniques.* These are used, especially during the early stages of therapy, to help the patient monitor his or her daily functioning. Common behavioral techniques include the intentional scheduling of activities that provide experiences of mastery and pleasure, cognitive rehearsal (i.e., imagining the step-by-step process involved in accomplishing tasks), self-reliance training (i.e., reassuming responsibility for routine, everyday tasks such as cleaning, cooking, shopping, etc.), role playing, and diversion techniques (i.e., physical activity, social contact, work, play, and visual imagery). Specific homework assignments relating to the issues discussed in the therapy session are assigned to patients and then reviewed in the next session. Examples with the medically ill might include recommendations to read a book or article related to the illness, to employ relaxation techniques to enhance sleep, or to encourage the patient to resume physical activities.

3. *Semantic techniques.* Through constant and specific questioning of the patient, the therapist elicits and tests the validity of automatic thoughts and underlying assumptions regarding the patient's view of reality. Patients thus learn to "question the evi-

dence" in support of a particular negative cognition or assumption, to provide "alternative explanations," and to "reattribute" unrealistic self-blame to other factors that may be causally pertinent. Patients are asked to keep a daily record of dysfunctional thoughts on which they record the automatic thoughts and accompanying emotions that occur in upsetting situations between sessions. As therapy progresses, patients learn to challenge their maladaptive negative thoughts with rational responses that are also recorded and analyzed in the next session.

Effectiveness of Cognitive Therapy

The effectiveness of cognitive therapy in the treatment of depression has been studied extensively among persons without a medical illness. Two recent meta-analyses have reported favorable results when cognitive therapy was compared with other treatments for depression (Dobson, 1989; Nietzel et al., 1987). Aggregating the results of 10 studies, Dobson (1989) reported that, on average, depressed patients treated with cognitive therapy became less depressed, based on the Beck Depression Inventory (BDI), than 98 percent of control patients (i.e., no-treatment or wait-listed). Moreover, in treatment comparisons, the average cognitive therapy patient had lower BDI scores than 67 percent of behavior therapy patients (nine studies), 70 percent of patients treated with a variety of other approaches (seven studies), and 70 percent of drug therapy patients (eight studies). These results are encouraging, although Dobson (1989) did not specify the type and severity of depression that was treated in the studies included in his meta-analysis. Shaw (1989) supported these findings in a review of 10 studies in which patients with unipolar depression were treated on an outpatient basis. He concluded that cognitive therapy, with or without pharmacotherapy, lowers the relapse rate of major depressive disorder. In the case of severe depression and, in the absence of any contraindications, he recommended that cognitive and drug therapies be used together to reduce depressive symptoms.

COGNITIVE TREATMENT OF DEPRESSION IN MEDICAL PATIENTS

In order to compare the two therapeutic techniques discussed in this chapter, the cognitive approach to treatment is illustrated here by hypothetically applying it to the case described in the section on psychodynamic therapy. It will be remembered that following the diagnosis of cancer, this 35-year-old woman was extremely anxious and agitated. The initial goal of cognitive therapy at this stage would be similar to that of psychodynamic therapy: to provide this patient with firm support and symptom relief. However, the means to achieve this goal are different with the two treatment approaches. A cognitive approach aims to normalize the nature and intensity of the patient's feelings by teaching her the connection between her thoughts (e.g., "I have lost all sense of myself"), and their accompanying emotions (e.g., despair) and behaviors (e.g., gastric upset). Teaching the connection between thoughts and feelings might be accomplished in early sessions by inquiring about her thoughts immediately prior to a visible change in affect, such as the onset of crying. Gentle challenges to the catastrophizing nature of the patient's cognitions at this stage, (e.g., "I have lost all sense of myself") may be helpful provided that they are framed so as not to invalidate her experience. Such approaches can also help the patient better manage her own responses to the threat that the illness represents. Setting an agenda for each session and prioritizing problem areas to be discussed orients the patient from the beginning to the process of cognitive therapy. In the early phase of treatment, goals may include reassurance that her reactions are manageable, and, moreover, that the therapist understands them and is not overwhelmed by them.

It may be difficult for cognitive therapists treating medical patients to distinguish cognitive distortions from unpleasant but realistic perceptions by the patient of the medical condition and its consequences. This distinction is less important in psychodynamic therapy which is more focused on subjective experience. However, disentangling objective from intrapsychic reality is necessary in cognitive therapy in order to correct cognitive distortions. In the young woman described, there was some basis in reality for her fears of dependency, illness, and even death. Indeed, with many medical conditions, even the most stringent adherence to treatment will not necessarily protect patients from the dire consequences that they fear. The sense of helplessness that some medical patients experience may have a firm basis in external reality. The common therapeutic question used by many cognitive therapists to confront a catastrophizing cognition—"What's the worst thing that can happen?"—may not elicit a reassuring response. Indeed, the realistic response by some medical patients could well be, "I could die." Debates between therapist and patient about the likelihood of such an extreme outcome can be unproductive and frustrating. It is more fruitful to identify the cognitive distortions that are associated with realistic fears, and that affect the emphasis of the cognitions. Guiding patients to focus on specific concerns, rather than on the more global threat represented by the illness, can also help to identify maladaptive thoughts that reinforce feelings of helplessness. A cognitive approach attempts to correct a catastrophizing cognition by encouraging the patient to question the evidence in support of it. By contrast, a psychodynamic approach would focus more on the subjective reality and the associated intrapsychic catastrophe that is feared.

In the middle phase of therapy, when the patient is more able to connect thoughts and feelings, she may have better access to the negative cognitions that accompany the illness. Specific maladaptive automatic thoughts (e.g., "I can't cope") are operationalized and examined in concrete terms (e.g., questioning whether or not the patient actually does have the resources necessary to cope with the situation at hand). The evidence to support particular cognitive distortions can also be examined at this time. This may help to identify that the patient's statement, "I have lost all control over my life," is an example of both overgeneralization (i.e., the loss of control over health is perceived to extend to all aspects of her life) and of all-or-nothing thinking (i.e., control is either complete or nonexistent). Then, through guided imagery and graduated behavioral tasks, the patient can be helped to regain a sense of mastery over many aspects of her life and of her illness. To demonstrate that emotional responses are often predictable, the therapist can teach the patient to monitor fluctuations in affect and to record the thoughts and behaviors that accompany and sustain such changes in mood. The principal goal of therapy at this stage is to help the patient overcome her sense of helplessness. This is accomplished through a variety of techniques that include identifying specific problems, setting priorities, labelling errors in thinking, and documenting progress on the targeted problems (Beck & Young, 1985).

As therapy progresses, other cognitive techniques can be employed to help the patient to focus on more complex problems that may include more than one dysfunctional thought, cognitive distortion, and/ or behavior. The patient also can be helped to uncover the underlying assumptions that might be at the root of her problems. For example, the patient perceived her therapist to be distant and unable to comfort her and this was the same way she had experienced her parents. The underlying assumption (i.e., "no one cares about me") led to the image of being "opened up," examined, and then left untreated. From the perspective of cognitive therapy, changing the underlying assumptions that interfere with her sense of mastery would diminish the vulnerability to depression. The cognitive view of underlying assumptions, as they apply to the therapist, is similar in some respects to the concept of transference as understood from a psychodynamic point of view.

In summary, the cognitive treatment of depression in the medically ill aims to help the patient to identify, test, and replace dysfunctional cognitions with more adaptive ones. The didactic aspects of this approach may be particularly useful at acute or crisis times in the patient's illness. Cognitive therapy is usually time-limited and thus may be appropriate for medical outpatients who face multiple demands on their time and financial resources.

EFFICACY OF INDIVIDUAL PSYCHOTHERAPY WITH THE MEDICALLY ILL

Both psychotropic medication and psychotherapy have been found to be effective in the treatment of depression; moreover, their effects have been found to be additive (APA Commission on Psychotherapies, 1982). Unfortunately, few outcome studies of psychotherapy for the treatment of depression in medically ill patients meet rigorous methodological criteria. Such criteria include the standardization of the treatment modality, the allocation of appropriate and competent therapists, the selection of patients with diagnoses based on structured diagnostic interviews and standardized criteria, and the employment of appropriate control groups and methods of evaluation (Elkin et al., 1988).

Those few studies that have been published suggest that psychotherapy may be of some benefit to medical patients in reducing depressive symptoms, although the results have been somewhat equivocal. For example, although some controlled studies of psychotherapy in cancer patients have reported a reduction in depressive symptoms in treated patients (Linn, Linn, & Harris, 1982; Maguire et al., 1980; Forester, Kornfeld, & Fleiss, 1985), another study found no significant change (Capone et al., 1980). Schiffer (1987) and Larcombe and Wilson (1984) reported the successful use of psychodynamically oriented psychotherapy and cognitive-behavior therapy, respectively, in the treatment of depressed patients with multiple sclerosis. Although the samples were small in the studies (20 patients in each), the results suggest that both of these therapeutic approaches may provide some benefit to such patients.

Finally, health care utilization studies provide another perspective on the benefits of psychological treatment. Gruen (1975) randomized 70 patients with a first heart attack into a treatment group or a control group. Treated patients were seen in daily psychotherapy to facilitate coping and to bolster personal resources. They found that the treated group demonstrated not only less depression but also fewer days in intensive care and in hospital, and fewer cardiac complications. Mumford, Schlesinger, and Glass (1982) reviewed 34 controlled studies of psychological interventions in patients recovering from surgery and heart attacks. They concluded that patients who are provided with information or support have been found to master the medical crisis better than patients who receive ordinary care. Furthermore, there was evidence from 13 studies that psychological interventions reduced the time of hospitalization, on average, by approximately two days. Borus et al. (1985) reported that medical patients with a diagnosed psychiatric disorder used less nonpsychiatric medical care following treatment of the mental disorder but that this apparent reduction in health care utilization was actually due to a shift of care from the primary to the specialist mental health sector. Further research is needed to evaluate the benefits of psychotherapy for depression in the medically ill in terms of its impact on subsequent health care utilization. However, current evidence is promising that psychotherapy not only has positive effects on emotional well-being, but also that it may help to diminish unnecessary medical hospitalization and treatment.

GROUP TREATMENT OF MEDICAL PATIENTS

There has been a trend in recent years toward the treatment of medical patients in groups. Group treatments tend to be designed to provide emotional support or education, to improve coping skills, to enhance treatment compliance, or to offer some combination thereof. Formats that have been employed in group treatment of the medically ill include standard group therapy, self-help psychoeducational groups, and more purely didactic approaches. Depending on the setting, treatment may be offered by professionals, peers, or by both. With respect to peer counselling, there has been a tremendous recent surge in the popularity of mutual aid/self-help groups. These groups are typically organized by and for the benefit of patients facing a particular disease, disability, or type of loss. They are not usually directed toward depression per se, but they may help patients to maintain a sense of mastery and prevent demoralization and despair.

Studies that have assessed the impact of group therapy on patients' mood are sparse indeed. Table 9.1 presents a review of seven studies that used various approaches to group treatment of medical patients. Studies were included here only if a control group and a standardized

TABLE 9.1. *Group Interventions*

Author(s) and Year	Participant Selection and Recruitment	Group Composition	Type of Treatment	Depression Measure	Results
Spiegel, Bloom, & Yalom (1981)	58 outpatients with metastatic breast cancer randomly assigned to experimental (n=34) and control (n=24) groups	Average of 7-10 members; weekly 90 minute sessions, open-ended	Open discussion	Profile of Mood States	E* showed greater decrease in total mood disturbance than C**; no difference in depression, self-esteem, or denial
Larcombe & Wilson (1984)	19 clinically depressed multiple sclerosis patients randomly assigned to E (n=9) and wait-listed C (n=10) groups	4 or 5 members; one 90 minute session/week, for 6 weeks	Cognitive-behavior therapy for depression	BDI[1] HAM-D[2] Mood ratings	E showed significant improvement on BDI, HAM-D, and daily mood compared with C
Horlick et al. (1984)	116 MI patients randomly assigned to E (n=83) and C (n=33) groups	Average of 4-8 members; one 90 minute session/ week, for 6 weeks	Education and discussion of 6 topics	MMPI[3]-Depression Scale	No differences between groups
Shearn & Fireman (1985)	81 rheumatoid arthritis patients randomly assigned to E1 (n=26), E2 (n=25), and C (n=30) groups	Average of 12-13 members/group; one 90 minute session/week, for 10 weeks	E1-Stress management E2-Mutual support	CES-D[4]	No differences between groups

Study	Sample	Duration/Frequency	Intervention	Measure	Results
Cohen et al. (1986)	96 arthritis patients randomly assigned to E1 (n=32), E2 (n=28), and C (n=36) groups	Average of 9-12 members/group; one 2 hour session per week, for 6 weeks	Education: E1-Peer led E2-Professionally led	CES-D	No differences between groups
Strauss et al. (1986)	57 rheumatoid arthritis outpatients randomly assigned to E1 (n=20), E2 (n=17), and C (n=20) groups	E1-weekly meetings for 6 months; E2-weekly meetings for 3 months	E1-Group psychotherapy E2-Assertion/relaxation	Aggregate score of psychological symptoms	No differences between groups
Maes & Schlosser (1988)	19 bronchial asthmatic outpatients with partners, matched by age/sex in one E and one C group	One 2-3 hour session/week, for 8 weeks	Rational emotive therapy	VROPSOM[5]	E<C on state depression, anger, anxiety, focus on asthma, and use of corticosteroid

* E=Experimental group
** C=Control group
[1] BDI=Beck Depression Inventory
[2] HAM-D=Hamilton Rating Scale for Depression
[3] MMPI=Minnesota Multiphasic Personality Inventory
[4] CES-D=Center for Epidemiologic Studies Depression Scale
[5] VROPSOM=see Rooijen (1977)

measure of depression were employed. In only two of these studies were interventions designed specifically to reduce depressive symptoms (Larcombe & Wilson, 1984; Maes & Schlosser, 1988), and in only one of these was there an initial assessment of depression using standardized diagnostic criteria (i.e., Feighner criteria) (Larcombe & Wilson, 1984). In both of the studies, depressive symptoms improved following a brief course of cognitive therapy. The goals of the remaining five studies included increasing patients' knowledge about the disease and its treatment, providing emotional support, and improving treatment adherence. Not surprisingly, given that patients were neither selected because of it nor treated for it, depression scores did not change as a result of the group intervention in any of these studies.

Clearly, more outcome studies are needed to assess the efficacy of specific types of group therapy to reduce depression in medical patients. Some preliminary findings suggest that cognitive therapy may be effective in the short term (Larcombe & Wilson, 1984; Maes & Schlosser, 1988), but follow-up studies using stringent diagnostic criteria are needed to assess long-term outcome. In this regard, some encouraging findings recently emerged from an eight-week psychoeducational group program for psychiatric outpatients with unipolar depression. In this nonmedical group, a social/cognitive intervention was associated with a reduction of depression by 85 percent at one month follow-up and 70 percent at six-month follow-up, using RDC criteria for depression (Hoberman, Lewinsohn, & Tilson, 1988). A similar approach to group therapy may also be appropriate for some medical patients, either to prevent depression or to treat patients with depressive symptoms that are not severe. As a rule, individual approaches are most appropriate with more severely depressed medical patients.

More research is also needed to determine which patients benefit from early intervention, and which treatments are most likely to be effective. For example, Gottlieb (1987) suggested that myocardial infarction patients who are most likely to benefit from group treatment are those with certain personality traits (e.g., neurotic introverts), those with premorbid tendencies toward pessimism and depression, and those who tend to rely on palliative modes of coping. In addition, men and women may differ in terms of which treatments are most acceptable or effective. For example, Euster (1984) suggested that men's groups should focus more on concrete rather than abstract concerns. The amount that individuals wish to know about their illness also influences the type of group that should be provided (Martelli et al., 1987). However, prospective research is needed to investigate such treatments and to document the psychosocial course of at-risk patients who are and who are not offered group therapy. Only then can it be determined whether such interventions offered early in the course of medical treatment can protect patients from developing depression as the medical illness progresses.

CONCLUSIONS

We have drawn attention in this chapter to several psychotherapeutic interventions that may be used to treat or prevent depression in the medically ill. Whereas pharmacological treatment is most effective for patients with more severe depressions, particularly those that are biologically autonomous, psychotherapy may be indicated for those who are less severely depressed or who are at risk of becoming depressed. In this regard, we view depression as a form of adaptive failure that may be most likely to occur in those who are unable to adapt flexibly to the complex demands and stresses of physical illness, who are less able to tolerate, regulate, and integrate depressive affect, and/or those who are predisposed for genetic or other reasons to become depressed.

The most important psychotherapeutic interventions may be empathic listening and the formation of a therapeutic relationship. Optimally, these functions can be performed by the primary care health practitioner. When this is not possible or when patients are more distressed, referral for formal psychotherapy may be indicated. With severely depressed patients, psychotherapy may need to be combined with pharmacotherapy.

We have discussed psychodynamic and cognitive approaches toward the treatment of milder forms of depression in the medically ill. Psychodynamic therapy emphasizes affective experiencing, emotionally-based insight, and the working through of depressive feelings in the context of the individuals' life history. Using this approach, depressive feelings are resolved not by correcting the associated cognitive distortions, but by treating the underlying psychological conflicts and deficits. This approach is less structured than cognitive therapy and may require more psychological-mindedness on the part of the patient. It may be less suitable for patients who prefer more structured situations, who have little access to their emotional life, or who are too depressed. Cognitive therapy emphasizes the correction of cognitive distortions that may lead to or perpetuate depression. This more structured approach may be most suitable with patients who are able to employ logical reasoning, who desire a more active stance by the therapist, and who have less capacity or interest in exploring the origins or nature of their emotional life. The selection of one or the other of these treatment approaches may be determined both by the experience and expertise of the therapist, and by the acceptability and suitability of the patient. In many cases, therapists will employ, to a greater or lesser extent, techniques from both modalities. We have also referred to psychoeducational, self-help, and group treatment approaches to depression in the medically ill. Although these approaches are used less often to treat more severe or clinical depression, they may help to sustain hope, raise morale, and to provide a sense of mastery, all of which serve to protect from depression.

REFERENCES

Adler, A. (1927). *Understanding Human Nature.* New York: Greenberg.

APA Commission on Psychotherapies (1982). Psychotherapy Research: Methodological and Efficacy Issues. APA Commission on Psychotherapies, American Psychological Association, pp. 161–164.

Arlow, J.A. (1987). The dynamics of interpretation. *Psychoanalytic Quarterly, 51,* 68–87.

Balint, M. (1957). *The Doctor, the Patient and the Illness.* New York: International Universities Press.

Basch, M.F. (1988). *Understanding Psychotherapy: The Science Behind the Art.* New York: Basic Books, Inc.

Beck, A.T., Rush, A.J., Shaw, B.F., & Emery, G. (1979). *Cognitive Therapy of Depression.* New York: Guilford Press.

Beck, A.T. & Young, J.E. (1985). Depression. In D.H. Barlow (Ed.), *Clinical Handbook of Psychological Disorders.* (pp. 206–244). New York: Guilford Press.

Beckham, E.E. & Leber, W.R. (1985). The comparative efficacy of psychotherapy and pharmacotherapy for depression. In E.E. Beckham & W.R. Leber (Eds.), *Handbook of Depression: Treatment, Assessment and Research.* (pp. 206–244). Homewood, Illinois: The Dorsey Press.

Beckman, H.B. & Frankel, R.M. (1984). The effect of physician behavior on the collection of data. *Annals of Internal Medicine, 101,* 692–696.

Borus, J.F., Olendzki, M.C., Kessler, L., Burns, B.J., Brandt, U.C., Broverman, C.A., & Henderson, P.R. (1985). The 'offset effect' of mental health treatment on ambulatory medical care utilization and charges: Month-by-month and grouped-month analyses of a five-year study. *Archives of General Psychiatry, 42,* 573–580.

Brenner, C. (1982). *The Mind in Conflict.* New York: International Universities Press.

Broadhead, W.E., Clapp-Channing, N.E., Finch, J.N., & Copeland, J.A. (1989).

Effects of medical illness and somatic symptoms on treatment of depression in a family medicine residency practice. *General Hospital Psychiatry, 11,* 194–200.

Brodsky, L. & Brodsky, V. (1984). Reconciling silent psychoses accompanying medical or surgical problems. *Psychosomatics, 25,* 191–196.

Capone, M.A., Good, R.S., Westie, K.S., & Jacobson, A.F. (1980). Psychosocial rehabilitation of gynecologic oncology patients. *Archives of Physical Medicine and Rehabilitation, 61,* 128–132.

Castelnuovo-Tedesco, P. (1965). *The Twenty Minute Hour: A Guide to Brief Psychotherapy for the Physician.* Boston: Little, Brown and Company.

Coen, S.J. (1986). The sense of defect. *Journal of the American Psychoanalytic Association, 34,* 47–67.

Cohen, J.L., van Houten Sauter, S., DeVellis, R.F., & McEvoy DeVellis, B. (1986). Evaluation of arthritis self-management courses led by laypersons and professionals. *Arthritis and Rheumatism, 29,* 388–393.

Conte, H.R., Plutchik, R., Wild, K.V., & Karasu, T.B. (1986). Combined psychotherapy and pharmacotherapy for depression: A systematic analysis of the evidence. *Archives of General Psychiatry, 43,* 471–479.

Cooper, A.M. (1986). Some limitations on therapeutic effectiveness: The "burnout syndrome" in psychoanalysts. *Psychoanalytic Quarterly, 55,* 576–598.

Cooper, A.M. (1989). Concepts of therapeutic effectiveness in psychoanalysis: A historical review. *Psychoanalytic Inquiry, 9,* 4–25.

Cooper, D.E. (1984). Group psychotherapy with the elderly: Dealing with loss and death. *American Journal of Psychotherapy, 38,* 203–214.

Demos, V. (1984). Empathy and affect: Reflections on infant experience. In J. Lichtenberg, M. Bornstein, & D. Silver (Eds.), *Empathy II.* (pp. 9–34). Hillsdale, New Jersey: The Analytic Press.

Dobson, K.S. (1989). A meta-analysis of the efficacy of cognitive therapy for depression. *Journal of Consulting and Clinical Psychology, 57,* 414–419.

Elkin, I., Pilkonis, P.A., Docherty, J.P., & Sotsky, S.M. (1988). Conceptual and methodological issues in comparative studies of psychotherapy and pharmacotherapy I: Active ingredients and mechanisms of change. *American Journal of Psychiatry, 145,* 909–917.

Emde, R.N. (1983). The prerepresentational self and its affective core. *Psychoanalytic Study of the Child, 38,* 165–192.

Euster, S. (1984). Adjusting to an adult family member's cancer. In H.B. Roback (Ed.), *Helping Patients and their Families Cope with Medical Problems.* (pp. 428–452). San Francisco: Jossey-Bass.

Firestein, S.K. (1978). *Termination in Psychoanalysis.* New York: International Universities Press.

Forester, B., Kornfeld, D.S., & Fleiss, J.L. (1985). Psychotherapy during radiotherapy: Effects on emotional and physical distress. *American Journal of Psychiatry, 142,* 22–27.

Frank, J.D. (1961). *Persuasion and Healing: A Comparative Study of Psychotherapy.* Baltimore: The Johns Hopkins University Press.

Freud, S. (1926). *Inhibitions, Symptoms and Anxiety.* London: The Hogarth Press and the Institute of Psychoanalysis, 1975.

Gedo, J.E. (1979). *Beyond Interpretation: Toward a Revised Theory of Psychoanalysis.* New York: International Universities Press.

Gottlieb, B.H. (1987). Marshalling social support for medical patients and their families. *Canadian Psychology, 28,* 201–217.

Gruen, W. (1975). Effects of brief psychotherapy during the hospitalization period on the recovery process in heart attacks. *Journal of Consulting and Clinical Psychology, 43,* 223–232.

Hoberman, H.M., Lewinsohn, P.M., & Tilson, M. (1988). Group treatment of depression: Individual predictors of outcome. *Journal of Consulting and Clinical Psychology, 56,* 393–398.

Holmes, J. (1988). Supportive analytical psychotherapy: An account of two cases. *British Journal of Psychiatry, 152,* 824–829.

Horlick, L., Cameron, R., Firor, W., Bhalerao, U., & Baltzan, R. (1984). The effects of education and group discussion in the post myocardial infarction patient. *Journal of Psychosomatic Research, 28,* 485–492.

Horney, K. (1950). *Neurosis and Human Growth: The Struggle Towards Self-Realization.* New York: W.W. Norton & Company.

Horowitz, M., Marmar, C., Krupnick, J., Wilner, N., Kaltreider, N., & Wallerstein, R. (1984). *Personality Styles and Brief Psychotherapy.* New York: Basic Books, Inc.

Karasu, T.B. (1986). Psychosomatic medicine and psychotherapy. *Psychiatric Annals, 16,* 522–525.

Kelly, G.A. (1955). *The Psychology of Personal Constructs.* New York: W.W. Norton & Company.

Kovacs, M. (1983). *Psychotherapies of Depression. Psychiatry Update: The American Psychiatric Association Annual Review, Vol. II.* Washington, D.C.: American Psychiatric Press.

Larcombe, N.A. & Wilson, P.H. (1984). An evaluation of cognitive-behavior therapy for depression in patients with multiple sclerosis. *British Journal of Psychiatry, 145,* 366–371.

Lazarus, R.S. (1979). Positive denial: The case for not facing reality. *Psychology Today, Nov.,* 44–60.

Levenson, J.L., Mishra, A., Hamer, R.M., & Hastillo, A. (1989). Denial and medical outcome in unstable angina. *Psychosomatic Medicine, 51,* 27–35.

Lichtenberg, J. (1983). *Psychoanalysis and Infant Research.* New York: The Analytic Press.

Linn, M.W., Linn, B.S., & Harris, R. (1982). Effects of counseling for late stage cancer patients. *Cancer, 49,* 1048–1055.

Luborsky, L. (1984). *Principles of Psychoanalytic Psychotherapy: A Manual for Supportive-Expressive Treatment.* New York: Basic Books, Inc.

Maes, S. & Schlosser, M. (1988). Changing health behaviour outcomes in asthmatic patients: A pilot intervention study. *Social Science and Medicine, 26,* 359–364.

Magruder-Habib, K., Zung, W.W.K., Feussner, J.R., Alling, W.C., Saunders, W.B., & Stevens, H.A. (1989). Management of general medical patients with symptoms of depression. *General Hospital Psychiatry, 11,* 201–206.

Maguire, P., Tait, A., Brooke, M., Thomas, C., & Sellwood, R. (1980). Effect of counselling on the psychiatric morbidity associated with mastectomy. *British Medical Journal, 281,* 1454–1456.

Malan, D.H. (1976). *The Frontier of Brief Psychotherapy: An Example of the Convergence of Research and Clinical Practice.* New York: Plenum Medical Book Co.

Malan, D.H., Heath, E.S., Bacal, H.A., & Balfour, F.H.G. (1975). Psychodynamic changes in untreated neurotic patients: II. Apparently genuine improvements. *Archives of General Psychiatry, 32,* 110–126.

Mann, A.H., Jenkins, R., & Belsey, E. (1981). The twelve-month outcome of patients with neurotic illness in general practice. *Psychological Medicine, 11,* 535–550.

Martelli, M.F., Auerbach, S.M., Alexander, J., & Mercuri, L.G. (1987). Stress management in the health care setting: Matching interventions with patient coping styles. *Journal of Consulting and Clinical Psychology, 55,* 201–207.

Michels, R. (1986). Oedipus and insight. *Psychoanalytic Quarterly, 55,* 599–617.

Mumford, E., Schlesinger, H.J., & Glass, G.V. (1982). The effects of psychological intervention on recovery from surgery and heart attacks: An analysis of the literature. *American Journal of Public Health, 72,* 141–151.

Muslin, H.L. (1984). Transformations of the self in cancer. *International Journal of Psychiatry in Medicine, 14,* 109–121.

Nietzel, M.T., Russell, R.L., Hemmings, K.A., & Gretter, M.L. (1987). The clinical significance of psychotherapy for unipolar depression: A meta-analytic approach to social comparison. *Journal of Consulting and Clinical Psychology, 55,* 156–161.

Paolino, T.J. (1981). *Psychoanalytic Psychotherapy: Theory, Technique, Therapeutic Relationship and Treatability.* New York: Brunner/Mazel.

Perry, S., Cooper, A.M., & Michels, R. (1987). The psychodynamic formulation: Its purpose, structure, and clinical application. *American Journal of Psychiatry, 144,* 543–550.

Rodin, G. (1984). Expressive psychotherapy in the medically ill: Resistances and possibilities. *International Journal of Psychiatry in Medicine, 14,* 99–108.

Rodin, G.M. (1988). Psychotherapy of patients with chronic medical disorders. In H.H. Goldman (Ed.), *Review of General Psychiatry.* (pp. 567–573). Connecticut: Lange Medical Publications.

Rooijen, L.V. (1977). Enige gegevens over de VROPSOM—lijsten voor de bepaling van depressie gevoelens. Onderzoeks-memorandum RN-PS 77-01. Vrije Universiteit Amsterdam, Amsterdam.

Schafer, R. (1985). The interpretation of psychic reality, developmental influences, and unconscious communication. *Journal of the American Psychoanalytic Association, 33,* 537–554.

Schiffer, R.B. (1987). The spectrum of depression in multiple sclerosis: An approach for clinical management. *Archives of Neurology, 44,* 596–599.

Schulberg, H.C., McClelland, M., & Gooding, W. (1987). Six month outcome for medical patients with major depressive disorders. *Journal of General Internal Medicine, 2,* 312–317.

Shaw, B.F. (1989). Cognitive-behavior therapies for major depression: Current status with an emphasis on prophylaxis. *Psychiatric Journal of the University of Ottawa, 14,* 403–408.

Shearn, M.A. & Fireman, B.H. (1985). Stress management and mutual support groups in rheumatoid arthritis. *American Journal of Medicine, 78,* 771–775.

Singer, M. (1988). Fantasy or structural defect: The borderline dilemma as viewed from analysis of an experience of nonhumanness. *Journal of the American Psychoanalytic Association, 36,* 31–59.

Sourkes, B.M. (1982). *The Deepening Shade: Psychological Aspects of Life-Threatening Illness.* Pittsburgh: University of Pittsburgh Press.

Spence, D.H. (1982). *Narrative Truth and Historical Truth: Meaning and Interpretation in Psychoanalysis.* New York: W.W. Norton & Company.

Spiegel, D., Bloom, J.R., & Yalom, I. (1981). Group support for patients with metastatic cancer: A randomized prospective outcome study. *Archives of General Psychiatry, 38,* 527–533.

Stern, D. (1985). *The Interpersonal World of the Infant.* New York: Basic Books, Inc.

Stolorow, R.D., Brandchaft, B., & Atwood, G. (1987). *Psychoanalytic Treatment: An Intersubjective Approach.* Hillsdale, New Jersey: The Analytic Press.

Strauss, G.D., Spiegel, J.S., Daniels, M., Spiegel, T., Landsverk, J., Roy-Byrne, P., Edelstein, C., Ehlhardt, J., Falke, R., Hindin, L., & Zackler, L. (1986). Group therapies for rheumatoid arthritis: A controlled study of two approaches. *Arthritis and Rheumatism, 29,* 1203–1209.

Strupp, H.H., Sandell, J.A., Jennings-Waterhouse, G., Samples-O'Malley, S., & Anderson, J.L. (1982). Psychodynamic therapy: Theory and research. In A.J. Rush (Ed.), *Short-Term Psychotherapies for Depression: Behavioral, Interpersonal, Cognitive and Psychodynamic Approaches.* (pp. 215–250). New York: Guilford Press.

Taylor, S.E. & Brown, J.D. (1988). Illusion and well-being: A social psychological perspective on mental health. *Psychological Bulletin, 103,* 193–210.

Viederman, M. & Perry III, S.W. (1980). Use of a psychodynamic life narrative in the treatment of depression in the physically ill. *General Hospital Psychiatry, 3,* 177–185.

Wallace IV, E.R. (1983). *Dynamic Psychiatry in Theory and Practice.* Philadelphia: Lea & Febiger.

10

Somatic Treatments

Current evidence suggests that depression is undertreated in medically ill patients. Surveys in general medical inpatients (Raft et al., 1975) and oncology patients (Derogatis et al., 1979; Jaeger et al., 1985; Goldberg & Mor, 1985) have documented that the frequency with which antidepressant medications are prescribed in these patients falls far short of the estimated prevalence of treatable depression. Undertreatment of depression has also been found in patients with endstage renal disease (Craven et al., 1987; Hong et al., 1987), diabetes mellitus (Lustman & Harper, 1987), and multiple sclerosis (Minden, Orav, & Reich, 1987). Most patients diagnosed with major depression in these studies were not being treated with antidepressant medication at the time of survey.

Some of the reasons that major depression is underdetected and undertreated in the medically ill are reviewed in Chapter 3, and therefore are noted only briefly here. Treatment may not be prescribed for clinically significant depression when it is interpreted as a normal reaction to disability. Also, physicians' unwillingness to stigmatize patients may contribute to the avoidance of "psychiatric" drugs. There may also be misinformation about the safety and efficacy of antidepressant drugs in the medically ill. A lack of appreciation of their efficacy and/or excessive concern regarding the side effects or toxicity of antidepressants are obstacles to their rational use in medical and other patients.

In this chapter, we discuss the indications, contraindications, and clinical use of pharmacotherapy and electroconvulsive therapy (ECT) for depression in the medically ill. The first section of the chapter outlines the indications and use of polycyclic antidepressants. Outcome studies of the use of these drugs for depression in the medically ill are reviewed. The remainder of the chapter discusses guidelines for the use of other somatic therapies including psychostimulants, monamine oxidase inhibitors, electroconvulsive therapy, and lithium. Emphasis is placed on interventions in the medically ill patient and on the interaction and influence of these medications with medical illness and its treatment.

POLYCYCLIC ANTIDEPRESSANTS

Indications

Polycyclic antidepressants remain the mainstay of biological treatment approaches for many patients with depression. Specific antidepressant treatment with these drugs is commonly considered for patients with a major depressive episode, particularly if associated with features of melancholia, atypical depression, or bipolar mood disorder (Bowden, 1985). Overall, 60 to 80 percent of medically well patients with major depressive disorders will demonstrate a positive clinical response to polycyclic antidepressants, compared with only 30 to 40 percent of patients who improve on placebo (Kessler, 1978). It appears that the more closely the depressive state approximates the syndrome of major depression with melancholia, the greater the likelihood that there will be a therapeutic response to antidepressants (Klein, 1974). Antidepressants may also be indicated in the management of situational or secondary major depressive disorder (Garvey et al., 1982; Hirschfeld et al., 1985; Black, Winokur, & Nasrallah, 1987), and may have a role in the management of selected patients with milder depressive syndromes such as dysthymic disorder or adjustment disorder with depressed mood (Stewart et al., 1981; Paykel, Freeling, & Hollyman, 1988). Some syndromes appear to be less responsive than others to antidepressants alone as the sole treatment modality. These syndromes include agitated depression first presenting in old age (Keller et al., 1983) and psychotic or delusional depression (Glassman & Roose, 1981; Charney & Nelson, 1981). Neuroleptic medications and/or ECT may be indicated for patients with psychotic or delusional depression (Glassman & Roose, 1981; Charney & Nelson, 1981).

These usual indications for antidepressant treatment are generally applicable to the patient with an associated physical illness. However, accurate assessment of the mood disorder and of the medical condition and its treatment is necessary for optimal management. Establishing the medical diagnosis allows the clinician to consider whether the depressive symptoms are a direct manifestation of organic factors (i.e., organic mood disorders). In such cases, amelioration of the depressive symptoms should first be attempted by optimizing medical treatment. When clinically feasible, drugs that are likely to be responsible for the depression should be decreased or discontinued. Similarly, depressive symptoms that are secondary to persistent physical distress (e.g., pain or nausea) may resolve with adequate analgesic or antiemetic treatment. As will be discussed further, characteristics of physical illness and its treatment may influence the timing and choice of antidepressant.

Since depressive symptoms are common with physical illness and are not necessarily pathological, other clinical features of the clinical situation may help to determine when to institute specific treatment for depression. In the medically ill patient, the following features, either alone or in combination, should suggest to the clinician that a depressive episode may be present and that specific antidepressant treatment may be indicated:

1. Depressive symptoms that are severe, persistent, or unresponsive to simple psychosocial interventions (Goldberg, 1981).
2. Depressive symptoms that interfere with medical interventions or otherwise contribute to a worsening of the medical illness.
3. Depressed mood, loss of interest, or demoralization that is not alleviated by improvement of the medical state.
4. Depressive symptoms in a patient with a subacute or inactive medical illness.
5. Depressive symptoms not temporally limited to a period of normal adjustment following a meaningful change in the medical state.

A trial of antidepressant medication may serve as a diagnostic aid when it is difficult to distinguish symptoms of a depressive syndrome from those due to the underlying medical condition. In particular, Bukberg, Penman, and Holland (1984) have argued that it may be extremely difficult to discriminate somatic symptoms of depression from those of medical illness, especially when the physical disability is grave. If the patient can tolerate the side effects of the medication, a trial of antidepressants may be justified in such cases. As discussed later in this chapter, the psychostimulant challenge test may be expedient to identify patients who are most likely to benefit from further antidepressant treatment. This is relevant because there is some risk that a trial of antidepressants will worsen the clinical state of patients with certain medical illnesses.

Efficacy

Only a small number of studies have specifically examined the efficacy and safety of polycyclic antidepressants for major depressive disorders in patients with concurrent medical conditions. To preserve sample homogeneity, the majority of outcome studies of antidepressants specifically excluded patients with physical illness from the study sample. Therefore, the conclusions of these reports are not necessarily generalizable to depression in the medically ill. The studies that have specifically examined the use of polycyclic antidepressants in patients with physical illness are briefly reviewed here.

In an early study, Porter (1970) administered imipramine (75 mg to 150 mg daily) to 26 depressed medical patients and 29 placebo-controls. No differences in subsequent depressive symptoms were found between the two groups. However, this study is limited in that no criteria for depression were specified, the investigators were not blind to the type of treatment that patients were receiving, and the duration of treatment was only three weeks. In contrast, Rifkin et al. (1985) conducted a randomized, double-blind, placebo-controlled trial of trimipramine in patients with both a major medical illness and major depression. They found significantly greater improvement in depression scores in the 17 patients who completed the three weeks of trimipramine treatment compared with the 25 patients who received the placebo for an equal length of time. Eight patients in the trimipramine group and three patients in the placebo group required discontinuation of their drug due to side effects. For the patients treated with trimipramine, depressive symptoms improved with or without any improvement in medical status. However, the mood of patients receiving the placebo improved only if and when their medical state improved.

In a study of poststroke major depression (based on Research Diagnostic Criteria), Lipsey et al. (1986) randomly assigned 34 patients either to treatment with nortriptyline or to a placebo control group. The duration of treatment ranged from four to six weeks and double-blind conditions were maintained throughout. Actively treated patients demonstrated a significantly greater improvement in depressive symptoms than did the control group. Serum levels of nortriptyline ranged from 50 to 140 ng/mL. Treatment was discontinued in six participants due to a variety of side effects that included oversedation (n=1), syncope (n=1), dizziness (n=1), and delirium (n=3). On balance, however, the authors concluded that nortriptyline was effective in the treatment of poststroke major depressive episodes.

This conclusion appears to be confirmed in a second study by Reding

et al. (1986), who treated 27 poststroke inpatients with either trazodone or placebo under double-blind conditions. In this study, only those patients who received active treatment and had a positive response to the Dexamethasone Suppression Test showed improvement in activities of daily living. Although consistent with the findings of Lipsey et al. (1986), it is difficult to generalize from this study because non-clinically depressed patients were also treated, and recovery from depression was not the primary outcome variable.

Two studies on the efficacy of tricyclic antidepressants in depressed patients with chronic obstructive pulmonary disease (COPD) have been reported. In the first, Light et al. (1986) reported no therapeutic effect for doxepin in a placebo-controlled trial in 12 patients. The authors explained their negative findings by suggesting that their sample consisted of patients with "secondary depression" who may have been less responsive to medication. However, as discussed in Chapter 1, the concept of "secondary depression" is ill-defined. A more likely explanation is that "cases" of depression in this study were based on Beck Depression Inventory scores of greater than 14, rather than on accepted diagnostic criteria, so that the patients treated did not necessarily have a true depressive syndrome. More favorable results were reported by Borson and McDonald (1989), who conducted a randomized trial of nortriptyline in 37 COPD patients diagnosed with major depression. They found improvement in significantly more patients in the treatment group than in the placebo control group.

Other studies of the efficacy of antidepressant medication in patients with cancer and with endstage renal disease have been encouraging. Costa, Mogos, and Toma (1985) entered 73 breast cancer patients with major depression into a placebo-controlled, double-blind study using mianserin. They found significant antidepressant effects in 36 patients receiving active treatment and noted that the side effects were well tolerated. In a study of postmastectomy patients, Maguire et al. (1980) found that a group who received counselling by a nurse-practitioner had no less depression than a control group who received no intervention. However, when the counselled patients were later treated with mianserin, the incidence of major depression in this group decreased three-fold compared with the control group.

Kennedy, Craven, and Rodin (1989) treated eight renal dialysis patients having DSM-III defined major depression with antidepressant medication (desipramine in six cases, and maprotiline and mianserin in one each). Five of the six patients who completed a four week open trial reported clinically significant improvement in their depressive syndromes, as measured by the Beck Depression Inventory and the

Hamilton Rating Scale for Depression. Patients received 75 to 100 mg of desipramine daily and serum levels were in the low therapeutic range. Desipramine was discontinued in one patient due to an allergic reaction, and this patient was subsequently treated successfully with maprotiline. Another patient discontinued mianserin because of complaints of oversedation but otherwise the side effects of these drugs were well tolerated.

Two studies have used naturalistic and retrospective designs to examine the usefulness of polycyclics in medical patients with depression. Black, Winokur, and Nasrallah (1987) reviewed the treatment and outcome of 1,087 patients with nonbipolar major depression. They concluded that patients with secondary depression were more likely to be undertreated and less likely to respond to adequate treatment than were primary depressives. In this sample, 76 percent of subjects had depression secondary to other psychiatric disorders, and in only 24 percent was depression secondary to a serious physical illness. However, as discussed in Chapter 1, these two types of secondary depression may have more differences than similarities, and the conclusions of this study do not necessarily apply to depression in the physically ill. Further to this point, this same group (Winokur, Black, & Nasrallah, 1988) subsequently reported that patients with depression secondary to physical illness were more likely to improve with treatment than were patients with depression secondary to psychiatric illness. These studies suggest that polycyclics may have a role in the treatment of depression secondary to physical illness, but this needs to be confirmed by research with homogeneous groups of depressed medical patients.

In another large scale study, Popkin, Callies, and Mackenzie (1985) reviewed the diagnosis and treatment of depression in 1,649 psychiatric consultations in a general hospital setting. They found 58 cases of treated depression in medical patients in which the following criteria were met: (1) a diagnosis of major depressive episode had been made by the consulting psychiatrist; (2) a polycyclic antidepressant was recommended and implemented; (3) a primary medical illness had been diagnosed; and (4) the outcome could be determined from the chart. They found that more than one-third of these patients demonstrated a positive clinical response to their antidepressant treatment and that, in 80 percent of these successful treatments, some improvement was observed within the first seven days of treatment. The reasons for treatment failure varied. In almost 25 percent of the sample, the antidepressant produced no therapeutic response. However, the conclusion of Popkin, Callies, and Mackenzie (1985) that antidepressants are less efficacious in medical than in psychiatric patients with depression may not be supported by their findings. The antidepressant was discontinued in more than 40 percent of the sample due to side effects, and there were medical contraindications to treatment in 8 percent. Physicians may have been reluctant to continue or to adjust the dosage of psychoactive drugs when side effects were reported. A greater number of patients might have improved had they been maintained on the antidepressant for a longer period, switched to a lower dose, or tried on an alternative antidepressant medication. Specific side effects may also be more common or more distressing for some medical patients. For example, Schwartz, Speed, and Clavier (1988) found that elderly men who were medically ill were particularly intolerant of antidepressants with high anticholinergic activity. As is discussed later in this chapter, the selection of an appropriate antidepressant for medical patients in terms of the risk of side effects may influence the success of treatment.

The preliminary evidence to date clearly suggests that many medically ill patients with major depressive disorder can benefit from antidepressant treatment. On the other hand, side effects may be a greater hindrance to treatment in these patients. It remains to be seen whether the efficacy of polycyclic antidepressants in the treatment of medical patients with major depression is similar to or different than that in psychiatric patients. A better response is likely for depression that is a first episode and not associated with other psychiatric disorders such as substance abuse. This circumstance is common in the medical setting. However, other features associated with a less favorable treatment response include persistent physical disability, socioeconomic complications of illness, and unalterable biological factors producing depression. The most reliable predictor of treatment outcome with antidepressants may be the extent to which the clinical picture approximates that of a major depressive episode with melancholia. Many cases of depression in the medical setting are relatively mild, even when DSM-III-R criteria for major depression are met. Several studies in the general practice setting have now shown that the treatment outcome of depression is strongly determined by the initial syndromal severity (Mann, Jenkins, & Belsey, 1981; Johnstone et al., 1980; Schulberg, McClelland, & Gooding, 1987). Thus, treatment studies that include many mildly depressed patients may show a lower response rate because of sample selection rather than because the medication is ineffective.

In the remainder of this section, we discuss guidelines for the use of polycyclic antidepressants in patients with active medical illness. The goal of these guidelines is to optimize the effectiveness of treatment, to minimize side effects, and to facilitate the completion of a clinical trial.

General Principles of Use

A reasonable rule of thumb for the institution of polycyclic antidepressants in patients with active medical illness is to begin with one-half the usual initiating dose and to raise the dose one-half as rapidly as one normally would. To minimize further the occurrence of some side effects, it may be beneficial in high-risk patients to prescribe divided daily doses rather than administering the total dose at bedtime. It has been reported that some medically ill patients appear to respond to antidepressants at doses ranging from one-half to three-quarters of the usual therapeutic dose recommended for these drugs. This observation has been reported in patients with advanced cancer (Goldberg, 1981; Massie & Holland, 1984), in general medical patients (Cavanaugh, 1984), and in renal dialysis patients (Kennedy, Craven, & Rodin, 1989). The mechanisms by which a therapeutic response to a lower dosage might occur are obscure. Pharmacokinetics may favor increased availability of the drug in some medical patients. Plasma levels would help to determine whether there is truly a response at lower serum levels or whether adequate serum levels are, in fact, achieved with lower oral doses. Unfortunately, many reports of antidepressant use in physically ill patients have failed to include plasma levels. Another explanation for a therapeutic response to a lower than usual dosage for antidepressant medication is that many patients will experience their first episode of depression following a major physical illness (Winokur, Black, & Nasrallah, 1988). Patients with a single episode of major depression respond more favorably to antidepressant treatment (Keller et al., 1983) than do patients with recurrent depression. This differential response may result from decreased genetic loading or from the absence of other predisposing factors.

Although some medical patients may respond to antidepressant medication at lower than usual doses, the dosage must always be titrated to the clinical response and to the occurrence of side-effects. The titration of the antidepressant dose may be facilitated by obtaining serum levels. Table 10.1 lists recommended clinical indications for antidepressant serum levels, as derived from reports by the American Psychiatric Association Task Force (1985) on the use of laboratory tests in psychiatry, and from a review of the subject by Potter (1984). Medical patients are best treated with the lowest effective dose, not only to reduce side effects but also to decrease the risk of medical

TABLE **10.1.** *Indications to Monitor Serum Antidepressant Levels**

No therapeutic response
Exaggerated side effects
Noncompliance
High risk (best treated with lowest possible dose)
    e.g., Advanced age
    Medical illness
    Polypharmacy/interacting drugs
Urgent need for therapeutic response
    Suicidality
    Need to limit hospital stay
        e.g., Employment or family support jeopardized
    Negative influence of depression on concurrent medical illness

---

* Desipramine, nortriptyline, and imipramine are the only antidepressants with therapeutic thresholds that are well enough defined to be used to optimize antidepressant response.

complications or drug interactions. Serum levels may help to optimize treatment expediently. This is particularly important when depressive symptoms such as loss of interest or appetite interfere with recovery or rehabilitation. Because well-defined therapeutic thresholds based on serum levels have been identified for desipramine, nortriptyline, and imipramine, these medications may be preferable for use when serum levels are desired.

Dosage considerations may be particularly important in elderly depressed patients with concurrent medical illness. These depressed patients have many physical conditions that may be exacerbated by tricyclic antidepressants (Koenig & Breitner, 1990). Further, elderly patients may be particularly susceptible to tricyclic side effects and, in some cases, may develop very high serum concentrations at average oral doses (Carr & Hobson, 1977). Although further substantiation is required, some reports suggest that lower doses are often effective in this group of patients (Jarvik et al., 1982; Lakshmanan, Mion, & Frengley, 1986).

Antidepressant response may occur as early as the first week that therapeutic levels are obtained, but more commonly a favorable response occurs during the second to fourth week. Some patients who have not yet responded after four weeks of treatment may still respond during the following two weeks. However, early improvement in most symptoms of the depressive syndrome is an indicator of the likelihood of an ultimate response (Small et al., 1981). It is important to assess the patient for full recovery from the depressive syndrome. Partial response may be an indication for higher drug levels, the addition of another agent to potentiate antidepressant activity (e.g., lithium), or a switch to an alternative antidepressant.

The risk of relapse of depression appears to be greatest during the first nine months following recovery (Keller et al., 1983). Data suggest that patients continued on antidepressant medication for six to 12 months following clinical recovery have a lower relapse rate than those whose medications are discontinued earlier (Klerman, 1978; Bialos et al., 1982). The rate of relapse of depression following treatment in medically ill patients has not been studied. However, because more time may be required to achieve therapeutic antidepressant levels in many of these patients, it may be prudent to maintain therapeutic levels for at least six months following full recovery. Earlier discontinuation of treatment, which may be requested by patients, is likely associated with greater risk of relapse, particularly if there is an exacerbation of medical difficulties. With discontinuation, polycyclic antidepressants should be tapered off over a few weeks to avoid the side effects of discontinuation, including nausea, insomnia, and a general feeling of being unwell (Mirin, Schatzberg, & Creasey, 1981). Early signs of relapse of depressive symptoms should also be assessed when antidepressants are discontinued.

Selection of Polycyclic for Use

A number of factors should be considered in antidepressant selection. A history of a therapeutic response to a particular antidepressant predicts future responsiveness to that drug (Pare & Mack, 1971). If plasma levels are desirable, the clinician may choose a drug for which therapeutic levels are well recognized (e.g., nortriptyline, imipramine, desipramine). For some severely ill patients, the availability of alternative preparations may influence the choice of antidepressants. Doxepin and amitriptyline are available in liquid form for easy administration via nasogastric or gastrostomy feeding tube. Clomipramine and amitriptyline are also available in parenteral form for patients with whom administration via the gastrointestinal tract is difficult or impossible.

Some reports suggest that intravenous antidepressants are relatively safe. Adams (1982a) administered amitriptyline intravenously to 100 depressed patients with advanced cancer, 16 of whom had coexisting cardiac problems. He infused 10 mg of amitriptyline in 100 ml of 5 percent dextrose solution over two hours at bedtime. The dose was increased by 10 mg each night until there was clinical improvement. Somewhat surprisingly, even at the maximum dose (i.e., 200 mg), no clinically significant cardiovascular abnormalities, unexpected deaths, acute episodes of hypotension, or electrocardiogram changes were found. Adams (1982b) also reported on the use of specially designed amitriptyline rectal suppositories in a 56-year-old woman with colonic cancer and bowel obstruction. He found that 50 mg bid provided sedation, improved sleep, and decreased symptoms of depression.

Side Effects

Although any of the above factors may substantially influence the choice of an antidepressant, in some cases the most important consideration is the side effect profile. The polycyclic side effect of sedation may be desirable when there is insomnia. Other side effects may be important to avoid (e.g., anticholinergic effects in elderly males with prostatic hypertrophy). Table 10.2 shows the most clinically relevant

TABLE **10.2.** *Clinically Relevant Side Effects*
of the Polycyclic Antidepressants

Anticholinergic effects
 Central
 Peripheral

Cardiovascular effects
 Orthostatic hypotension
 Cardiac conduction disturbances
 Rhythm disturbances
 Left ventricular dysfunction

Central Nervous System effects
 Tremor
 Lowering of the seizure threshold

Other Effects
 Noradrenergic effects
 Antiserotonergic effects
 Antihistaminic effects
 Analgesia and migraine prophylaxis

TABLE 10.3. *Side Effects of Commonly Used Antidepressant Medications*

| Medication | Adult Dose Range mg/day* | Side Effects | | |
		Sedation	Anti-Cholinergic	Noradrenergic
Amitriptyline	100-300	+++	+++	++
Clomipramine	100-350	++	++	++
Desipramine	100-300	–	+	+++
Doxepin	75-300	+++	++	+
Imipramine	100-300	++	++	++
Maprotiline	75-250	–	+	++
Nortriptyline	50-150	++	+	++
Protriptyline	30-100	++	+++	+++
Trazodone	250-600	+++	–	–
Trimipramine	150-300	+++	++	+

* Certain medically ill patients may be unable to tolerate these doses and may respond with lower doses.

adverse effects of the polycyclic antidepressants. The side effects of these antidepressants, which are discussed in detail in the following sections, include anticholinergic, cardiovascular, and central nervous system effects. Table 10.3 shows the relative likelihood of side effects with some common antidepressants.

Anticholinergic Effects

Anticholinergic effects are the most common cause of adverse side-effects with the polycyclic antidepressants. Milder side-effects such as drying of glandular secretions, constipation, or urinary hesitancy may be annoying for the younger patient without concurrent medical illness, but, together with other anticholinergic side effects, result in serious complications for the elderly. Table 10.4 lists the effects of anticholinergic activity in various organ systems.

All of the polycyclic antidepressants, with the exception of trazodone, have clinically significant anticholinergic effects. It should also be noted that fluoxetine is a recently marketed antidepressant that has no anticholinergic effects. The relative magnitude of these effects are listed in Table 10.3. An antidepressant with lower anticholinergic activity is

TABLE **10.4.** *Peripheral Anticholinergic Effects*

Peripheral Organ System	Anticholinergic Effect
Smooth muscle of the eye	Mydriasis
Salivary glands	Decreased saliva
Sweat glands	Decreased sweat
Skin	Increased blood flow/temperature
Heart	Tachycardia
Lower esophageal sphincter	Decreased tone
Stomach	Decreased secretion of enzymes
Upper and lower bowel	Decreased motility
Lower urinary sphincter	Increased tone
Respiratory system	Thickened secretions

preferred for treatment of major depression in patients with medical conditions that might be adversely affected by anticholinergic activity. Desipramine, nortriptyline, maprotiline, or trazodone are reasonable choices in this situation. The adverse consequences of anticholinergic effects may also be minimized by a number of treatment strategies. These include: optimizing treatment of the medical condition prior to institution of the antidepressant; beginning the antidepressant at a low dose; increasing its dose slowly and monitoring closely for side effects; consulting with other physicians; and instructing the patient to notify the treating physician if a worsening of medical state occurs.

Table 10.5 lists some of the medical conditions that may be adversely affected by the anticholinergic activity of the polycyclic antidepressants. For each condition, the risks and precautions of using these drugs are delineated.

The anticholinergic activity of antidepressant drugs is sometimes desirable as it may ameliorate the symptoms of some medical conditions. As early as 1965, Strang reported a double-blind, placebo controlled study demonstrating that patients with Parkinson's disease responded favorably to treatment with tricyclic antidepressants. Other medical conditions in which improvement of physical symptoms may occur due to antidepressant treatment include peptic ulceration, asthma, irritable bowel syndrome, ventricular dysrhythmias, and stable angina. The dose of other medications may need to be reduced when tricyclic antidepressants are administered to patients being treated for any of these conditions.

TABLE 10.5.   *Medical Conditions That May Be Adversely Affected by Anticholinergic Drugs*

Medical Condition	Risk	Precautions
Narrow angle glaucoma	Precipitation of acute glaucoma	Administer polycyclics only after control of glaucoma with cholinergic eyedrops*
Obstructive repiratory disease e.g., COPD Cystic fibrosis Chronic bronchitis	Thickened secretions, increased cough, increased risk of infection	Increased physiotherapy and medical management
Unstable angina Uncontrolled congestive heart failure	Tachycardia	Avoid polycyclics until condition well controlled
Hiatus hernia	Relaxation of lower esophageal sphincter with exacerbation of hernia, reflux esophagitis	Optimize medical management
Mechanical or functional ileus	Prolonged recovery time	Avoid polycyclics until resolved
Benign prostatic hypertrophy	Urinary retention	Prostate surgery
Urinary retention	Prolonged recovery time	Avoid polycyclics until resolved**
Organic mental disorder	Exacerbation of confusion, delirium	Temporarily discontinue
Other anticholinergic drug use	Delirium, peripheral side effects	Minimize or discontinue if possible

* (Ban, Guy & Wilson, 1984)
** If urinary retention is primarily the result of polycyclic antidepressant use, in/out urinary catheterization may be required in addition to bethanicol (urecholile) 25 mg tid.

Fluoxetine is a strongly antiserotonergic antidepressant that has minimal anticholinergic side effects (Koenig & Breitner, 1990). Therefore, it may be considered for the depressed medical patient who is at risk from these effects. Although fluoxetine is not associated with many of the anticholinergic and other side effects of tricyclic antidepressants, it has its own side effect profile; nausea, headache, nervousness, and insomnia are all common (Wernicke, 1985). We are presently unaware of any systematic report on the treatment of major depression in medical patients with fluoxetine. However, its proven efficacy in nonmedical patients and its unique side effect profile suggest that in future it may have a primary place in the treatment of depressed medical patients.

Orthostatic Hypotension

Orthostatic hypotension refers to an acute fall in blood pressure upon assumption of an upright posture, due to a loss of vasoconstrictor reflexes in the resistance and capacitance vessels of the lower extremities. This may result from interference with either central or peripheral neuronal activity. However, the exact mechanism by which polycyclic antidepressants produce orthostatic hypotension is still unclear.

In a retrospective examination of inpatient charts, Glassman et al. (1979) found that almost 20 percent of patients treated with polycyclic antidepressants had symptoms of orthostatic hypotension severe enough to warrant an alteration of treatment. They reported that tricyclic-induced orthostatic hypotension may result in serious injury from falls, particularly in the elderly who may be at risk for hip fractures, in patients with thrombocytopenia who are at risk for intracerebral hemorrhage, and with other medical conditions in which there is increased risk of injury from a fall. Muller, Goodman, and Bellet (1961) reported two cases of myocardial infarction resulting from tricyclic antidepressant-induced orthostatic hypotension. However, in an exhaustive review of this literature, Glassman and Carino (1984) concluded that it remains unclear whether myocardial infarction is, in fact, a complication of antidepressant-induced hypotension. They note that tricyclic antidepressants have been widely used in France for the treatment of stable angina, with no apparent increase in the rate of myocardial infarction. In their review of the cardiovascular side effects of the tricyclic antidepressants, Glassman and Bigger (1981) concluded that orthostatic hypotension was the most serious, common cardiovascular complication.

Common causes of orthostatic hypotension in the medically ill include: prolonged bed rest (particularly in the elderly); dehydration and hypovolemia; vasodilator therapy for hypertension or angina; and autonomic hypotension secondary to diabetes, alcoholism, or chemotherapy-induced neuropathy. Antidepressants are likely to exacerbate preexisting orthostatic hypotension whatever its cause. In treating these patients with a tricyclic antidepressant, precautions should be undertaken to ensure that postural symptoms do not result in a fall.

There is evidence that some tricyclics are less likely than others to cause orthostatic hypotension. Roose et al. (1981) found that patients who could not tolerate imipramine because of orthostatic hypotension did not develop clinically significant postural symptoms when switched to nortriptyline. Thayssen et al. (1981) also found that nortriptyline produced less orthostatic hypotension than imipramine. Cavanaugh (1984) reported little difficulty with orthostatic hypotension when treating medically ill patients with desipramine. Overall, orthostatic hypotension appears to occur more frequently and more severely with the tertiary amines (i.e., amitriptyline, imipramine, doxepin) than with the secondary amines (i.e., nortriptyline, desipramine) or with maprotiline and trazodone.

Orthostatic hypotension with tricyclic antidepressants also appears to be a frequent occurrence in patients with preexisting cardiovascular disease. Muller, Goodman, and Bellet (1961) found that patients over 60 years of age with cardiovascular disease were three times more likely to demonstrate clinically significant orthostatic hypotension when treated with tricyclic antidepressants than patients under 60 years of age without cardiovascular disease. Glassman et al. (1983) found clinically significant orthostatic hypotension in up to 50 percent of patients with preexisting impairment in left ventricular function who were being treated with imipramine. Roose et al. (1987) found that 7 percent of 122 imipramine-treated patients with previously normal electrocardiograms required discontinuation of their antidepressant due to orthostatic hypotension. This was necessary in none of the nortriptyline-treated patients with normal pretreatment electrocardiograms. However, almost one-third of subjects in this study with cardiac conduction defects developed orthostatic hypotension severe enough to require discontinuation of the imipramine. This was necessary in only one of 20 similar patients treated with nortriptyline. The authors concluded that orthostatic hypotension was significantly more frequent with imipramine than with nortriptyline, whether or not there was preexisting cardiovascular disease. Bucknall et al. (1988) compared mianserin and trazodone in a placebo-controlled, double-blind crossover study of the cardiovascular effects of these drugs in 16 patients with preexisting cardiovascular disease. No hemodynamic deterioration occurred in 14 of the 16 patients. One patient developed severe postural hypotension with trazodone and one had an exacerbation of transient ischemic attacks with both drugs.

Glassman et al. (1979) found that the pretreatment drop in lying to standing blood pressure was a good predictor of the extent of postural hypotension that would occur after initiation of antidepressants. Although subsequent studies have not replicated this finding (Thayssen et al., 1981; Jarvik et al., 1983; Neshkes et al., 1985), it is wise to record baseline postural drop in blood pressure prior to the institution of antidepressants. In patients with preexisting cardiovascular disease, a pretreatment electrocardiogram is also indicated. Repeated measures of postural drop may be required during the early phase of treatment, and in-hospital monitoring may be indicated for some high-risk patients. Also, a number of precautionary measures are available to minimize the risk of orthostatic hypotension. When fitted correctly, Jobst venous pressure support stockings may minimize postural drop, as may the administration of fluorocortisone. Jefferson (1983) has utilized methylphenidate in conjunction with tricyclic antidepressants to help maintain blood pressure. Finally, if orthostatic hypotension is still problematic in spite of these measures, an alternative approach to the treatment of the depressive syndrome should be considered.

Cardiac Conduction Effects

Polycyclic antidepressants affect the electrical conduction system of the heart by slowing conduction in the HIS bundle and Purkinje fibers. The electrocardiogram effects include increased PR, QRS, and QT intervals, and decreased T-wave amplitude. Conduction abnormalities appear to be most common with antidepressants with the greatest anticholinergic activity. Kantor et al. (1975) have reported imipramine-induced complete heart block in a single case study. However, other studies have shown that, although these drugs do have effects on the cardiac conduction system, they are seldom, if ever, the sole cause of symptomatic conduction disturbances (Giardina et al., 1979).

Roose et al. (1987) have reported on cardiac complications of 196 patients with major depression who were treated with either imipramine or nortriptyline. This study included patients with and without preexisting cardiac disease. Forty-one patients in their study sample had prolonged PR interval and/or bundle branch block (BBB) prior to initiation of the antidepressant. They found no serious conduction abnormalities during polycyclic treatment in patients with no preexisting conduction defects. Of the 10 patients with a first-degree atrioventricular block before treatment, none developed further conduction complications with therapeutic concentrations of either imipramine or nortriptyline. However, of the 24 patients with BBB who reached therapeutic drug levels, the following complications occurred: two of the imipramine-treated patients developed 2:1 AV block which reverted to sinus rhythm when treatment was stopped; an additional two imipramine-treated patients developed a greater than 25 percent increase in QRS duration; one nortriptyline-treated patient developed sinus arrest and required permanent pacemaker insertion; and 1 nortriptyline-treated patient had a repeat myocardial infarction. These findings suggest that depressed patients with BBB are at increased risk of developing high degree AV block when treated with polycyclic antidepressants. Rudorfer and Young (1980) also found that tricyclic antidepressants may exacerbate preexisting ventricular conduction defects. Stoudemire and Atkinson (1988) have noted that these antidepressants may contribute to clinical deterioration in patients with congenital long QT syndrome, Torsade de Pointes syndrome, and Wolff-Parkinson-White syndrome.

Dietch and Fine (1990) reported the results of nortriptyline treatment for depression in ten elderly patients with cardiac conduction defects. Conduction abnormalities included first degree atrioventricular block, left anterior hemiblock, and either left or right bundle branch block. Six of the ten patients showed clinical improvement in depression and none suffered adverse clinical effects that could be attributed to the nortriptyline. In particular, no clinically relevant electrocardiogram changes were observed. Based on their own findings and those in the literature, these authors concluded that there is minimal risk of serious exacerbations of conduction abnormalities when tricyclic antidepressants are used in patients with isolated first-degree atrioventricular block or hemiblock. Bundle branch block and bifascicular block present greater risks that require careful monitoring but are not absolute contraindications to antidepressant treatment.

Roose et al. (1987) suggested that depending upon the clinical likelihood of conduction defects, ECG, 24-hour-rhythm monitoring, and blood pressure recordings should be determined before initiation of tricyclics. Patients with preexisting heart block should be closely monitored by ECG, to identify pathological change in rhythm, and by determining plasma levels of polycyclics. If severe conduction delay (i.e., sick sinus syndrome) occurs, pacemaker insertion may be indicated prior to reinstitution of antidepressants. Alexopoulos & Shamoian (1982) suggest that the safe use of tricyclics in patients with cardiac pacemakers requires:

1. awareness of the presence of heart disease and the type and properties of the pacemaker used
2. that the pacemaker's proper function be established before initiating treatment
3. smaller than usual doses and increments of doses of tricyclics, especially in older patients

4. avoidance of very high plasma levels of tricyclics
5. frequent monitoring of pulse and ECG, with particular attention paid to the QRS duration.

Arrhythmic Effects

Several studies have shown that imipramine and nortriptyline act similar to group-I antiarrythmic agents (e.g., quinidine and procainamide) (Giardina et al., 1979; Giardina, Bigger, & Johnson, 1981). There may be an increased frequency of premature ventricular contractions (PVCs) during the early phase of treatment due to the predominent noradrenergic activity of these drugs. Electrocardiographic monitoring is mandatory during the antidepressant loading phase in patients with frequent PVCs, multifocal PVCs, bigeminy, or trigeminy. However, although the risk of PVCs is increased risk during the loading phase, the quinidine-like activity of these drugs should eventually decrease the PVCs to below their pretreatment level. At this time, other group-I agents may be decreased or even discontinued.

Contractility Effects

At least two studies have specifically examined the effect of tricyclic antidepressants on cardiac contractility. Glassman et al. (1983) performed radionuclide angiography before and after the institution of imipramine in 15 elderly male patients with major depression. The average daily dose of imipramine in this study was 223 mg per day and plasma levels approached 400 ng/mL. No significant angiographic changes were found in patients on therapeutic doses of imipramine. However, almost one-half of these patients discontinued treatment due to symptomatic postural hypotension.

In a double-blind study using radionuclide ventriculograms to assess ventricular function, Veith et al. (1982) treated 24 patients with cardiac disease with major depression, based on Research Diagnostic Criteria. Patients were treated with imipramine, doxepin, or placebo. They found that the tricyclics had no significant adverse effect on left ventricular ejection contraction, either at rest or at maximal exercise. In addition, premature ventricular contractions were reduced by imipramine. Although postural blood pressure changes were not significantly different among groups, symptomatic postural hypotension did develop in one patient taking imipramine and in three patients taking doxepin. One patient who received doxepin experienced a syncopal episode.

These and other studies have failed to demonstrate clinically significant contractility effects with antidepressant treatment, even in patients with preexisting cardiovascular disease. Nevertheless, it is obviously prudent to treat any manifestations of cardiac decompensation, prior to the institution of antidepressants.

Myocardial Infarction

Raskind et al. (1982) examined the effects of imipramine in 12 patients with recent myocardial infarctions diagnosed with major depression, based on Research Diagnostic Criteria. They found that imipramine treatment was associated with a reduction in ventricular arrhythmias. Electrocardiographic changes reflecting prolonged conduction time occurred, but no clinically relevant conduction disturbances were found. Although it was necessary to discontinue the drug in one man due to postural hypotension, they concluded that the treatment of depression with imipramine is safe and effective in patients with previous myocardial infarction. However, they cautioned that the patients they studied were not at the highest risk because at least four months had passed since their myocardial infarction and they did not have clinically significant conduction defects, unstable cardiac arrhythmias, or poorly controlled congestive heart failure. No systematic data exist regarding the earliest time at which it is safe to begin antidepressant treatment for depression associated with myocardial infarction. According to conventional clinical wisdom, polycyclics are contraindicated within six weeks of such an event. However, when there are persistently prolonged QT intervals following myocardial infarction, there is still a higher risk of ventricular fibrillation with these drugs, even after this period of time. Tricyclics may prolong the QT interval further and are contraindicated in patients with QT interval prolongation (Stoudemire & Atkinson, 1988). Infrequently, polycyclic antidepressants cause sinus tachycardia. This complication should be recognized early in patients with coronary artery disease and should be treated with an appropriate antiarrhythmic medication.

Hypertension

Although polycyclic antidepressants sometimes cause hypertension, the tricyclic antidepressants do not commonly cause any clinically significant changes in blood pressure readings, other than postural hypotension. Other issues regarding hypertension and depression should be noted. First, depression may arise as a complication of antihypertensive treatment. Reserpine has been shown to cause depression in about 15 percent of patients who take this drug on a long-term basis (Simpson, 1973). Methyldopa, clonidine, guanethidine, and propranolol have also been implicated in causing depression, although the evidence is much less persuasive than with reserpine (Paykel, Flemingero, & Watson, 1982; Glassman & Carino, 1984). The diagnosis of an organic mood disorder should always be considered in patients who present with major depression while receiving these antihypertensive agents. Second, tricyclic antidepressants should be avoided when the antihypertensives guanethidine or clonidine are being administered, since the interaction of the tricyclics with these medications may lead to a decreased antihypertensive effect. Finally, diuretic therapy or strict low-salt diets may lead to depletion of intravascular volume and to a substantial increase in the likelihood of orthostatic hypotension during treatment with tricyclic antidepressants. Precautions previously noted regarding orthostatic hypotension also apply to these patients.

Sedation

Many of the tricyclic antidepressants produce at least some sedation, partly related to their antihistamine I activity. This effect begins within one to two hours following administration of a dose and it lasts for several hours. Sedation is greatest when the antidepressant is first initiated or when the dose is raised. However, the level of sedation usually abates somewhat over three to four days, as tolerance to this effect of the drug develops. Sedation is greater with the dimethylated antidepressants (e.g., amitriptyline, doxepin, imipramine) and with trazodone than with monomethylated drugs (nortriptyline, protriptyline); it is almost nonexistent with desipramine. Sedation may be problematic for some patients who experience lethargy after awakening in the morning. The operation of motor vehicles or heavy machinery should be undertaken only with great caution during the initial administration of a sedating antidepressant. However, sedation is often a welcome side effect in depressed patients with sleep disturbance, and therefore these drugs (e.g., amitriptyline or doxepin, in doses ranging from 10–50 mg qhs) may be given at bedtime.

Appetite Stimulation and Weight Gain

Antidepressants may stimulate appetite and weight gain. The anti-serotonergic property of these drugs is likely involved in producing these side effects, although the regulation of appetite and weight is complex and antidepressants also influence other neurotransmitters. The occurrence of weight gain appears to be somewhat idiosyncratic, in that some patients may gain up to two pounds a week for several weeks whereas others demonstrate no change in weight (Cole & Bodkin,

1990). There is presently no means to predict which patients will become obese while taking tricyclic antidepressants. When weight gain does occur, switching to another antidepressant (e.g., desipramine, fluoxetine) may halt the increase, but significant weight loss is often not achieved (Cole & Bodkin, 1990). Weight gain may be a desirable side effect for some medical patients (e.g., with metastatic carcinoma). Appetite stimulation with amitriptyline or imipramine has also been found to be clinically beneficial for some hemodialysis patients (Zetin et al., 1982).

Movement Disorders

The antidepressant amoxapine, which is the demethylated version of the neuroleptic loxapine, has significant potential for dopamine blockade. Not surprisingly, akathisia, dystonic reactions, and dyskinesia have all been reported with this drug (Ross, Walker, & Peterson, 1983; Steele, 1982; Lesser, 1983). Therefore, its utilization is best avoided in patients with Parkinson's disease or other neurological disorders that involve extrapyramidal movement changes. In addition, amoxapine may also be undesirable in oncology patients who receive, with their chemotherapy, antinauseants that have significant potential for dopamine blockade. The concomitant use of amoxapine may increase the risk of extrapyramidal movement disorders in these patients.

Lowering of Seizure Threshold

There is evidence that all polycyclic antidepressants lower the seizure threshold (Edwards, 1979). Maprotiline in particular has been associated with grand mal seizures (Edwards, 1979; Holliday, Brasfield, & Powers, 1982; Molnar, 1983) and is best avoided in patients with a propensity for seizures. The tricyclic antidepressants compete with the anticonvulsant diphenylhydantoin for metabolism via the hepatic microzomal enzyme system. Thus, the concomitant administration of these drugs may result in higher serum levels of the anticonvulsant so that doses of the latter must usually be decreased. The use of polycyclics must be carefully monitored in patients with seizure disorders, and plasma levels of both the antidepressant and anticonvulsants should be obtained.

Interactions

The tricyclic antidepressants interact with a large number of medications that are commonly prescribed for medically ill patients. No effort is made here to list all potential interactions, but the possibility

TABLE **10.6.** *Drug Interactions: Tricyclic Antidepressants (TCA)*

Interacts with	Effect	Mechanism
Direct-acting sympathomimetics (epinephrine, norepinephrine)	Hypertension, arrhythmias	Inhibition of neuronal uptake mechanisms
Anticonvulsants	Decreased effect of TCA	Increased TCA metabolism
CNS depressants: alcohol, anaesthetics, barbiturates, benzodiazepines	Increased CNS depression, hypotension	Additive CNS depressive effects, and adrenergic blockade and direct vasodilation
Alcohol Barbiturates Chloral hydrate Lithium carbonate	Decreased TCA effect	Lowered TCA serum concentration, enhanced TCA metabolism
Diazepam Antipsychotics Antiparkinsonian drugs Antisecretory drugs	Increased TCA effect, confusion, delirium, tachycardia, urinary retention, ileus	Decreased TCA metabolism, anticholinergic toxicity
Phenothiazines	Enhanced effects of both drugs	Decrease metabolism of each other
Antihypertensives: guanethidine, clonidine, hydrochloride, bethanidine sulfate, debrisoquin sulfate	TCA block antihypertensive effects; hypertension may occur	TCA inhibit nerve uptake of these antihypertensive drugs
Antiarrhythmic drugs: quinidine, procainamide, hydrochloride, disopyramide, lidocaine, propranolol hydrochloride, etc.	Myocardial depression, decreased contractility, dysrhythmias	Additive quinidine-like effects on myocardium and conduction system
Monoamine oxidase inhibitors (MAOI) (including the chemotherapeutic agent procarbazine)	Increased TCA effect; increase or decrease in blood pressure	Monoamine oxidase inhibition with reuptake blockade

for drug interactions should always be considered. Table 10.6 lists some drug interactions that are commonly encountered with polycyclic antidepressants.

PSYCHOSTIMULANTS

The psychostimulants have had a long and controversial history in psychiatry (Chiarello & Cole, 1987). They are specifically indicated for attention deficit disorder and narcolepsy. In a 1987 review of the use of psychostimulants in psychiatry, Chiarello and Cole examined 12 studies in which outcomes were clearly classified as either improved, not improved, or worse with regard to the depressive disorder, after treatment with psychostimulants. Although they noted that there were substantial methodological flaws in all of the studies, they concluded that many depressed patients showed a positive response for varying periods of time. Satel and Nelson (1989) concluded in a critical review of the use of psychostimulants for depression that psychostimulants were of little benefit in primary depression, but might have more clinical utility with apathetic or depressed geriatric patients, or with the physically ill. Table 10.7 lists some of the uses of psychostimulants, as applied to depression in the medically ill. Psychostimulants are an attractive treatment option for depression in the physically ill because they do not cause many of the side effects associated with the polycyclics, and because their onset of action is rapid. In the remainder of this

TABLE **10.7.** *Potential Indications for Psychostimulants in Depressed Medically Ill Patients*

To predict antidepressant response (Methylphenidate challenge test) (Hackett & Draper, 1978; Katon & Raskind, 1980)

Refractory depression (Klein et al., 1980)

Potentiation of other antidepressants

Short term treatment of situational depressions and states of demoralization following severe physical illness (Klein et al., 1980)

Apathy and withdrawal in elderly patients without severe senile dementia (Clark & Mankikar, 1979; Branconnier & Cole, 1980)

Problematic hypotension with polycyclics (Jefferson, 1983)

---

section, we describe the psychostimulants that are in common use and we discuss the evidence to support their role in the management of depression in the medically ill patient.

Dextroamphetamine and methylphenidate are the two psychostimulants most commonly prescribed for the treatment of depression in the medically ill. Dextroamphetamine is rapidly absorbed from the small intestine and has a rapid onset of action, with peak plasma levels reached within three hours. Elimination of this drug occurs via complex pathways of biotransformation and renal excretion. The plasma half-life is approximately 12 hours. Methylphenidate has similar pharmacokinetic properties but is a relatively mild stimulant compared with dextroamphetamine. The reported effects of these drugs include increased motor behavior, enhanced arousal, and improved mood and energy. The side effects include tachycardia and blood pressure elevation, palpitations, cardiac tachyarrhythmias, jitteriness, insomnia, and anorexia. Methylphenidate has also been reported to stimulate appetite in depressed, medically ill patients (Fernandez et al., 1987).

Although psychostimulants have significant potential for abuse and dependency in humans, this has not proved to be a significant problem in the treatment of depression. Tolerance to the anorexic effects of these drugs has been documented, but not to the central stimulant properties, or, as Chiarello and Cole (1987) reported, to the antidepressant effect of these drugs. Acute withdrawal following prolonged, high-dose administration may result in depression, fatigue, or an acute paranoid psychosis (Britton et al., 1978).

Efficacy and Safety

Katon and Raskind (1980) reported that methylphenidate was safe and effective in three elderly patients who had experienced problematic urinary retention or orthostatic hypotension with tricyclics, or had cardiac contraindications to their use (i.e., atrioventricular block and bundle branch block). Kaufmann and Murray (1982) also reported the successful treatment of depression with dextroamphetamine in three medically ill patients who were either unresponsive to tricyclics or who were unable to tolerate the side effects. Kaufmann et al. (1984b) similarly reported three cases in which methylphenidate was successfully used to treat major depression following cardiac surgery. Tricyclic antidepressants were contraindicated in these patients due to third degree atrioventricular block managed with a temporary pacemaker, difficult-to-treat congestive heart failure, and left bundle branch block with rapid atrial fibrillation. Kaufmann et al. (1984a) reported on the use

324 /   DEPRESSION IN THE MEDICALLY ILL

of psychostimulants for major depression in five patients hospitalized on medical or surgical floors with significant medical illness. Tricyclics had been previously tried but were discontinued in four of these patients because of side effects; these drugs were not tried in one of the five because there was cardiovascular disease that was considered to be a relative contraindication to tricyclic use. All patients responded well to psychostimulants without worsening of their medical condition.

A small number of reported treatment studies of psychostimulants involve larger samples of depressed medical patients. Woods et al. (1986) reported a retrospective survey of all 66 medical or surgical patients who were treated with psychostimulants for depression in Massachusetts General Hospital over a four-year period. The psychiatric diagnoses included major depressive episode, adjustment disorders with depressed mood, and major depressive episodes with dementia. Following treatment with psychostimulants, 73 percent of the patients showed at least some improvement in depressive symptoms, and 48 percent showed marked to moderate improvement. Of those who improved, 93 percent showed signs of improvement during the first two days of treatment. The side effects, which were minimal, included sinus tachycardia and diaphoresis, nausea, maculopapular rash in one patient each, and increased confusion in two patients with preexisting dementia. Depressive symptoms relapsed in five patients during treatment with the psychostimulant, but in no case was the psychostimulant medication associated with an overall worsening of the medical condition.

Fernandez et al. (1987) described the use of methylphenidate in 30 oncology patients with depressive symptoms. Methylphenidate was selected in preference to tricyclics in these patients for one or more of the following reasons: a rapid response was urgently required; the risk of side effects from tricyclics was considered to be increased; or tricyclics were contraindicated for cardiac problems including high degree atrioventricular block and adriamycin-induced cardiotoxicity. The depressive disorders diagnosed by two psychiatrists (based on DSM-III criteria) included major depressive episode, adjustment disorder with depressed mood, and dementia. The patients were treated with 30 mg per day of methylphenidate administered in divided doses during the early part of the day. Adjustments of 5 to 10 mg per dose were made following an observation period of two to three days. Seventy-seven percent of these patients demonstrated marked or moderate improvement in depressive symptoms, usually evident by the fourth day of treatment. The patients were continued on methylphenidate for at least two weeks. Patients who demonstrated an exacerbation of depressive symptoms when the dose was decreased were kept on the medication at doses of 5 to 10 mg daily for up to one year. No problems with abuse or tolerance were noted, and the authors reported that the side effects were minimal and that none were life-threatening. All patients who benefitted reported appetite stimulation.

Lingam et al. (1988) retrospectively reviewed 25 patients with post-stroke major depression treated with methylphenidate. The psychiatric diagnosis was made by clinical interview based on DSM III criteria. At least 10 mg of methylphenidate was administered twice daily to these patients for at least five days. It was reported that 52 percent of the patients recovered completely, usually with mood improvement evident within 48 hours. Twelve percent experienced side effects, but in no case did these side effects require treatment discontinuation. None of the patients demonstrated a clinically significant increase in blood pressure, a side effect that could be hazardous in poststroke patients. Of the 12 nonresponders, seven showed at least some improvement of mood symptoms during treatment with the psychostimulants. Although significant cardiac and other serious medical problems were present in all patients at the time of treatment, anticholinergic side effects and orthostatic hypotension were not observed with the stimulants. The absence of these side effects is a considerable advantage in these high-risk medical patients.

In summary, case reports, retrospective surveys, and open clinical trials suggest that psychostimulants are useful in the treatment of depressive disorders in the medically ill. In particular, they may be indicated for situational depressions, states of demoralization following significant physical illness, or when tricyclics are relatively contrain-dicated on medical grounds. The potentially rapid onset of action is particularly advantageous in clinical situations that require patient participation (e.g., recovery and rehabilitation poststroke). However, definite conclusions about the efficacy of psychostimulants in the treat-ment of depression cannot be drawn from the literature published to date. Many of the studies included a wide range of depressive disorders such as major depressive episode, adjustment disorder with depressed mood, and other states of demoralization or situational depressions that do not clearly fit current diagnostic criteria for major depression. In addition, many of these studies rely, for diagnosis, on clinical assessments by treating clinicians, rather than on standardized inter-views and measures. To date, no controlled studies on the use of psychostimulants in the medically ill have been reported.

Until methodologically valid, controlled studies have been under-taken, recommendations for the use of psychostimulants to treat depressed medically ill patients should be considered tentative. Given the apparent usefulness of these medications in some patients and the attractive side effect profile, controlled studies are certainly warranted.

Methylphenidate Challenge Test

The methylphenidate challenge test, carried out either by oral or intravenous administration, has been used to predict a therapeutic response to tricyclic antidepressants. Oral doses of the psychostimulant administered over an extended period of time appear to predict tricyclic antidepressant response better than intravenous administration over a shorter period of time (Goff, 1986). Sabelli et al. (1983) and others have provided evidence that suggests that the methylphenidate challenge test may specifically predict response to desipramine.

A commonly used form of the test involves administering 5 mg of methylphenidate at 0800 and 1200 hours for two consecutive days. Improvement in mood and other psychological and somatic symptoms of the depressed syndrome indicate a positive response, suggesting that further treatment with a tricyclic or with methylphenidate itself may be beneficial. This test has been utilized to differentiate depression from an enfeebling medical condition that produces symptoms resembling depression. Sustained improvement with a psychostimulant suggests that a substantial component of the symptoms represents reversible depression that would benefit from continued treatment (Hackett & Draper, 1978; Katon & Raskind, 1980). However, although a positive response to the methylphenidate challenge test suggests that antidepressant treatment should be continued, a negative response does not unequivocally rule out the possibility of benefit from such treatment.

MONOAMINE OXIDASE INHIBITORS

The monoamine oxidase inhibitors (MAOIs) that are used as antidepressants include both the hydrazines (e.g., phenelzine, isocarboxazid) and nonhydrazines (e.g., tranylcypromine). Some patients with major depressive episodes unresponsive to treatment with a polycyclic antidepressant may recover with an MAOI treatment (Lydiard, 1985). In particular, a depressive syndrome associated with prominent phobic anxiety, feelings of inadequacy, emotional instability, moodiness, irritability, and somatic complaints may respond to an MAOI as well as, or better than, to a polycyclic antidepressant (Robinson et al., 1973). The MAOIs fell out of common use during the early 1970s due to reports of hypertensive crises. However, concern about this side effect has diminished somewhat since it is now apparent that it may be avoided by eliminating tyramine-containing foodstuffs from the diet (Tollefson, 1983).

Lehmann (1982) reported on the successful use of MAOIs in elderly patients, many of whom had concurrent medical illness. However beneficial and safe for use in selected medical patients who are instructed in the appropriate dietary precautions, a number of concerns about MAOIs remain. Severe or chronic physical illness may itself impose multiple restrictions on diet and/or lifestyle, so that further dietary limitations may be undesirable. Also, the adverse consequences of a hypertensive crisis may be great in patients with preexisting cardiovascular disease. MAOIs may complicate metabolic control in patients with diabetes, because the hydrazines potentiate and prolong insulin-induced hypoglycemia, and the nonhydrazines delay the time of recovery from it (Cooper & Ashcroft, 1966). Thus, when an MAOI is added to the regimen of diabetic patients, the dosage of insulin often needs to be reduced. It should also be noted that the MAOIs may cause orthostatic hypotension. However, unlike the more rapid onset of this side effect with tricyclics, orthostatic hypotension with the MAOIs may not occur until several weeks following the institution of treatment (Kronig et al., 1983). MAOIs are problematic in patients who are likely to require surgery because of the increased risk of cardiovascular complications. These drugs should be discontinued at least two weeks prior to elective surgery. Because of all of the side effects noted, MAOIs should generally be reserved for patients proven to be unresponsive to other antidepressant treatment.

In patients with rheumatoid arthritis, MAOIs may have positive side effects. Lieb (1983) presented several cases in which rheumatic symptoms were alleviated with tranylcypromine. These changes were evident, at least in part, on objective parameters that would not be expected to improve solely as a result of mood elevation. Lieb (1983) has suggested that tranylcypromine alleviates symptoms by inhibiting the release of arachadonic acid from cells and thereby inhibiting prostaglandin E2 synthesis, which is involved in the pathogenesis of rheumatoid arthritis.

LITHIUM CARBONATE

Lithium carbonate may be utilized as the antidepressant of first choice in the treatment of major depressive episode associated with bipolar affective disorder. Tricyclics can be added to augment treatment in refractory patients (Katona, 1988), but they are not usually the first choice in patients with bipolar affective disorder because of the risk of precipitating mania. Carbamazepine has also been successfully used to manage lithium-unresponsive mania and to maintain patients with lithium-unresponsive bipolar disorder (Post et al., 1983).

Because of potential somatic effects with long-term lithium use, any patient started on lithium should first be evaluated with at least the following laboratory tests: thyroid function studies; electrocardiogram, in patients over the age of 40; urinalysis; serum creatinine; and serum electrolytes. These tests should be repeated every two to four months for as long as the patient is being treated with lithium. Specific precautions are indicated for lithium treatment in patients with renal, thyroid, cardiovascular, or dermatologic disease. The administration of lithium to persons with these illnesses has been the subject of two extensive reviews (Amdisen & Hildebrandt, 1988; DasGupta & Jefferson, 1990). DasGupta and Jefferson (1990) also provided a listing of prescription drugs that interact with lithium. The use of lithium is discussed here only briefly as it applies to selected medical patients.

Lithium and Renal Disease

Lithium causes a renal concentration defect leading to low urinary concentration, polyuria, and polydipsia in from 10 percent to 20 percent of patients treated with it. Although these effects were first considered to be purely functional and reversible (c.f., DasGupta & Jefferson, 1990), subsequent reports suggest prolonged changes in renal function (Rabin et al., 1979; Bucht & Wahlin, 1980) or morphology (Bendz, 1983). The most common renal structural changes documented are interstitial fibrosis, tubular atrophy, and glomerular sclerosis (Bendz, 1983). However, others have questioned whether long-term lithium use causes structural changes in the kidney in patients with no preexisting renal pathology (Hetmar et al., 1987). Some suggest that lithium has no demonstrable effects on glomerular filtration (Grof et al., 1980; Grof & O'Sullivan, 1984) unless the glomeruli are already impaired (Grof & O'Sullivan, 1984). Extreme care should be taken to avoid toxic levels of lithium in patients with compromised renal function. Frequent monitoring of serum creatinine and electrolytes, and of creatinine clearance are necessary to prevent this occurrence.

Although endstage renal disease managed with renal dialysis has been considered to be a relative contraindication to the use of lithium, there have been several reports of successful lithium management of bipolar affective disorder in patients on dialysis (Procci, 1977; Port, Kroll, & Rosenzweig, 1979; Zetin et al., 1981). Since lithium is excreted unmetabolized by the kidney, these patients require a much lower dose than those with normal renal function. Zetin et al. (1981) reported the treatment of three dialysis patients with 600 mg of lithium administered once only following each of three dialysis treatments per week. Therapeutic serum levels were maintained in these patients without any clinical evidence of toxicity. Flynn et al. (1987) have reported a case in which lithium was administered intraperitoneally to a patient on continuous ambulatory peritoneal dialysis.

Lithium has also been safely administered to endstage renal disease patients who have received a kidney transplant (Blazer, Petrie, & Wilson, 1976; Koecheler et al., 1986). However, it is important to note that transplant recipients may require dialysis for one to two weeks after transplantation, and that the time required for renal function to stabilize is variable (DasGupta & Jefferson, 1990). Koecheler et al. (1986) recommend that the usual low lithium dose administered to dialysis patients be continued at that level after transplantation, until serum creatinine stabilizes. Measurement of lithium concentration is indicated three times weekly during this period. Monitoring renal function is crucial during this time, as the commonly used immunosuppressant cyclosporine may cause renal impairment or failure.

Lithium and Thyroid Disease

The effects of lithium on thyroid function have been well-documented. Slightly decreased levels of T4 and elevated levels of TSH are very common and goiter develops in about 4 percent of persons on long-term lithium therapy (DasGupta & Jefferson, 1990). Discontinuation of lithium and/or thyroid hormone treatment will usually lead to shrinkage of the goiter. Clinical hypothyroidism has been reported in from 15 to 25 percent of patients on chronic lithium treatment (Rosenthal & Goodwin, 1982). Some of these patients have preexisting autoimmune thyroiditis (Smigan et al., 1984; Calabrese et al., 1985). Lithium-induced inhibition of T-cell suppressor function may result in increased antibody titers. This condition may resolve with discontinuation of lithium; otherwise, thyroid replacement therapy may be necessary. Although rare, hyperthyroidism has been reported in patients taking lithium (Amdisen & Andersen, 1982; Yassa, Saunders, & Nastase, 1988). However, a cause and effect relationship between lithium treatment and subsequent hyperthyroidism has not been clearly demonstrated. When this complication occurs during lithium administration, treatment of clinical hyperthyroidism is indicated, but discontinuation of lithium is unnecessary.

Lithium and Other Medical Conditions

Lithium may cause clinically insignificant T-wave flattening or inversion on the electrocardiogram (Bucht et al., 1984). In a small number of patients, it has been associated with sinus node dysfunction (Hagman, Arnman, & Ryden, 1979; Brady & Horgan, 1988). Following myocardial infarction, the clinician must weigh the advantages and disadvantages of discontinuing lithium carbonate, even temporarily. DasGupta and Jefferson (1990) suggest that if the risk of early relapse of a mood episode is low, temporary discontinuation of lithium is indicated during the recovery phase following myocardial infarction to avoid increasing the risk of conduction disturbances. However, because a manic episode might substantially interfere with cardiac recovery, lithium should be continued following infarction if the risk of this is high. For patients undergoing coronary artery bypass graft, lithium should be discontinued prior to surgery and then restarted at a lower dose when the patient is able to tolerate oral intake (DasGupta & Jefferson, 1990). Lithium levels should be closely monitored following surgery because of fluid shifts and frequent medication changes. If postoperative delirium occurs, lithium should be discontinued until the mental status becomes normal.

The dermatologic effects of lithium have implications for some medical patients. Lithium has been reported to precipitate or to aggravate acneiform lesions (Lambert & Dalac, 1987) and psoriasis (Carter, 1972; Skoven & Thormann, 1979; Deandrea et al., 1982). Skin lesions may be difficult to treat in lithium-treated patients (Remmer & Falk, 1986; DasGupta & Jefferson, 1990). Psoriasis, in particular, may be largely unresponsive to standard treatment and discontinuation of lithium may be necessary for some patients with this complication. However, a trial of the drug may be undertaken in psoriasis patients, for whom it is otherwise clinically indicated, since psoriasis is not always exacerbated with lithium.

Lithium levels are affected by a number of medications that are commonly prescribed for medical patients (DasGupta & Jefferson, 1990). Increased lithium levels will be found with diuretics including the thiazides, loop diuretics (e.g., furosemide, ethacrinic acid), potassium-sparing diuretics (e.g., spironolactone, triamterene), and those with effects upon the distal tubule. Decreased lithium levels will be found with osmotic diuretics (e.g., mannitol, urea), carbonic anhydrase inhibitors (e.g., acetazolamide), and diuretics with effects upon the proximal tubule. Phenylbutazone and indomethacin decrease lithium clearance and substantially increase serum levels. Similarly, cyclosporine decreases the excretion of lithium and, thereby, leads to increased serum concentrations (Vincent, Weimar, & Schalekamp, 1987). If lithium administration is absolutely required in patients who are concurrently receiving these medications, intensive monitoring of dose and serum levels is required. Similar precautions must be undertaken for patients who are on very low salt diets. All fluid and electrolyte imbalances should be corrected prior to the institution of lithium.

ELECTROCONVULSIVE THERAPY

Electroconvulsive therapy is efficacious in the treatment of major depression, particularly if melancholic features are present (Crowe, 1984). It may be indicated for patients with a major depressive episode that is refractory to other treatment or is life-threatening (e.g., because of dangerous suicidal activity, refusal of fluid intake, or exacerbation of a serious medical condition). The technique of ECT involves the controlled application of an electrical stimulus to the brain, which produces a generalized tonic clonic seizure. It has been determined that repeated seizures are the therapeutic ingredient of ECT (Janicak et al., 1985). Patients undergoing ECT receive general anaesthesia with pentobarbital sodium, and muscle paralysis with succinylcholine. Yudofsky (1981) has suggested that reports of improved safety with this procedure are due to its increased use in the general hospital setting where better facilities are available to manage medical complications. The full technique of the ECT is not reviewed here, and the interested reader is referred to any one of a number of reviews on the treatment (e.g., Crowe, 1984; Selvin, 1987).

Historically, preexisting skeletal, cardiovascular, or central nervous system disease were considered to be contraindications to the use of ECT (Maltbie et al., 1980). These conditions, including space-occupying central nervous system lesions, are no longer regarded as absolute contraindications. Maltbie et al. (1980) found a successful outcome in 21 percent of 35 case reports of ECT in patients with intracranial tumors. These authors suggested that although there is increased risk with ECT in patients with intracranial tumors, this risk may be acceptable in certain clinical circumstances. Carter (1977) suggested that steroids (e.g., dexamethasone), which reduce peribrain tumor edema, might help to prevent the neurological complications that may result from ECT in these patients.

Gerring and Shields (1982) found that 28 percent of patients undergoing modified ECT suffered from cardiac arrhythmias or transient ischemia following treatment. All of the patients with these complications had preexisting cardiovascular disease. These authors suggested there is a higher risk of cardiovascular complications from ECT in those with angina, past myocardial infarction, congestive heart failure, arrhythmias, rheumatic heart disease, hypertension, or abnormal baseline electrocardiograms. They proposed the following guidelines for cardiac patients being treated with ECT: medical clearance by an internist or cardiologist, frequent monitoring of serum electrolytes; tailoring of the anaesthetic regimen to the cardiac status; and adequate treatment of hypertension prior to ECT. ECT should be avoided, they suggest, in patients with previous hemorrhagic strokes.

Dec, Stern, and Welch (1985) found no persistent electrocardiographic changes or elevations in CPK or SGOT following 85 electroconvulsive treatments in 29 patients, even though 24 percent of these patients had preexisting cardiovascular disease including cardiac conduction defects, recent myocardial infarction, and depressed ventricular function. They suggested that the safety of ECT was enhanced by the careful evaluation before and after the procedure. Propranolol has been utilized to minimize the pressor response to ECT in patients with coronary artery disease (Anton, Uy, & Redderson, 1977; Jones & Knight, 1981). However, Decina et al. (1984) have cautioned against this procedure, following their experience with a hypotensive patient with diabetes and ischemic heart disease who suffered from a cardiac arrest during electroconvulsive treatment, having been premedicated with propranolol.

There are a variety of other effects of ECT in individuals with different medical conditions. ECT may lead to either hyperglycemia or hypoglycemia when administered to patients with insulin dependent diabetes mellitus (Finestone & Weiner, 1984). Also, changes in the anaesthetic regimen will be required for patients with succinylcholine sensitivity, malignant hyperthermia, or porphyria. ECT may be used in patients with cardiac pacemakers, but only with close involvement of a cardiologist and precautionary monitoring (Bidder, 1981). ECT has now been successfully used to treat major depression in patients with a wide variety of physical illnesses, including Parkinson's disease (Yudofsky, 1979; Levy, Savit, & Hodes, 1983), multiple sclerosis (Gallineck & Kalinowsky, 1958) and other illnesses (Bidder, 1981). We emphasize that there must be a careful evaluation of the potential consequences when ECT is considered in a medically compromised depressed patient. However, when extreme care is taken, ECT may be successfully administered to patients with severe and complicated physical illness (e.g., Dubovsky et al., 1985).

CONCLUSIONS

Somatic treatments, including polycyclic antidepressants, psychostimulants, lithium, and electroconvulsive therapy, may be indicated for medically ill patients with major depressive disorder. However, research is indicated to establish the treatment of first choice and the efficacy of interventions for depressed medical patients. Many physical conditions are now regarded as relative rather than absolute contraindications to these treatments. Characteristics of the depressive syndrome, the concurrent medical illness, and the side effect profile must all be taken into account, and close collaboration between the psychiatrist and other health professionals involved in the patient's medical care is important.

The results are somewhat conflicting regarding the efficacy of tricyclic antidepressants for depression in medical patients. The findings have been most encouraging for patients diagnosed with major depression and treated in prospective studies. Inappropriate case selection and insufficient effort to minimize side effects and complications may have contributed to the negative findings of other studies. The psychostimulants have shown benefit in clinical samples of depressed medical patients, but studies that are better controlled with longer term follow-up are needed.

REFERENCES

Adams, F. (1982a). Cardiovascular effects of phenelzine and amitriptyline (letter to the editor). *Journal of Clinical Psychiatry, 43,* 472.
Adams, F. (1982b). Amitriptyline suppositories (letter to the editor). *New England Journal of Medicine, 306,* 996.
Alexopoulos, G.S. & Shamoian, C.A. (1982). Tricyclic antidepressants and cardiac patients with pacemakers. *American Journal of Psychiatry, 139,* 519–520.
Amdisen, A. & Andersen, C.J. (1982). Lithium treatment and thyroid function: A survey of 237 patients in long-term lithium treatment. *Pharmacopsychiatry, 15,* 149–155.
Amdisen, A. & Hildebrandt, J. (1988). Use of lithium in the medically ill. *Psychotherapy and Psychosomatics, 49,* 103–119.

American Psychiatric Association Task Force (1985). Tricyclic antidepressants — Blood level measurements and clinical outcome: An APA Task Force Report. Task force on the use of laboratory tests in psychiatry. *American Journal of Psychiatry, 142,* 155-162.

Anton, A.H., Uy, D.S., & Redderson, C.L. (1977). Autonomic blockade and the cardiovascular and catecholamine response to electroshock. *Anaesthesia and Analgesics, 56,* 46-54.

Ban, T.A., Guy, W., & Wilson, W.H. (1984). The psychopharmacological treatment of depression in the medically ill patient. *Canadian Journal of Psychiatry, 29,* 461-466.

Bendz, H. (1983). Kidney function in lithium-treated patients: A literature survey. *Acta Psychiatrica Scandinavica, 68,* 303-324.

Bialos, D., Giller, E., Jatlow, P., Docherty, J., & Harkness, L. (1982). Recurrence of depression after discontinuation of long-term amitriptyline treatment. *American Journal of Psychiatry, 139,* 325-329.

Bidder, T.G. (1981). Electroconvulsive therapy in the medically ill patient. *Psychiatric Clinics of North America, 4,* 391-405.

Black, D.W., Winokur, G., & Nasrallah, A. (1987). Treatment and outcome in secondary depression: A naturalistic study of 1,087 patients. *Journal of Clinical Psychiatry, 48,* 438-441.

Blazer, D.G., Petrie, W.M., & Wilson, W.P. (1976). Affective psychoses following renal transplant. *Diseases of the Nervous System, 37,* 663-667.

Borson, S. & McDonald, G.J. (1989). Depression and chronic obstructive pulmonary disease. In R.G. Robinson & P.V. Rabins (Eds.), *Depression and Coexisting Disease.* (pp. 40-60). New York: Igaku-Shoin.

Bowden, C.L. (1985). Current treatment of depression. *Hospital and Community Psychiatry, 36,* 1192-1200.

Brady, H.R. & Horgan, J.H. (1988). Lithium and the heart: Unanswered questions. *Chest, 93,* 166-169.

Branconnier, R.J. & Cole, J.O. (1980). The therapeutic role of methylphenidate in senile organic brain syndrome. *Proceedings of the Annual Meeting of the American Psychopathological Association, 69,* 183-196.

Britton, D.R., El-Wardany, Z.S., Brown, C.P., & Bianchine, J.R. (1978). Clinical pharmacokinetics of selected psychotropic drugs. In L. Iverson, S. Iverson, & S. Snyder (Eds.), *Handbook of Psychopharmacology (Vol. 13).* (pp. 299-344). New York: Plenum Press.

Bucht, G., Smigan, L., Wahlin, A., & Eriksson, P. (1984). ECG-changes during lithium therapy: A prospective study. *Acta Medica Scandinavica, 216,* 101-104.

Bucht, G. & Wahlin, A. (1980). Renal concentrating capacity in long-term lithium treatment after withdrawal of lithium. *Acta Medica Scandinavica, 207,* 309-314.

Bucknall, C., Brooks, D., Curry, P.V., Bridges, P.K., Bouras, N., & Ankier, S.I. (1988). Mianserin and trazodone for cardiac patients with depression. *European Journal of Clinical Pharmacology, 33,* 565-569.

Bukberg, J., Penman, D., & Holland, J.C. (1984). Depression in hospitalized cancer patients. *Psychosomatic Medicine, 46,* 199–212.

Calabrese, J.R., Gulledge, A.D., Hahn, K., Skwerer, R., Kotz, M., Schumacher, O.P., Gupta, M.K., Krupp, N., & Gold, P.W. (1985). Autoimmune thyroiditis in manic-depressive patients treated with lithium. *American Journal of Psychiatry, 142,* 1318–1321.

Carr, A.C. & Hobson, R.P. (1977). High serum concentrations of antidepressants in the elderly. *British Medical Journal, 4,* 1151.

Carter, C. (1977). Neurological considerations with ECT. *Convulsive Therapy Bulletin Tardive Dyskinesia Notes, 2,* 16–19.

Carter, T.N. (1972). The relationship of lithium carbonate to psoriasis. *Psychosomatics, 13,* 325–327.

Cavanaugh, S.V.A. (1984). Diagnosing depression in the hospitalized patient with chronic medical illness. *Journal of Clinical Psychiatry, 45,* 13–16.

Charney, D.S. & Nelson, J.C. (1981). Delusional and nondelusional unipolar depression: Further evidence for distinct subtypes. *American Journal of Psychiatry, 138,* 328–333.

Chiarello, R.J. & Cole, J.O. (1987). The use of psychostimulants in general psychiatry: A reconsideration. *Archives of General Psychiatry, 44,* 286–295.

Clark, A.N. & Mankikar, G. (1979). D-amphetamine in elderly patients refractory to rehabilitation procedures. *Journal of the American Geriatrics Society, 27,* 174–177.

Cole, J.O. & Bodkin, J.A. (1990). Antidepressant drug side effects. *Journal of Clinical Psychiatry, 51,* 21–26.

Cooper, A.J. & Ashcroft, G. (1966). Potentiation of insulin hypoglycemia by MAOI antidepressant drugs. *Lancet, 1,* 407–409.

Costa, D., Mogos, I., & Toma, T. (1985). Efficacy and safety of mianserin in the treatment of depression in women with cancer. *Acta Psychiatrica Scandinavica [Suppl], 320,* 85–92.

Craven, J.L., Rodin, G.M., Johnson, L., & Kennedy, S.H. (1987). The diagnosis of major depression in renal dialysis patients. *Psychosomatic Medicine, 49,* 482–492.

Crowe, R.R. (1984). Electroconvulsive therapy—A current perspective. *New England Journal of Medicine, 311,* 163–167.

DasGupta, K. & Jefferson, J.W. (1990). The use of lithium in the medically ill. *General Hospital Psychiatry, 12,* 83–97.

Deandrea, D., Walker, N., Mehlmauer, M., & White, K. (1982). Dermatological reactions to lithium: A critical review of the literature. *Journal of Clinical Psychopharmacology, 2,* 199–204.

Dec, D.W., Stern, T.A., & Welch, C. (1985). The effect of electroconvulsive therapy on serial electrocardiograms and serum cardiac enzyme values. *Journal of the American Medical Association, 253,* 2525–2529.

Decina, P., Malitz, S., Sackeim, H.A., Holzer, J., & Yudofsky, S. (1984). Cardiac arrest during ECT modified by B-adrenergic blockade. *American Journal of Psychiatry, 141,* 298–300.

Derogatis, L.R., Feldstein, M., Morrow, G., Schmale, A., Schmitt, M., Gates, C., Murawski, B., Holland, J., Penman, D., Melisaratos, N., Enelow, A.J., & Adler, L.M. (1979). A survey of psychotropic drug prescriptions in an oncology population. *Cancer, 44,* 1919-1929.

Dietch, J.T. & Fine, M. (1990). The effect of nortriptyline in elderly patients with cardiac conduction disease. *Journal of Clinical Psychiatry, 51,* 65-67.

Dubovsky, S.L., Gay, M.A.A., Franks, R.D., & Haddenhorst, A. (1985). ECT in the presence of increased intracranial pressure and respiratory failure: Case report. *Journal of Clinical Psychiatry, 46,* 489-491.

Edwards, J.G. (1979). Antidepressants and convulsions. *Lancet, 2,* 1368-1369.

Fernandez, F., Adams, F., Holmes, V.F., Levy, J.K., & Neidhart, M. (1987). Methylphenidate for depressive disorders in cancer patients. *Psychosomatics, 28,* 455-461.

Finestone, D.H. & Weiner, R.D. (1984). Effects of ECT on diabetes mellitus: An attempt to account for conflicting data. *Acta Psychiatrica Scandinavica, 70,* 321-326.

Flynn, C.T., Chandran, P.K.G., Taylor, M.J., & Shadur, C.A. (1987). Intraperitoneal lithium administration for bipolar affective disorder in a patient on continuous ambulatory peritoneal dialysis. *International Journal of Artificial Organs, 10,* 105-107.

Gallineck, A. & Kalinowsky, L.B. (1958). Psychiatric aspects of multiple sclerosis. *Diseases of the Nervous System, 19,* 77-80.

Garvey, M.J., Tuason, V.B., Johnson, R.A., & Valentine, R. (1982). RDC depressive subtypes: Are they valid? *Journal of Clinical Psychiatry, 43,* 442-444.

Gerring, J.P. & Shields, H.M. (1982). The identification and management of patients with a high risk for cardiac arrhythmias during modified ECT. *Journal of Clinical Psychiatry, 43,* 140-143.

Giardina, E.G.V., Bigger, J.T., Glassman, A.H., Perel, J.M., & Kantor, S.J. (1979). The electrocardiographic and antiarrhythmic effects of imipramine hydrochloride at therapeutic plasma concentrations. *Circulation, 60,* 1045-1052.

Giardina, E.G.V., Bigger, J.T., & Johnson, L.L. (1981). The effect of imipramine and nortriptyline on ventricular premature depolarizations and left ventricular function. *Circulation, 64,* 316-318.

Glassman, A.H. & Bigger, J.T. (1981). Cardiovascular effects of therapeutic doses of tricyclic antidepressants. *Archives of General Psychiatry, 38,* 815-820.

Glassman, A.H., Bigger, J.T., Giardina, E.V., Kantor, S.J., Perel, J.M., & Davies, M. (1979). Clinical characteristics of imipramine-induced orthostatic hypotension. *Lancet, 1,* 468-472.

Glassman, A.H. & Carino, J.S. (1984). Use of antidepressants in the geriatric population. In H.C. Stancer, P.E. Garfinkel, & V.M. Rakoff (Eds.), *Guidelines for the Use of Psychotropic Drugs: A Clinical Handbook.* (pp. 19-30). New York: Spectrum Publications, Inc.

Glassman, A.H., Johnson, L.L., Giardina, E.G.V., Walsh, T., Roose, S.P., Cooper, T.B., & Bigger Jr., J.T. (1983). The use of imipramine in depressed patients with congestive heart failure. *Journal of the American Medical Association, 250,* 1997-2001.

Glassman, A.H. & Roose, S.P. (1981). Delusional depression: A distinct clinical entity? *Archives of General Psychiatry, 38,* 815-820.

Goff, D.C. (1986). The stimulant challenge test in depression. *Journal of Clinical Psychiatry, 47,* 538-543.

Goldberg, R.J. (1981). Management of depression in the patient with advanced cancer. *Journal of the American Medical Association, 246,* 373-376.

Goldberg, R.J. & Mor, V. (1985). A survey of psychotropic use in terminal cancer patients. *Psychosomatics, 26,* 745-751.

Grof, P., MacCrimmon, D.J., Smith, E.K.M., Daigle, L., Varma, R., Saxena, B., Keitner, G., & Kenny, J. (1980). Long-term lithium treatment and the kidney. *Canadian Journal of Psychiatry, 25,* 535-543.

Grof, P. & O'Sullivan, K. (1984). Somatic side effects of long-term lithium treatment. In H.C. Stancer, P.E. Garfinkel, & V.M. Rakoff (Eds.), *Guidelines for the Use of Psychotropic Drugs: A Clinical Handbook.* (pp. 105-118). New York: Spectrum Publications, Inc.

Hackett, T.P. & Draper, E. (1978). *The Use of Stimulant Drugs in General Hospital Psychiatry.* Audio-digest tape, Glendale, California. Audio-Digest Foundation, Vol. 7, 12.

Hagman, A., Arnman, K., & Ryden, L. (1979). Syncope caused by lithium treatment: Report on two cases and a prospective investigation of the prevalence of lithium-induced sinus node dysfunction. *Acta Medica Scandinavica, 205,* 467-471.

Hetmar, O., Brun, C., Clemmesen, L., Ladefoged, J., Larsen, S., & Rafaelsen, O.J. (1987). Lithium: Long-term effects on the kidney: II. Structural changes. *Journal of Psychiatric Research, 21,* 279-288.

Hirschfeld, R.M.A., Klerman, G.L., Andreasen, N.C., Clayton, P.J., & Keller, M.B. (1985). Situational major depressive disorder. *Archives of General Psychiatry, 42,* 1109-1114.

Holliday, W., Brasfield, K.H., & Powers, B. (1982). Grand mal seizures induced by maprotiline. *American Journal of Psychiatry, 139,* 673-674.

Hong, B.A., Smith, M.D., Robson, A.M., & Wetzel, R.D. (1987). Depressive symptomatology and treatment in patients with end-stage renal disease. *Psychological Medicine, 17,* 185-190.

Jaeger, H., Morrow, G.R., Carpenter, P.J., & Brescia, F. (1985). A survey of psychotropic drug utilization by patients with advanced neoplastic disease. *General Hospital Psychiatry, 7,* 353-360.

Janicak, P.G., Davis, J.M., Gibbons, R.D., Ericksen, S., Chang, S., & Gallagher, P. (1985). Efficacy of ECT: A meta-analysis. *American Journal of Psychiatry, 142,* 297-302.

Jarvik, L.F., Mintz, J., Steuer, J., & Gerner, R. (1982). Treating geriatric depression: A 26-week interim analysis. *Journal of the American Geriatrics Society, 30,* 713-717.

338 / DEPRESSION IN THE MEDICALLY ILL

Jarvik, L.F., Read, S.L., Mintz, J., & Neshkes, R.E. (1983). Pretreatment of orthostatic hypotension in geriatric depression: Prediction of response to imipramine and doxepin. *Journal of Clinical Psychopharmacology, 3,* 368-371.

Jefferson, J.W. (1983). Treating affective disorders in the presence of cardiovascular disease. *Psychiatric Clinics of North America, 6,* 141-155.

Johnstone, E.C., Cunningham Owens, D.G., Frith, C.D., McPherson, K., Dowie, C., Riley, G., & Gold, A. (1980). Neurotic illness and its response to anxiolytic and antidepressant treatment. *Psychological Medicine, 10,* 321-328.

Jones, R.M. & Knight, P.R. (1981). Cardiovascular and hormonal responses to electroconvulsive therapy: Modification of an exaggerated response in an hypertensive patient by beta-receptor blockade. *Anaesthesia, 36,* 795-799.

Kantor, S.J., Bigger Jr., J.T., Glassman, A.H., Macken, D.L., & Perel, J.M. (1975). Imipramine-induced heart block: A longitudinal case study. *Journal of the American Medical Association, 231,* 1364-1366.

Katon, W. & Raskind, M. (1980). Treatment of depression in the medically ill elderly with methylphenidate. *American Journal of Psychiatry, 137,* 963-965.

Katona, C.L.E. (1988). Lithium augmentation in refractory depression. *Psychiatric Developments, 2,* 153-171.

Kaufmann, M.W., Cassem, N.H., Murray, G.B., & Jenike, M. (1984a). Use of psychostimulants in medically ill patients with neurological disease and major depression. *Canadian Journal of Psychiatry, 29,* 46-49.

Kaufmann, M.W., Cassem, N., Murray, G., & MacDonald, D. (1984b). The use of methylphenidate in depressed patients after cardiac surgery. *Journal of Clinical Psychiatry, 45,* 82-84.

Kaufmann, M.W. & Murray, G.B. (1982). The use of d-amphetamine in medically ill depressed patients. *Journal of Clinical Psychiatry, 43,* 463-464.

Keller, M.B., Lavori, P.W., Lewis, C.E., & Klerman, G.L. (1983). Predictors of relapse in major depressive disorder. *Journal of the American Medical Association, 250,* 3299-3044.

Kennedy, S.H., Craven, J.L., & Rodin, G.M. (1989). Major depression in renal dialysis patients: An open trial of antidepressant therapy. *Journal of Clinical Psychiatry, 50,* 60-63.

Kessler, K.A. (1978). Tricyclic antidepressants: Mode of action and clinical use. In M.A. Lipton, A. DiMascio, & K.F. Killam (Eds.), *Psychopharmacology: A Generation of Progress.* (pp. 1289-1302). New York: Raven Press.

Klein, D., Gittelman-Klein, R., Quitkin, F., & Rifkin, A. (1980). *Diagnosis and Drug Treatment of Psychiatric Disorders: Adults and Children.* Baltimore: Williams & Wilkins.

Klein, D.F. (1974). Endogenomorphic depression: A conceptual and terminological revision. *Archives of General Psychiatry, 31,* 447-454.

Klerman, G.L. (1978). Long-term treatment of affective disorders. In M.A.

Lipton, A. DiMascio, & K.F. Killam (Eds.), *Psychopharmacology: A Generation of Progress.* (pp. 1303–1311). New York: Raven Press.

Koecheler, J.A., Canafax, D.M., Simmons, R.L., & Najarian, J.S. (1986). Lithium dosing in renal allograft recipients with changing renal function (letter). *Drug Intelligence and Clinical Pharmacy, 20,* 623–624.

Koenig, H.G. & Breitner, J.C.S. (1990). Use of antidepressants in medically ill older patients. *Psychosomatics, 31,* 22–32.

Kronig, M.H., Roose, S.P., Walsh, B.T., Woodring, S., & Glassman, A.H. (1983). Blood pressure effects of phenelzine. *Journal of Clinical Psychopharmacology, 3,* 307–310.

Lakshmanan, M., Mion, L.C., & Frengley, J.D. (1986). Effective low-dose tricyclic antidepressant treatment for depressed geriatric rehabilitation patients. *Journal of the American Geriatrics Society, 34,* 421–426.

Lambert, D. & Dalac, S. (1987). Skin, hair and nails. In F.N. Johnson (Ed.), *Depression and Mania: Modern Lithium Therapy.* (pp. 232–234). Oxford: Irl Press.

Lehmann, H. (1982). Affective disorders in the aged. *Psychiatric Clinics of North America, 5,* 27–44.

Lesser, I. (1983). Case report of withdrawal dyskinesia associated with amoxapine. *American Journal of Psychiatry, 140,* 1358–1359.

Levy, L.A., Savit, J.M., & Hodes, M. (1983). Parkinsonism: Improvement by electroconvulsive therapy. *Archives of Physical Medicine and Rehabilitation, 64,* 432–433.

Lieb, J. (1983). Remission of rheumatoid arthritis and other disorders of immunity in patients taking monoamine oxidase inhibitors. *International Journal of Immunopharmacology, 5,* 353–357.

Light, R.W., Merrill, E.J., Despars, J., Gordon, G.H., & Mutalipassi, L.R. (1986). Doxepin treatment of depressed patients with chronic obstructive pulmonary disease. *Archives of Internal Medicine, 146,* 1377–1380.

Lingam, V.R., Lazarus, L.W., Groves, L., & Oh, S.H. (1988). Methylphenidate in treating poststroke depression. *Journal of Clinical Psychiatry, 49,* 151–153.

Lipsey, J.R., Spencer, W.C., Rabins, P.V., & Robinson, R.G. (1986). Phenomenological comparison of poststroke depression and functional depression. *American Journal of Psychiatry, 143,* 527–529.

Lustman, P.J. & Harper, G.W. (1987). Nonpsychiatric physicians' identification and treatment of depression in patients with diabetes. *Comprehensive Psychiatry, 28,* 22–27.

Lydiard, R.B. (1985). Tricyclic resistant depression: Treatment resistance or inadequate treatment. *Journal of Clinical Psychiatry, 46,* 412–416.

Maguire, G.P., Tait, A., Brooke, M., Thomas, C., Howat, J.M.T., Sellwood, R.A., & Bush, H. (1980). Psychiatric morbidity and physical toxicity associated with adjuvant chemotherapy after mastectomy. *British Medical Journal, 281,* 1179–1180.

Maltbie, A.A., Wingfield, M.S., Volow, M.R., Weiner, R.D., Sullivan, J.L., &

Cavenar Jr., J.O. (1980). Electroconvulsive therapy in the presence of brain tumor: Case reports and an evaluation of risk. *Journal of Nervous and Mental Disease, 168,* 400–405.

Mann, A.H., Jenkins, R., & Belsey, E. (1981). The twelve month outcome of patients with neurotic illness in general practice. *Psychological Medicine, 11,* 535–550.

Massie, M.J. & Holland, J.C. (1984). Diagnosis and treatment of depression in the cancer patient. *Journal of Clinical Psychiatry, 45,* 25–28.

Minden, S.L., Orav, J., & Reich, P. (1987). Depression in multiple sclerosis. *General Hospital Psychiatry, 9,* 426–434.

Mirin, S.M., Schatzberg, A.F., & Creasey, D.E. (1981). Hypomania and mania after withdrawal of tricyclic antidepressants. *American Journal of Psychiatry, 138,* 87–89.

Molnar, G. (1983). Seizures associated with high maprotiline serum concentrations. *Canadian Journal of Psychiatry, 28,* 555–556.

Muller, O.F., Goodman, N., & Bellet, S. (1961). The hypotensive effect of imipramine hydrochloride in patients with cardiovascular disease. *Clinical Pharmacology and Therapeutics, 2,* 300–307.

Neshkes, R.E., Gerner, R., Jarvik, L.F., Mintz, J., Joseph, J., Linde, S., Aldrich, J., Conolly, M.E., Rosen, R., & Hill, M. (1985). Orthostatic effect of imipramine and doxepin in depressed geriatric outpatients. *Journal of Clinical Psychopharmacology, 5,* 102–106.

Pare, C.M.B. & Mack, J.W. (1971). Differentiation of two genetically specific types of depression by the response to antidepressant drugs. *Journal of Medical Genetics, 8,* 306–309.

Paykel, E.S., Flemingero, R.F., & Watson, J.P. (1982). Psychiatric side effects of antihypertensive drugs other than reserpine. *Journal of Clinical Psychopharmacology, 2,* 14–39.

Paykel, E.S., Freeling, P., & Hollyman, J.A. (1988). Are tricyclic antidepressants useful for mild depression? A placebo controlled trial. *Pharmacopsychiatry, 21,* 15–18.

Popkin, M.K., Callies, A.L., & Mackenzie, T.B. (1985). The outcome of antidepressant use in the medically ill. *Archives of General Psychiatry, 42,* 1160–1163.

Port, F.K., Kroll, P.D., & Rosenzweig, J. (1979). Lithium therapy during maintenance hemodialysis. *Psychosomatics, 20,* 130–132.

Porter, A.M.W. (1970). Depressive illness in a general practice: A demographic study and a controlled trial of imipramine. *British Medical Journal, 1,* 773–778.

Post, R.M., Uhde, T.W., Ballenger, J.C., & Squillace, K.M. (1983). Prophylactic efficacy of carbamazepine in manic-depressive illness. *American Journal of Psychiatry, 140,* 1602–1604.

Potter, W.Z. (1984). Clinical pharmacokinetics of antidepressants. In H.C. Stancer, P.E. Garfinkel, & V.M. Rakoff (Eds.), *Guidelines for the Use of Psychotropic Drugs: A Clinical Handbook.* (pp. 119–137). New York: Spectrum Publications, Inc.

Procci, W.R. (1977). Mania during maintenance hemodialysis successfully treated with oral lithium carbonate. *Journal of Nervous and Mental Disease, 164,* 355–358.

Rabin, E.Z., Garston, R.G., Weir, R.V., & Posen, G.A. (1979). Persistent nephrogenic diabetes insipidus associated with long-term lithium carbonate treatment. *Canadian Medical Association Journal, 121,* 194–198.

Raft, D., Davidson, J., Toomey, T.C., Spencer, R.F., & Lewis, B.F. (1975). Inpatient and outpatient patterns of psychotropic drug prescribing by nonpsychiatrist physicians. *American Journal of Psychiatry, 132,* 1309–1312.

Raskind, M., Veith, R., Barnes, R., & Gumbrecht, G. (1982). Cardiovascular and antidepressant effects of imipramine in the treatment of secondary depression in patients with ischemic heart disease. *American Journal of Psychiatry, 139,* 1114–1117.

Reding, M.J., Orto, L.A., Winter, S.W., Fortuna, I.M., Di Ponte, P., & McDowell, F.H. (1986). Antidepressant therapy after stroke: A double-blind study. *Archives of Neurology, 43,* 763–765.

Remmer, H.I. & Falk, W.E. (1986). Successful treatment of lithium-induced acne. *Journal of Clinical Psychiatry, 47,* 48.

Rifkin, A., Reardon, G., Siris, S., Karagji, B., Kim, Y.S., Hackstaff, L., & Endicott, N. (1985). Trimipramine in physical illness with depression. *Journal of Clinical Psychiatry, 46,* 4–8.

Robinson, D.S., Nies, A., Revaris, C.L., & Lamborn, K.R. (1973). The monoamine oxidase inhibitor, phenelzine, in the treatment of depressive-anxiety states: A controlled clinical trial. *Archives of General Psychiatry, 29,* 407–413.

Roose, S.P., Glassman, A.H., Giardina, E.G.V., Walsh, B.T., Woodring, S., & Bigger, J.T. (1987). Tricyclic antidepressants in depressed patients with cardiac conduction disease. *Archives of General Psychiatry, 44,* 273–275.

Roose, S.P., Glassman, A.H., Siris, S.G., Walsh, B.T., Bruno, R.L., & Wright, L.B. (1981). Comparison of imipramine and nortriptyline-induced orthostatic hypotension: A meaningful difference. *Journal of Clinical Psychopharmacology, 1,* 316–319.

Rosenthal, N.E. & Goodwin, F.K. (1982). The role of the lithium ion in medicine. *Annual Review of Medicine, 33,* 555–568.

Ross, D.R., Walker, J.I., & Peterson, J. (1983). Akathisia induced by amoxapine. *American Journal of Psychiatry, 140,* 115–116.

Rudorfer, M.V. & Young, R.C. (1980). Desipramine: Cardiovascular effects and plasma levels. *American Journal of Psychiatry, 137,* 984–986.

Sabelli, H.C., Fawcett, J., Javaid, J.I., & Bagri, S. (1983). The methylphenidate test for differentiating desipramine-responsive from nortriptyline-responsive depression. *American Journal of Psychiatry, 140,* 212–214.

Satel, S.L. & Nelson, J.C. (1989). Stimulants in the treatment of depression: A critical overview. *Journal of Clinical Psychiatry, 50,* 241–249.

Schulberg, H., McClelland, M., & Gooding, W. (1987). Six month outcomes for medical patients with major depressive disorders. *Journal of General Internal Medicine, 2,* 312–317.

Schwartz, J., Speed, N., & Clavier, E. (1988). Antidepressant side effects in the medically ill: The value of psychiatric consultation. *International Journal of Psychiatry in Medicine, 18,* 235–241.

Selvin, B.L. (1987). Electroconvulsive therapy – 1987. *Anesthesiology, 67,* 367–385.

Simpson, F.O. (1973). Editorial: Hypertension and depression and their treatment. *Australian and New Zealand Journal of Psychiatry, 7,* 133–137.

Skoven, I. & Thormann, J. (1979). Lithium compound treatment and psoriasis. *Archives of Dermatology, 115,* 1185–1187.

Small, J.G., Milstein, V., Kellams, J.J., & Small, I.F. (1981). Comparative onset of improvement in depressive symptomatology with drug treatment, electroconvulsive therapy, and placebo. *Journal of Clinical Psychopharmacology, 1,* 62S–69S.

Smigan, L., Wahlin, A., Jacobsson, L., & von Knorring, L. (1984). Lithium therapy and thyroid function tests: A prospective study. *Neuropsychobiology, 11,* 39–43.

Steele, T.E. (1982). Adverse reactions suggesting amoxapine-induced dopamine blockade. *American Journal of Psychiatry, 139,* 1500–1501.

Stewart, J.W., Quitkin, F., Liebowitz, M.R., McGrath, P.J., & Klein, D.F. (1981). Efficacy of desipramine in mildly depressed patients: A double-blind placebo controlled trial. *Psychopharmacology Bulletin, 17,* 136–138.

Stoudemire, A. & Atkinson, P. (1988). Use of cyclic antidepressants in patients with cardiac conduction disturbances. *General Hospital Psychiatry, 10,* 389–397.

Strang, R.R. (1965). Imipramine in treatment of Parkinsonism: A double-blind placebo study. *British Medical Journal, 2,* 33–34.

Thayssen, P., Bjerre, M., Kragh-Sorenson, P., Miller, M., Petersen, O.L., Kristensen, C.B., & Gram, L.F. (1981). Cardiovascular effects of imipramine and nortriptyline in elderly patients. *Psychopharmacology, 74,* 360–364.

Tollefson, G.D. (1983). Monoamine oxidase inhibitors: A review. *Journal of Clinical Psychiatry, 44,* 280–288.

Veith, R.C., Raskind, M.A., Caldwell, J.H., Barnes, R.F., Gumbrecht, G., & Ritchie, J.L. (1982). Cardiovascular effects of tricyclic antidepressants in depressed patients with chronic heart disease. *New England Journal of Medicine, 306,* 954–959.

Vincent, H.H., Weimar, W., & Schalekamp, M.A.D. (1987). Effect of cyclosporine in fractional excretion of lithium and potassium in kidney transplant recipients. *Kidney International, 31,* 1048.

Wernicke, J.F. (1985). The side effect profile and safety of fluoxetine. *Journal of Clinical Psychiatry, 46,* 59–67.

Winokur, G., Black, D.W., & Nasrallah, A. (1988). Depressions secondary to other psychiatric disorders and medical illnesses. *American Journal of Psychiatry, 145,* 233–237.

Woods, S.W., Tesar, G.E., Murray, G.B., & Cassem, N.H. (1986). Psychostimulant treatment of depressive disorders secondary to medical illness. *Journal of Clinical Psychiatry, 47,* 12–15.

Yassa, R., Saunders, A., & Nastase, C. (1988). Lithium-induced thyroid disorders: A prevalence study. *Journal of Clinical Psychiatry, 49,* 14–16.

Yudofsky, S.C. (1979). Parkinson's disease, depression, and electroconvulsive therapy: A clinical and neurobiologic synthesis. *Comprehensive Psychiatry, 20,* 579–581.

Yudofsky, S.C. (1981). Electroconvulsive therapy in general hospital psychiatry: A focus on new indications and technologies. *General Hospital Psychiatry, 3,* 292–296.

Zetin, M., Frost, N.R., Brumfield, D., & Stone, R.A. (1982). Amitriptyline stimulates weight gain in hemodialysis patients. *Clinical Nephrology, 18,* 79–82.

Zetin, M., Plon, L., Vaziri, N., Cramer, M., & Greco, D. (1981). Lithium carbonate dose and serum level relationships in chronic hemodialysis patients. *American Journal of Psychiatry, 138,* 1387–1388.

Conclusions

We have chosen to write about depression in the medically ill because it is the most common psychological disturbance associated with medical illness, and because it is often undetected and/or untreated. We hope, however, that this focus on depression does not convey the impression that the mental state associated with medical illness is necessarily gloomy or bleak. In fact, what is most striking in medical and other settings is the remarkable capacity of human beings to adapt to adversity of all kinds.

Depressed mood is a normal human response to the sense of injury, loss, uncertainty, and vulnerability that may be associated with a serious medical condition. In the majority of cases, depressive symptoms are not persistent and they subside when there has been sufficient time for psychological adaptation to the condition to take place. However, the discomfort, disfigurement, disability, and altered life circumstances associated with a medical illness are risk factors for depression, particularly in individuals with a premorbid disposition. In addition, the biological disturbances associated with a number of medical conditions may contribute to depression by either specific or nonspecific mechanisms.

It has been our goal throughout this text to maintain a perspective that balances the scientific and the humanistic. In the health care setting, one of these approaches is too often emphasized at the expense of the other. The clinician who is trained only to search narrowly for organic disease is prone to the error of "medicalizing" illness and missing the texture and drama of human experience. Such narrow approaches tend to place emphasis on diseases rather than on the patients who suffer from them. From such a perspective, the sorrow associated with the loss of health or of life opportunities may be viewed in purely diagnostic terms that inevitably dehumanize the sufferer. On the other hand, a humanistic approach that ignores the presence of treatable psychiatric illness may deprive patients of the possibility of relief through specific and effective interventions.

It has now been clearly documented that there is considerable physical disability associated with depression alone (Wells et al., 1989). Thus, depression may aggravate or compound the disability associated with a medical condition. Furthermore, most treatment studies have shown that depression in medically ill patients responds favorably to therapeutic interventions. Unfortunately, clinically significant depression is often overlooked in the medical setting and depressed medical patients frequently receive inadequate treatment for their mood disturbances. We have reviewed in the text some of the reasons for missed clinical diagnoses of depression and some of the myths that are still common among practicing physicians regarding psychotherapeutic and pharmacologic treatments in the medically ill.

We have drawn attention to both the personal vulnerabilities which may predispose to depression with physical illness and also to the individual and interpersonal strengths that may protect patients from clinical depression. The personality and premorbid predisposition to depression, the capacity to marshal support from the environment, and the actual availability of support all may contribute to the psychological state. Some of the factors that protect a person from depression are illustrated by historical data based on one of psychiatry's most famous patients. Sigmund Freud's chronic illness, which eventually took his life, has been documented by several biographers including Max Schur (1972), who was his personal physician during the last 11 years of his life, Ernest Jones (1957), his most extensive biographer, and most recently, by Sharon Romm (1983), a plastic surgeon who wrote a detailed account of his clinical condition. As these authors documented, at the age of 66, Freud noted a lesion in his mouth which proved to be oral cancer. He did not accept the initial attempts of his physicians to conceal the diagnosis from him (Romm, 1983), and he was subsequently treated with both surgery and radiotherapy. Partly as a result of these treatments, Freud experienced considerable pain and discomfort for the rest of his life.

There is no evidence that Freud complained of depressive feelings related to his illness when it was first diagnosed. In fact, it was not until the death of a favorite grandchild several years later, due to miliary tuberculosis, that Freud wrote that he had become depressed for the first time in his life (Jones, 1957). In retrospect, it may have been that depressive feelings triggered by his illness could emerge only in displaced form in relation to the deceased grandchild or when compounded by another significant adverse event. However, there is no evidence that Freud ever became clinically depressed and, indeed, some of his most creative papers were written during the years in which he suffered greatly from his condition. His strength of character, his personal investment in his scientific career and in the value of psychoanalysis, and the surfeit of family, friends, and admirers around him, likely protected him from the fate of persistent depression. He came grudgingly to accept his illness, which he referred to ironically as "my dear old cancer with whom I have been sharing my existence for 16 years" (Schur, 1972, p. 520). Eventually, however, he could no longer exclude the illness from his awareness and the discomfort became intolerable. When Freud could no longer take nutrition and was in great pain, he wrote in a letter that his "world" was "a small island of pain floating on an ocean of indifference" (Schur, 1972, p. 524). Whether this numbed state reflected the effects of denial, emotional blunting, or the physical effects of his disease and the medication is not clear. However, on September 21, 1939, when Freud found his suffering unbearable and unrelenting, he asked his physician, Max Schur, to relieve his misery, saying, "You promised me then not to forsake me when my time comes. Now it's nothing but torture and makes no sense any more" (Schur, 1972, p. 529).

Whether Freud's state at the end of his life was in any respect akin to depression is now impossible to determine. This diagnosis must, of course, be considered when any patient requests that his or her life be taken. Further, the physical weakness, lethargy, and blunting of emotional responsiveness associated with progressive disease may be difficult to distinguish from depression. However, Freud's physician assumed, likely correctly, that Freud's request to end his life arose out of a rational awareness of his progressive disease and of the inevitability of his further suffering and eventual demise. Freud's ongoing relationship with his physician and with others may well have prevented him from entering a state of alienation and despair. His personal strength and the support he experienced from others undoubtedly eased his passage through the final stages of illness and may have protected him from overt depression. The presence or absence of these protective factors, may be important predictors of depression and of other psychiatric morbidity in the medically ill and others exposed to stressful life circumstances.

The occurrence of depression in the medically ill is most often the result of multiple biological and psychological stressors that may lead to depression depending upon such variables as the adaptive capacities of the individual, the premorbid propensity to depression, the social environment, and the nature and course of the medical condition. Treatment of depression is important not only because the affective disturbance may impair quality of life, but also because psychiatric intervention in this context may decrease medical morbidity, reduce unnecessary health care utilization, and prolong survival. We hope that this text has helped to illuminate the experience of depression in medical patients and will encourage a scientific basis for the understanding and treatment of depression in this context.

REFERENCES

Jones, E. (1957). *Sigmund Freud: Life and Work, Volume III.* London: The Hogarth Press.
Romm, S. (1983). *The Unwelcome Intruder: Freud's Struggle with Cancer.* New York: Praeger Publishers.
Schur, M. (1972). *Freud: Living and Dying.* London: The Hogarth Press.
Wells, K.B., Stewart, A., Hays, R.D., Burnam, A., Rogers, W., Daniels, M., Berry, S., Greenfield, S., & Ware, J. (1989). The functioning and well-being of depressed patients: Results from the Medical Outcomes Study. *Journal of the American Medical Association, 262,* 914–919.

Name Index

Subject Index

Depression *(continued)*
defining valid clinical categories of,
    29–30
as discrete categorical state, 29
"endogenous" versus "reactive," 30
identification of consistent biological
    alterations in, 90
importance of recognizing and treating,
    74–75
medical illness and, xi–xiv
misconceptions about, xiii
overdiagnosis of, 8–9
primary, 30
research on, xv–xvi
as response to existing calamity,
    170–171
secondary, 30
secondary to medical illness, 31
secondary to psychiatric illness, 31
somatization and, 105–110
Depression in the medically ill,
    distinguishing symptoms of, 28–29
Depression-pain syndrome, 115
"Depression-withdrawal," 105–106
Depressive states, self-esteem and, 186
Depressive symptom measures, 53–55
Depressive symptoms in the medically
    ill, 4–29
age and, 27–28
description of measures, 4–7
factors associated with, 23–28
other factors in determining, 27–28
gender and, 27
illness severity and, 23–27
prevalence of, 10–23
    in general medical inpatients, 14–15t
    in patients with specific medical
      illness, 16–21t
    in primary care or general medical
      outpatient settings, 12–13t
Dexamethasone suppression test (DST),
    90–96, 249, 303
administration of, 91
development of, 91
studies using, 92–96
usefulness of, 91
Dextroamphetamine, 323
Diabetes. *See* Insulin Dependent Mellitus
Diagnostic and Statistical Manual of
    Mental Disorders (DSM-III), 32–34
criteria for MDE, 34
limitations of, 43
standard diagnostic interviews, 32–34
Diagnostic and Statistical Manual of
    Mental Disorders, Third Edition,
    Revised (DSM-III-R), 32–43

definition of MDE, 34
disorders with depression as
    predominant feature, 33t
limitations of, 43
on somatic symptoms, 40–41
standard diagnostic interviews, 32–34
Diagnostic Interview Schedule (DIS), 33,
    34, 40, 53, 83, 113, 141
Dialysis patients
depression and, 38
fatigue in, 111
Didactic techniques, in cognitive therapy,
    284
Differential emotions theory, 174
Digitalis intoxication, 255
"Dimensional" measures, 4
DIS. *See* Diagnostic Interview Schedule
Disease-specific research, xvi
Distancing, 205
Doxepin, 308
Drugs, depression and, 238
DSM-III. *See* Diagnostic and Statistical
    Manual for Mental Disorders
DSM-III-R. *See* Diagnostic and Statistical
    Manual of Mental Disorders, Third
    Edition, Revised
DST. *See* Dexamethasone suppression
    test
Dynamics of depression, 191–194
case example, 191–193
Dysfunctional attitudes, 198
Dysphoria, 268
"Dysregulation hypothesis," 176
Dysthymic disorder, 42
Dysthymic pain disorder, 115, 116

EBV. *See* Epstein-Barr virus
ECT. *See* Electroconvulsive therapy
Electroconvulsive therapy, 331–333
Emotional experience, 169
Emotional symptoms
communicating, 75
reluctance to report, 78
Emotion-focused strategies, 173
Emotions, definition of, 173
Endocrine abnormalities, 249–252
Endocrine changes, 176
Endogenous depression, 30
Endstage renal disease (ESRD), 26, 328
depression and, 24, 38, 137
prevalence rates for major depression
    in, 53
suicide and, 152
Endstage Renal Disease Severity Index
    (ESRD-SI), 26
Enterovirus, 112

About the Authors

Gary Rodin, M.D., is Psychiatrist-in-Chief at The Toronto Hospital, Associate Professor in the Department of Psychiatry at the University of Toronto, and a practicing psychoanalyst.

John Craven, M.D., is Director of the Psychosomatic Medicine Program at The Toronto Hospital, Assistant Professor in the Department of Psychiatry at the University of Toronto, and a consulting psychiatrist with the Toronto Multiorgan Transplant Program.

Christine Littlefield, Ph.D., is a Health Psychologist at The Toronto Hospital, Assistant Professor in the Department of Psychiatry at the University of Toronto, and a Longterm Research Fellow with the Ontario Mental Health Foundation.